VOLUME EIGHTY EIGHT

Advances in PHARMACOLOGY

From Structure to Clinical Development: Allosteric Modula of G Protein-Coupled Receptors

VOLUME EIGHTY EIGHT

ADVANCES IN PHARMACOLOGY

From Structure to Clinical Development: Allosteric Modulation of G Protein-Coupled Receptors

Edited by

CHRISTOPHER J. LANGMEAD

Drug Discovery Biology, Monash Institute of Pharmaceutical Sciences, Monash University, Parkville, VIC, Australia

Serial Editor

S.J. ENNA

University of Kansas Medical Center, Kansas City, KS, United States

Managing Editor

LYNN LeCOUNT

University of Kansas Medical Center, School of Medicine, Kansas City, KS, United States

ELSEVIER

ACADEMIC PRESS
An imprint of Elsevier

Academic Press is an imprint of Elsevier
50 Hampshire Street, 5th Floor, Cambridge, MA 02139, United States
525 B Street, Suite 1650, San Diego, CA 92101, United States
The Boulevard, Langford Lane, Kidlington, Oxford OX5 1GB, United Kingdom
125 London Wall, London, EC2Y 5AS, United Kingdom

First edition 2020

ISBN: 978-0-12-820187-9
ISSN: 1054-3589

For information on all Academic Press publications
visit our website at https://www.elsevier.com/books-and-journals

Publisher: Zoe Kruze
Editorial Project Manager: Shellie Bryant
Production Project Manager: Denny Mansingh
Cover Designer: Greg Harris

Typeset by SPi Global, India

Contents

Contributors

Kirstie A. Bennett
Sosei Heptares, Cambridge, United Kingdom

Alice E. Berizzi
IGF, CNRS, INSERM, Univ. de Montpellier, Montpellier, France

Sophie J. Bradley
The Centre for Translational Pharmacology, Institute of Molecular, Cell and Systems Biology, College of Medical, Veterinary and Life Sciences, University of Glasgow, Glasgow, United Kingdom

John A. Christopher
Sosei Heptares, Cambridge, United Kingdom

Cyril Goudet
IGF, CNRS, INSERM, Univ. de Montpellier, Montpellier, France

Debbie L. Hay
School of Biological Sciences; Maurice Wilkins Centre for Molecular Biodiscovery, University of Auckland, Auckland, New Zealand

Sarah Hesse
The Centre for Translational Pharmacology, Institute of Molecular, Cell and Systems Biology, College of Medical, Veterinary and Life Sciences, University of Glasgow, Glasgow, United Kingdom

Joseph D. Ho
Lilly Biotechnology Center, San Diego, CA, United States

Kari A. Johnson
Department of Pharmacology, Uniformed Services University of the Health Sciences, Bethesda, MD, United States

Terry Kenakin
Department of Pharmacology, University of North Carolina School of Medicine, Chapel Hill, NC, United States

Julie Kniazeff
Institut de Génomique Fonctionnelle (IGF), Université de Montpellier, CNRS, INSERM, Montpellier, France

Andrew J. Lawrence
Florey Institute of Neuroscience and Mental Health, University of Melbourne, Parkville, VIC, Australia

Claudia Llinas del Torrent
Laboratori de Medicina Computacional Unitat de Bioestadistica, Facultat de Medicina, Universitat Autonoma de Barcelona, Bellaterra, Spain

David M. Lovinger
Laboratory for Integrative Neuroscience, National Institute on Alcohol Abuse and Alcoholism, US National Institutes of Health, Rockville, MD, United States

Leonardo Pardo
Laboratori de Medicina Computacional Unitat de Bioestadistica, Facultat de Medicina, Universitat Autonoma de Barcelona, Bellaterra, Spain

Laura Pérez-Benito
Computational Chemistry, Janssen Research & Development, Janssen Pharmaceutica N. V., Beerse, Belgium

Augen A. Pioszak
Department of Biochemistry and Molecular Biology, The University of Oklahoma Health Sciences Center, Oklahoma City, OK, United States

Miriam Scarpa
The Centre for Translational Pharmacology, Institute of Molecular, Cell and Systems Biology, College of Medical, Veterinary and Life Sciences, University of Glasgow, Glasgow, United Kingdom

Guy Servant
Firmenich Inc., San Diego, CA, United States

Nicole Servant
Eurofins DiscoverX, San Diego, CA, United States

Kyle W. Sloop
Diabetes and Complications, Lilly Research Laboratories, Indianapolis, IN, United States

Benjamin G. Tehan
OMass Therapeutics, Oxford, United Kingdom

Gary Tresadern
Computational Chemistry, Janssen Research & Development, Janssen Pharmaceutica N. V., Beerse, Belgium

Leigh C. Walker
Florey Institute of Neuroscience and Mental Health, University of Melbourne, Parkville, VIC, Australia

Francis S. Willard
Quantitative Biology, Lilly Research Laboratories, Indianapolis, IN, United States

Mark Williams
Firmenich Inc., San Diego, CA, United States

Lan Zhang
Firmenich Inc., San Diego, CA, United States

Preface

The phenomenon of allosteric transitions within proteins was elegantly described in the 1960s by Monod, Wyman, and Changeux. However, the concept of allosteric modulation of G protein-coupled receptors (GPCRs) remained little more than a pharmacological curiosity until the 1990s when functional cell-based assays overtook traditional radioligand binding methods as the high-throughput screening method of choice, revealing a multiplicity of GPCR-interacting ligands. As we enter 2020, it is timely to consider the progress made toward the discovery, mechanistic understanding, and development of allosteric modulators of GPCRs as new therapeutics.

The term *allosteric*, from the Greek *allos* (other) and *stereos* ("solid" or "shape"), defines binding sites (and their ligands) that are topographically distinct from that utilized by the endogenous agonist for a receptor (the *orthosteric* site). As such, allosteric modulation confers a unique set of properties onto a GPCR, including probe dependence (different responses depending on the cobound orthosteric ligand), saturability of effect (driven by the level of cooperativity between the two cobound ligands), and often enhanced receptor selectivity.

The past two decades have seen the advent of hundreds of discovery projects targeting allosteric modulators of GPCRs. A critical element of success has been developing improved methods for understanding the (at times complex) mechanistic pharmacology of this class of ligand. This spans from exploiting recent advances in GPCR computational and structural biology through to considering how the inherent properties of allosteric ligands translate into efficacy in disease states, both in animal models and patients.

With 4 allosteric GPCR drugs now approved, and a further 22 in active clinical development (Table 1), it is an opportune time to review the landscape. What we have learnt, and what remains unanswered in our understanding of GPCR allosteric modulation—and how we can bring these concepts to the development of improved therapeutics?

This volume includes contributions from experts across the field of GPCR allosterism, spanning the spectrum from computational chemistry through to evaluation of allosteric modulators in preclinical models of disease. In Chapter 1, Gary Tresadern (Janssen) and colleagues outline ligand- and receptor model-based computational approaches that have been used for drug discovery targeting metabotropic glutamate (mGlu) receptors.

Table 1 Allosteric modulators of GPCRs either approved or in active clinical development (as of March 2020; data from Cortellis Competitive Intelligence database search[a]).

Drug	Main indication(s)	GPCR target	Mode[b]	Clinical Phase
Maraviroc	HIV infection	Chemokine CCR5	NAM	Launched
Evocalcet	Hypercalcemia; secondary hyperparathyroidism	Calcium sensing receptor	PAM	Launched
Etelcalcetide	Secondary hyperparathyroidism	Calcium sensing receptor	PAM	Launched
Cinacalcet	Hypercalcemia; secondary hyperparathyroidism	Calcium sensing receptor	PAM	Launched
Cenicriviroc	NAFLD/NASH[c]; primary sclerosing cholangitis	Chemokine CCR2/CCR5	NAM	Phase III
SK-1403	Secondary hyperparathyroidism	Calcium sensing receptor	PAM	Phase III
LY-3154207	Alzheimer's disease; Parkinson's disease	Dopamine D_1 receptor	PAM	Phase II
ASP4345	Schizophrenia	Dopamine D_1 receptor	PAM	Phase II
Dipraglurant-ER[d] Dipraglurant-IR[d]	Dystonia L-DOPA-induced dyskinesia	Metabotropic Glu5 receptor	NAM	Phase II
Foliglurax	Parkinson's disease	Metabotropic Glu4 receptor	PAM	Phase II
RVT-1502	Insulin-dependent and non-insulin-dependent diabetes	Glucagon receptor	NAM	Phase II
Mavoglurant	Obsessive compulsive disorder	Metabotropic Glu5 receptor	NAM	Phase II
ADX-71149	Epilepsy	Metabotropic Glu2 receptor	PAM	Phase II
ASP-8302	Bladder disease	Muscarinic M_3 receptor	PAM	Phase II

Table 1 Allosteric modulators of GPCRs either approved or in active clinical development (as of March 2020; data from Cortellis Competitive Intelligence database search[a]).—cont'd

Drug	Main indication(s)	GPCR target	Mode[b]	Clinical Phase
Vicriviroc	Colorectal cancer	Chemokine CCR5	NAM	Phase II
Nimacimab	NAFLD/NASH[c]	Cannabinoid CB_1 receptor	NAM[e]	Phase II
HME-0266	Movement disorders	Metabotropic Glu5 receptor	NAM	Phase I
JNJ-55375515	Neurological disease; psychiatric disorder	Metabotropic Glu2 receptor	NAM	Phase I
SX-682	Various cancers	Chemokine CXCR1/2 receptor	NAM	Phase I
VU-319	Mild cognitive impairment	Muscarinic M_1 receptor	PAM	Phase I
LY-3154885	Parkinson's disease dementia	Dopamine D_1 receptor	PAM	Phase I
CVL-231	Schizophrenia	Muscarinic M_4 receptor	PAM	Phase I
ASP-8062	Drug dependence	$GABA_B$ receptor	PAM	Phase I
HTL-14242	Multiple CNS indications	Metabotropic Glu5 receptor	NAM	Phase I

[a]Search in Cortellis Competitive Intelligence for drugs with "*Any Action (G protein coupled receptor modulator) AND Any Text (allosteric)*" filtered for "*Highest Status*", "*Launched; Phase 1 Clinical; Phase 2 Clinical; Phase 3 Clinical,*" with manual curation for missing, duplicated or incorrectly annotated entries.
[b]PAM, positive allosteric modulator; NAM, negative allosteric modulator.
[c]NAFLD, nonalcoholic fatty liver disease; NASH, nonalcoholic steatohepatitis.
[d]IR, immediate release formulation; ER, extended release formulation.
[e]Monoclonal antibody.

In Chapter 2, Kirstie Bennett, John Christopher and Benjamin Tehan (Sosei-Heptares) elegantly describe computational and medicinal chemistry, along with structural biology approaches, to the identification of novel mGlu5 negative allosteric modulators.

In Chapter 3, Guy Servant (Firmenich) and colleagues provide an overview of the broad range of allosteric modulators that have been discovered and developed for the human sweet taste receptor, and apply state-of-the-art analytical models to better understand their function. Completing the set of chapters on molecular understanding of allostery at Class C GPCRs, in Chapter 4, Julie Kniazeff (IGF, CNRS) outlines mechanisms of modulation the $GABA_B$ receptor, which encompass not only small molecule ligands, but also allosteric interactions that occur across the obligate dimer and higher order oligomers. In Chapter 5, Augen Pioszak (University of Oklahoma) and Debbie Hay (University of Auckland) extend the notion of allosteric modulation of GPCRs by endogenous protein partners by exploring the effect of receptor activity modifying proteins (RAMPs) on the function of calcitonin and calcitonin-like Class B GPCRs. In Chapter 6, Alice Berizzi and Cyril Goudet (IGF, CNRS) outline the opportunities to interrogate receptor function and GPCR allostery by using photo-switchable ligands, which have most notably been applied to Class C GPCRs, but have broad applicability to interrogate physiology of any receptor. In Chapter 7, Francis Willard, Joseph Ho and Kyle Sloop (Lilly) describe the discovery of a small molecule allosteric modulator of the Class B glucagon-like peptide-1 receptor, BETP, and its utility in terms of understanding receptor function and tractability as a drug target for medicinal chemistry.

In Chapter 8, Kari Johnson (Uniformed Services University of the Health Sciences) and David Lovinger (NIAAA) summarize the Class C mGlu receptor family as drug targets for the treatment of alcohol use disorder, outlining the preclinical evidence base, most notably for mGlu2 and mGlu5 receptors. In a similar vein, Leigh Walker and Andrew Lawrence (Florey Institute of Neuroscience and Mental Health) highlight recent advances in allosterically targeting the muscarinic M_1, M_4 and M_5 receptor subtypes in the context of alcohol and other substance use disorders in Chapter 9. Miriam Scarpa, Sarah Hesse and Sophie Bradley (University of Glasgow) complete the volume with a summary of the progress toward the development of selective muscarinic M_1 receptor ligands as an approach to both symptomatic and disease modification in Alzheimer's disease in Chapter 10.

I am enormously grateful to all of the authors who so willingly gave up their time to contribute to this venture. It is only through projects such as this that we have the opportunity to take a broad view of the field, assess our progress, and establish what will still have to achieve. The road to the discovery and development of better GPCR therapeutics may be a long and challenging one, but it is no doubt slightly shorter and easier to traverse thanks to the colleagues who have assembled this volume. I would like also to thank Sam Enna and Lynn LeCount, who not only provided me the opportunity to edit the book, but have been unfailingly helpful through its production. Final thanks must go to my wife Lorraine, who is unswerving in her support of me and my work. I could not do it without you.

Christopher J. Langmead
Drug Discovery Biology, Monash Institute of Pharmaceutical Sciences,
Monash University, Parkville, VIC, Australia
March 4, 2020

CHAPTER ONE

The computational modeling of allosteric modulation of metabotropic glutamate receptors

Laura Pérez-Benito[a], Claudia Llinas del Torrent[b], Leonardo Pardo[b], Gary Tresadern[a,*]
[a]Computational Chemistry, Janssen Research & Development, Janssen Pharmaceutica N. V., Beerse, Belgium
[b]Laboratori de Medicina Computacional Unitat de Bioestadística, Facultat de Medicina, Universitat Autonoma de Barcelona, Bellaterra, Spain
*Corresponding author: e-mail address: gtresade@its.jnj.com

Contents

Abstract

Allosteric modulation of GPCRs, especially metabotropic glutamate (mGlu) receptors, has become an important strategy for drug discovery. Positive and negative allosteric modulators (PAM, NAM) are widely reported for the mGlu receptor family with leads mostly originating by high-throughput screening followed by iterative medicinal chemistry. The progression of the field from mutagenesis and homology modeling to elaborate structure-enabled drug discovery is described. We detail how computational methods have delivered new chemical matter and revealed the functional details of PAM and NAM activity. The breakthrough in mGlu receptor 7-transmembrane (7TM) crystal structures enabled recent combined modeling and experimental studies to

Advances in Pharmacology, Volume 88
ISSN 1054-3589
https://doi.org/10.1016/bs.apha.2020.02.004

confirm common binding sites, interactions and the origins of ligand effect on functional activity. Focusing on allosteric modulation of the $mGlu_2$ and $mGlu_5$ receptors, similarities are seen that still accommodate the known differences in binding sites and SAR. This work reveals the promise of a methodical computational approach built upon deep analysis of 7TM receptor simulations and interpretation of results in the context of our current understanding of receptor function. A crucial aspect was the close collaboration between modeling and experiment necessary to build and interrogate the hypotheses.

Abbreviations

7TM 7-transmembrane
BW Ballesteros–Weinstein
CNS central nervous system
CRD cysteine rich domain
Cryo-EM cryogenic electron microscopy
ECD extracellular domain
ECL extracellular loop
GPCR G protein-coupled receptor
GTP Guanosine-5′-triphosphate
ICL intracellular loop
MD molecular dynamics
mGlu metabotropic glutamate
NAM negative allosteric modulator
PAM positive allosteric modulator
PCM proteochemometric
PDB protein data bank
QSAR quantitative structure–activity relationship
SAM silent allosteric modulator
SAR structure–activity relationship
SDM site-directed mutagenesis
TM transmembrane
VFT venus fly-trap

1. Introduction

G protein-coupled receptors (GPCRs) are the largest and most diverse family of membrane proteins that are present in almost every eukaryotic organism. They are highly diversified in mammalian genomes with current estimates of about 800 genes (2–3% of the human proteome) (Fredriksson & Schiöth, 2005). Based on sequence similarity methods, GPCRs are classified into subfamilies that include classes A (rhodopsin-like, >700 receptors including >400 olfactory receptors), B (secretin or B1 family, 41 receptors; adhesion or B2 family, 34 receptors), C (including metabotropic glutamate, 22 receptors), and F (frizzled, 11 receptors) (Alexander et al., 2017; Pándy-Szekeres et al., 2018). This diversity permits GPCRs to transduce exogenous signals of external origin such as light, odors or pheromones and endogenous signals such as neurotransmitters, (neuro)peptides, proteases, glycoprotein hormones and ions, among others, to the cytoplasmic side of the cell membrane (Kristiansen, 2004). Significant advances in crystallization of GPCRs (Day et al., 2007; Serrano-Vega, Magnani, Shibata, & Tate, 2008), together with cryogenic electron microscopy (cryo-EM) (Renaud et al., 2018) have allowed many receptor structures to be solved (Munk et al., 2019). Today, structures of classes A (Palczewski et al., 2000), B (Zhang et al., 2017), C (Koehl et al., 2019), and F (Wang et al., 2013) are available, bound to either agonists, antagonists, inverse agonists, or allosteric modulators (Kruse et al., 2013; Rasmussen et al., 2007, 2011), in the form of monomers or homo-oligomers (Huang, Chen, Zhang, & Huang, 2013; Manglik et al., 2012), in complex with G-proteins (Krishna Kumar et al., 2019; Maeda, Qu, Robertson, Skiniotis, & Kobilka, 2019; Rasmussen et al., 2011), β-arrestin (Kang et al., 2015), or GRK5 (Komolov et al., 2017). All these structures share the common architecture of seven transmembrane domains (TMs, which also terms this family of proteins as 7TM receptors) connected to each other with three extracellular (ECL) and three intracellular loops (ICL), a disulfide bridge between ECL2 and TM3, and a cytoplasmic C-terminus containing an α-helix (helix 8) parallel to the cell membrane.

Our understanding of the details of GPCR signaling has advanced greatly. In a simple manner, receptors exist as a population of different conformations: resting, active, inactive, and various intermediates that are connected through an energy landscape (Fig. 1). The transition probability among conformations depends on their energy difference and the energy barrier between them. Ligands or coupling proteins bind preferentially to specific state(s), increasing the proportion of those states, leading to more signaling of the corresponding pathway. Thus, the diverse pharmacology of specific GPCRs can be understood: basal activity arising from a small population of receptors in an active state even in the absence of agonist (black line in Fig. 1); inverse agonists (in red) preferring inactive states (red line); agonists (in green) favoring and stabilizing intermediate states, and the final formation of the agonist-receptor-active G protein complex further increasing activity (green line) (Nygaard et al., 2013). Specifically, for class A GPCRs, ligand binding occurs in the extracellular part of

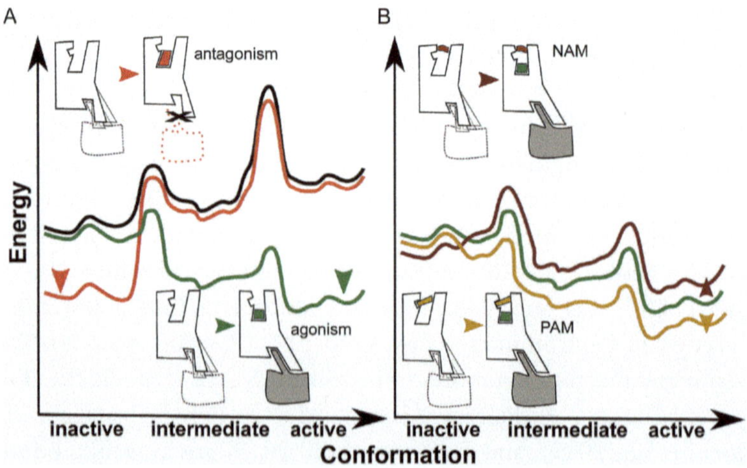

Fig. 1 Dynamic properties of GPCRs based on a schematic view of class A receptors. (A) Energy landscape of a GPCR in the unliganded form (black line), after the action of an inverse agonist/antagonist (in red) or an agonist (in green). (B) Energy landscape of a GPCR in the presence of a negative allosteric modulator (NAM, in brown) and a positive allosteric modulator (PAM, in yellow).

the transmembrane (TM) region, stabilizing the activated conformational states of the 7TM core (Fig. 2). As will be described in more detail later, GPCRs can also bind allosteric ligands in different sites where they can augment or inhibit orthosteric activity, as indicated in Fig. 1B. These sites can be different between GPCR classes, for instance a class B allosteric site is known toward the intracellular side of the receptor, whereas for class C the orthosteric site is in the extracellular domain and the allosteric site(s) within the 7TM core.

Structural breakthroughs have revealed the molecular mechanisms of agonist-induced receptor activation, this includes observing the specific ligand interactions that preferentially stabilize active states and promote functional activity. In this regard, agonist binding at the extracellular orthosteric binding site triggers local structural changes that are varied and include a hydrogen bond interaction between agonists and $S^{5.46a}$ (Rasmussen et al., 2011; Warne et al., 2011), the movement of $W^{6.48a}$ (Xu et al., 2011), or a conformational toggle switch of the side chain of the amino acid at position 3.36a (Pellissier et al., 2009) (Fig. 2). Thus, these changes occur in the immediate proximity of the ligand, but they must translate into larger-scale helix movements at the intracellular site (Rasmussen et al., 2011). Further comparison of active-like and inactive-like complexes has shown this proceeds via movement of TM5

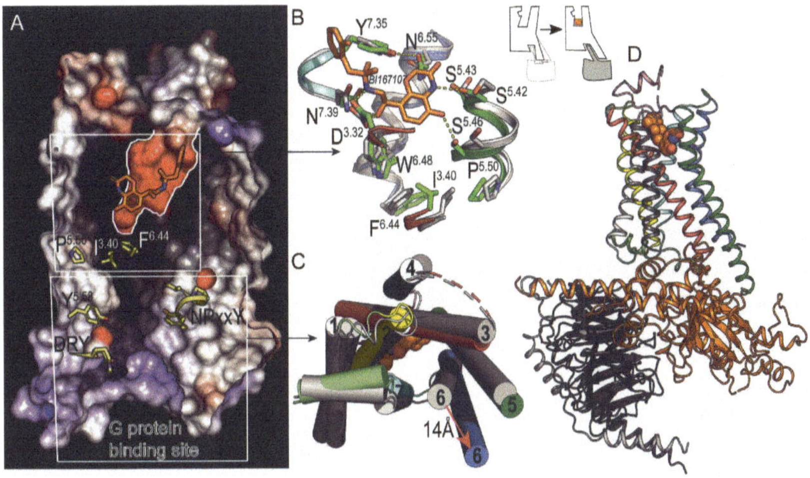

Fig. 2 Schematic view of the details associated with class A GPCR activation. (A) Cross-section through a prototypical class A GPCR, highlighting the agonist (orange sticks) occupying the orthosteric site (delineated by a white line), the PIF motif located below the orthosteric binding cavity, and the side chains of the highly conserved NPxxY and DRY motifs and $Y^{5.58a}$ that transmit the signal from the PIF motif to the G protein binding site. (B) Detailed view of the β_2-adrenergic receptor bound to the full agonist BI-167107 (in orange) (PDB ID: 3P0G). The hydrogen bond interaction between full agonists and $S^{5.46}$ stabilizes a receptor conformation that includes an inward movement of TM5 at $P^{5.50a}$, rotation of TM3 due to a steric clash with the bulky hydrophobic $I^{3.40a}$ side chain, and an outward movement of $F^{6.44a}$ in TM6 relative to the inactive (shown in white for comparison purposes), Carazolol-bound structure (PDB ID: 2RH1). (C and D) These small local structural changes near the binding site (panel B) are translated into larger-scale helix movements at the intracellular side. The structure of β_2- in complex with G_s (PDB ID: 3SN6) shows, relative to the inactive structure (in white) an outward movement of TM6 (panel C), opening an intracellular cavity required for the binding of the G-protein (panel D).

at $P^{5.50a}$, rotation of TM3 due to a steric clash with the bulky hydrophobic side chain at position 3.40a (Sansuk et al., 2011), and an outward movement of $F^{6.44a}$ in TM6 (Fig. 2). These key highly conserved amino acids, located below the orthosteric binding cavity and above the G protein binding cavity, have been named as the "P-I-F" motif (Wacker et al., 2013), the "transmission switch" (Venkatakrishnan et al., 2013), the "triad core" (Huang et al., 2015), or the connector region (Weis & Kobilka, 2018). The arrangement of these side chains is transmitted to the intracellular side via the highly conserved NPxxY and DRY motifs and $Y^{5.58a}$ (Weis & Kobilka, 2018). This leads to outward movement of TMs 5 and 6 (~14 Å) and the opening of an intracellular cavity that is required for the binding of the C-terminal α5 helix of the G-protein (Fig. 2). Due to the conservation of these amino acids, and despite the structurally diverse type of extracellular signals, the propagation of the signal from the orthosteric binding site to the intracellular amino acids of the TM bundle converge upon structurally conserved mechanisms of effector activation (Venkatakrishnan et al., 2016). Thus, different specific contacts, interactions, and conformational effects arise between ligand and the protein binding site initiating pathways that converge at the "transmission switch" with the final steps on the intracellular side sharing many common structural features. We have proposed that these features are also present in families B (Cordomí et al., 2015; Spyridaki et al., 2014) and C GPCRs (Llinas del Torrent, Casajuana-Martin, Pardo, Tresadern, & Pérez-Benito, 2019; Pérez-Benito et al., 2017).

Considering the vast amount of cellular processes regulated by GPCRs (Wootten, Christopoulos, Marti-Solano, Babu, & Sexton, 2018) it is unsurprising that they form one of the most important pharmaceutical drug-target classes with around 35% of marketed drugs acting through this superfamily of proteins (Sriram & Insel, 2018). However, these drugs target <10% of all known GPCRs (Hauser, Attwood, Rask-Andersen, Schiöth, & Gloriam, 2017; Wise, Gearing, & Rees, 2002). One of the reasons being that the orthosteric binding sites for a particular endogenous ligand across a GPCR subfamily are often highly conserved, making it difficult to achieve high selectivity for specific receptor subtypes (Foster & Conn, 2017). Thus, novel approaches to modulate GPCRs have emerged (Cooke & Congreve, 2016). These new approaches are varied and include the discovery of bitopic ligands that bind the orthosteric site as well as a less conserved site at the extracellular entrance (Lane, Sexton, & Christopoulos, 2013; Shonberg, Kling, Gmeiner, & Löber, 2015), multivalent ligands that target physiologically relevant GPCR homo/hetero-oligomers (Pérez-Benito et al., 2018; Pulido et al., 2018), or allosteric ligands that bind at allosteric sites and act in conjunction with the endogenous ligand (Christopoulos, 2014). Allosteric modulators are categorized as negative (NAM) or positive (PAM) depending on their ability to decrease or increase the action (affinity and/or efficacy) of the orthosteric ligand by destabilizing or stabilizing intermediate and active conformations (Fig. 1B). Ago-PAMs are allosteric modulators than in addition to increasing the potency and/or efficacy of orthosteric agonists, can induce receptor activation by themselves. Finally, silent allosteric modulators (SAMs) have also been identified that bind as neutral allosteric ligands with no effect on orthosteric affinity or efficacy.

There are numerous allosteric binding sites seen in the published crystal structures of classes A, B, C, and F of GPCRs in complex with small-molecule allosteric modulators, Fig. 3, see (Lu & Zhang, 2019) for a recent review. In addition to the prevailing site in the 7TM domain near the extracellular side (classes A, C, and F), other binding sites are also observed in the 7TM domain near the intracellular side (classes A and B), or at the extra-helical part facing the membrane bilayer (classes A and B). We are

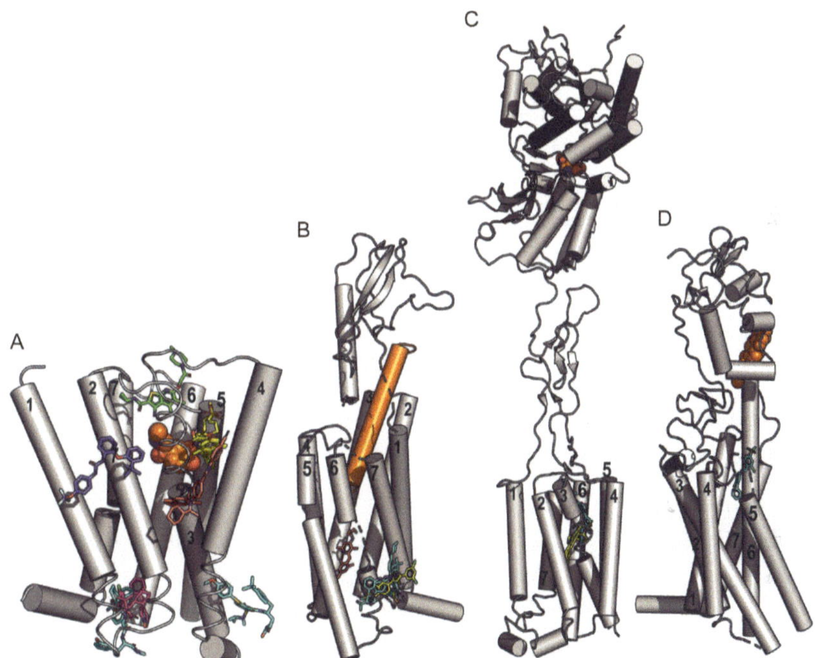

Fig. 3 The allosteric binding sites of GPCRs. (A) A schematic view of the 7TM domain of a class A receptor (white cylinders), showing the orthosteric ligand (adrenaline in orange spheres, PDB ID: 4LDO) and the binding of allosteric modulators to the muscarinic M2 receptor (green, 4MQT), the β_2-adrenergic receptor (cyan, 5X7D and 6N48), CCR2 and CCR9 (magenta, 5T1A and 5LWE), GPR40 (yellow, 4PHU and 5TZR), PAR2 (pink, 5NDZ), and P2Y1 (blue, 4XNV). (B) The backbone of a class B receptor (GLP-1 receptor in white, 5VAI), showing the orthosteric ligand (GLP-1 peptide in orange cylinder) and the binding of allosteric modulators to GCGR (yellow, 5EE7), CRF$_1$R (pink, 4K5Y) and GLP-1R (cyan, 5VEX and 5VEW). (C) The backbone of a class C receptor (mGlu$_5$ receptor in white, 6N52, only a monomer is depicted for clarity), showing the orthosteric ligand (glutamate in orange spheres, 3LMK) and the binding of allosteric modulators to mGlu$_1$ (cyan, 4OR2) and mGlu$_5$ receptors (yellow, 4OO9 and 5CGD). (D) The backbone of a class F receptor (SMO receptor in white, 5L7D), showing the orthosteric ligand (cholesterol in orange spheres, 5L7D) and the binding of the allosteric modulator Vismodegib to the same receptor (cyan, 5L7I).

also starting to understand the mechanistic aspects of canonical allosteric ligands. For instance, the crystal structure of the muscarinic M2 receptor simultaneously bound to an orthosteric agonist and a PAM (Kruse et al., 2013) shows that the allosteric modulator binds at the extracellular vestibule identified in binding pathway simulations (Dror et al., 2011; González, Perez-Acle, Pardo, & Deupi, 2011) inducing a slight contraction of the binding pocket, enhancing the potency without modifying the efficacy of the orthosteric agonist (Kruse et al., 2013). In contrast, a crystal structure of the β_2-adrenergic receptor also in complex with an orthosteric agonist and a PAM shows that the allosteric modulator binds on the receptor's inner surface in a pocket created by ICL 2 and TMs 3 and 4, stabilizing the loop in an α-helical conformation required to engage the G protein (Liu et al., 2019). In between these two contrasting binding modes, PAMs of class C GPCRs bind within the 7TM domain and function in a similar manner as class A orthosteric agonists (Llinas del Torrent, Casajuana-Martin, et al., 2019; Pérez-Benito et al., 2017) (see below). Thus, the mechanisms by which PAMs elicit their function over the whole GPCR family is, in contrast to orthosteric agonists, highly diverse.

2. Introduction to class C GPCRs

Glutamate is the major excitatory neurotransmitter in the central nervous system (CNS) and acts via ionotropic glutamate receptors and GPCRs named metabotropic glutamate (mGlu) receptors (Conn & Pin, 1997). Eight mGlu receptor subtypes and multiple splice variants have been cloned and classified into three groups based upon sequence homology, pharmacological profile and preferential signal transduction pathways: Group I ($mGlu_1$ and $mGlu_5$), group II ($mGlu_2$ and $mGlu_3$) and group III ($mGlu_4$, $mGlu_6$, $mGlu_7$ and $mGlu_8$) (Pin, Galvez, & Prézeau, 2003).

The mGlu receptors are an important target family for drug discovery (Niswender & Conn, 2010). Indications cover a variety of CNS illnesses such as schizophrenia (Conn, Lindsley, & Jones, 2009; Stansley & Conn, 2018), anxiety and stress-related disorders (Peterlik, Flor, & Uschold-Schmidt, 2016), and epilepsy (Celli et al., 2019) to name just a few. While there has been some success targeting the extracellular orthosteric site, for instance the work on constrained glutamate analogues from Eli Lilly laboratories (Monn et al., 2015), most current efforts focus on allosteric modulation at the 7TM domain, an allosteric binding site positionally homologous to the ancestrally conserved class A orthosteric binding site (Fig. 3) (Conn, Christopoulos, & Lindsley, 2009; Foster & Conn, 2017; Sheffler, Gregory, Rook, & Conn, 2011).

The design of allosteric modulators offers several advantages. First, allosteric ligands do not activate receptors alone but modulate signaling in the presence of the endogenous ligand, responding with physiological changes in agonist concentration. In turn, allosteric modulators are less likely to cause receptor desensitization (Gjoni & Urwyler, 2008; Pin, Parmentier, & Prézeau, 2001; Urwyler, 2011). Furthermore, it can be easier to identify selective ligands as allosteric sites are often less conserved across a family of receptors than the orthosteric counterpart. Also, some orthosteric binding sites may have properties that hinder the identification of drug-like ligands, for instance the glutamate amino acid site in mGlu receptors, or the peptide binding sites of class B GPCRs.

Within the mGlu receptor family, the $mGlu_1$, $mGlu_2$ and $mGlu_5$ receptors are by far the most explored from both a biology and chemistry point of view, with the most reported synthetic ligands, while group III receptors such as $mGlu_4$ and $mGlu_7$ are receiving increasing attention (Llinas del Torrent, Pérez-Benito, & Tresadern, 2019). The intense interest in the $mGlu_2$ receptor for instance has seen over a dozen pharmaceutical companies including Astra-Zeneca, Bristol Myers Squibb, Janssen, Lilly, Merck, Organon, Pfizer, Roche, Sanofi, Taisho, etc. publishing and patenting multiple chemical series of allosteric modulators (Trabanco & Cid, 2013; Trabanco, Cid, Lavreysen, Macdonald, & Tresadern, 2011). While no mGlu receptor targeted drugs have reached market, various compounds have been evaluated in human clinical trials with $mGlu_5$ NAM fenobam showing anxiolytic effects, another $mGlu_5$ NAM ADX10059 showing a positive outcome for gastroesophageal reflux disease (GERD), and the $mGlu_{2/3}$ agonist LY2140023 (an agonist prodrug) for the treatment of schizophrenia. To date, two $mGlu_2$ receptor PAMs, AZD8529 (Fig. 4) from AstraZeneca and JNJ-40411813 (also known as ADX71149, Fig. 4) from Janssen Pharmaceuticals and Addex Therapeutics have been tested in clinic for indications including schizophrenia, major depressive disorder with anxious distress (Trabanco, Bartolomé, & Cid, 2019). Likewise, several $mGlu_5$ NAMs have been evaluated in clinic for indications such as Parkinson's, treatment resistant depression, and fragile X syndrome (Barnes, Sheffler, Semenova, Cosford, & Bespalov, 2018).

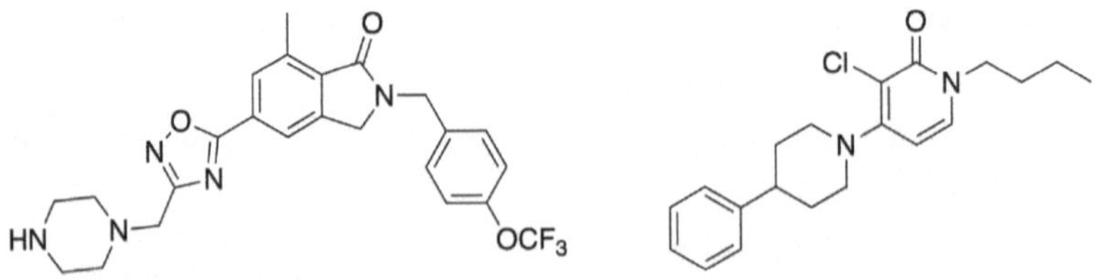

AZD8529 JNJ-40411813 (ADX71149)

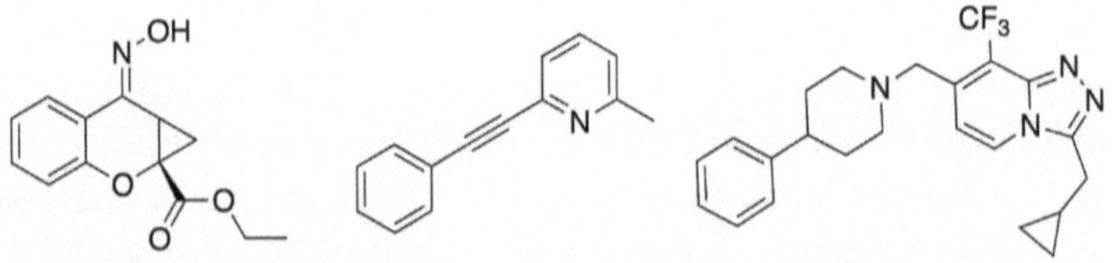

CPCCOEt MPEP JNJ-46281222

Fig. 4 Chemical structures of selected mGlu receptor allosteric modulators.

3. Structural aspects of mGlu receptors

Class C mGlu receptors are structurally more complex than the other GPCR classes (Pin & Bettler, 2016). First, they form obligate cysteine-linked homodimers (Romano, Yang, & O'Malley, 1996). Second, each protomer is formed by a large and characteristic extracellular Venus fly-trap (VFT) domain that binds orthosteric ligands (i.e., the endogenous glutamate agonist), a 7TM domain, and a cysteine rich domain (CRD) that connects these two domains (Niswender & Conn, 2010), Fig. 5. Crystal structures of the homodimeric extracellular VFT domains of $mGlu_1$ receptor in the empty (inactive or open conformation) and glutamate-bound (active or closed conformation) forms were disclosed in 2000 (Kunishima et al., 2000). Thus, these bi-lobed structures show that glutamate binding stabilizes both the active dimer and the closed protomer in dynamic equilibrium (Fig. 5A and B). In addition, the homodimeric extracellular VFT and CRD domains are known for $mGlu_3$ receptor since 2007 (Muto, Tsuchiya, Morikawa, & Jingami, 2007). Since these pioneering structures, the VFT domains of mGlu's 1, 2, 3, 5, 7 and 8 have been reported. Similar bi-lobed protomer architectures of the heterodimeric $GABA_{B1}$ and $GABA_{B2}$ in the empty, agonist-bound and antagonist-bound forms, have confirmed that class C activation requires the agonist-induced closed

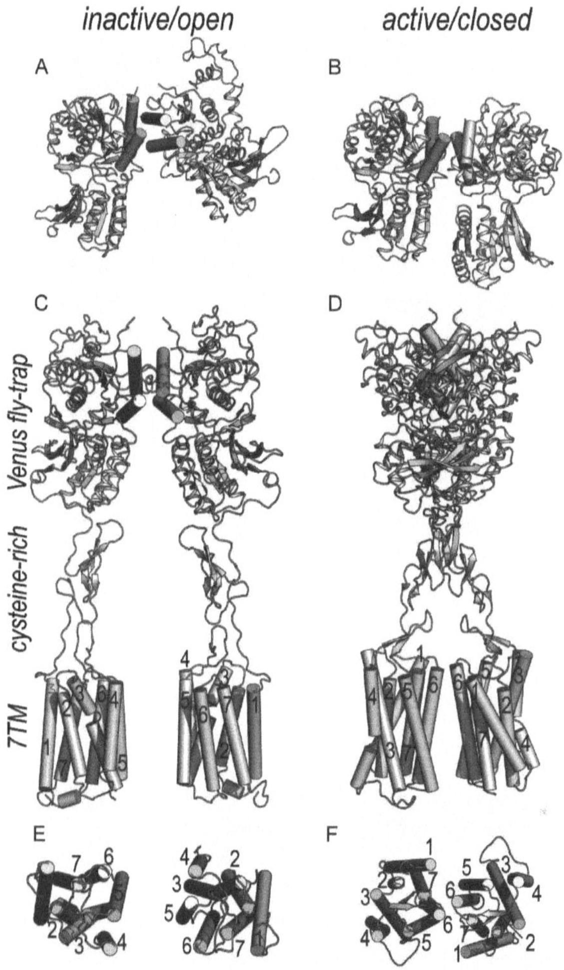

Fig. 5 Crystal structures of mGlu receptors. (A and B) Structures of the homodimeric extracellular VFT domains of $mGlu_1$ receptor in the empty (inactive/open conformation) (PDB ID: 1EWT) and glutamate-bound (active/closed conformation) (1EWK). The helix interface between protomers of the VFT domains is shown as cylinders. (C and D) Cryo-EM structure of a full-length $mGlu_5$ receptor, capturing both apo inactive/open (6N52) and active/closed (6N51) conformations. (E and F) Top views of the 7TM domains showing the reorientation of their interface. Both protomers are colored in light blue and gray.

conformation of the VFT domains (Geng, Bush, Mosyak, Wang, & Fan, 2013). More recently, the structures of the 7TM domain of the $mGlu_1$ receptor (Wu et al., 2014) and the $mGlu_5$ receptor (Doré et al., 2014) have also been reported. These structures have allowed structure-based sequence alignments between the TM helices of classes A and C and propose a cross-class GPCR residue numbering (Isberg et al., 2015) based on a modified Ballesteros–Weinstein (BW) scheme (Ballesteros & Weinstein, 1995).

A major breakthrough for the understanding of mGlu receptor function is the very recent cryo-EM structure of a full-length $mGlu_5$ receptor, capturing both apo inactive/open and active/closed conformations (Koehl et al., 2019) (Fig. 5C–F). Like the previous $mGlu_1$ receptor structures of the VFT domain (Fig. 5A and B), the action of an orthosteric agonist to the $mGlu_5$ receptor leads to an intersubunit reorientation, from inactive/open to active/closed conformations, bringing the bottom lobes together (Fig. 5C and D). Activation results in compacting of the $mGlu_5$ dimer, bringing the CRDs into proximity, and in-turn enabling the 7TM domains to reposition closer to initiate signaling (Figs. 5C and D). The inactive state shows a TM5–TM5 interface but with substantial separation between the 7TM domains (Fig. 5E). Activation leads to a 20° rotation of each 7TM domain, resulting in a close contact TM6–TM6 dimer interface as was previously proposed (Xue et al., 2015) (Fig. 5F). ECL2 makes crucial interactions with CRD suggesting a structural explanation for the allostery observed between the extracellular and 7TM domains (Doornbos et al., 2015).

4. Mutagenesis and structure-based modeling of mGlu receptor allosteric modulators

For a detailed report of the varied computational molecular modeling approaches applied to the mGlu receptors, the reader is referred to a recent review (Llinas del Torrent, Pérez-Benito, & Tresadern, 2019). Here, we highlight studies performed in tandem with experiment to understand the location and function of the PAM and NAM binding site. Many of the joint experimental/modeling reports involved structural homology modeling of the receptor performed with site directed mutagenesis (SDM) experiments. In most cases, this work precedes the publication of the mGlu receptor 7TM X-ray structures in 2014.

The late 1990s saw the first $mGlu_1$ selective non-competitive antagonists binding at an alternative allosteric site. SDM identified $mGlu_1$ receptor amino acids involved in the recognition of ligands such as CPCCOEt (Fig. 4), suggesting an overlapping binding site in the 7TM domain of the receptor (Litschig et al., 1999; Pagano et al., 2000) (Fig. 6A and B). In 2003, Malherbe et al. used SDM and a homology model of the $mGlu_5$ receptor to pinpoint aromatic residues in TM6 important for NAM

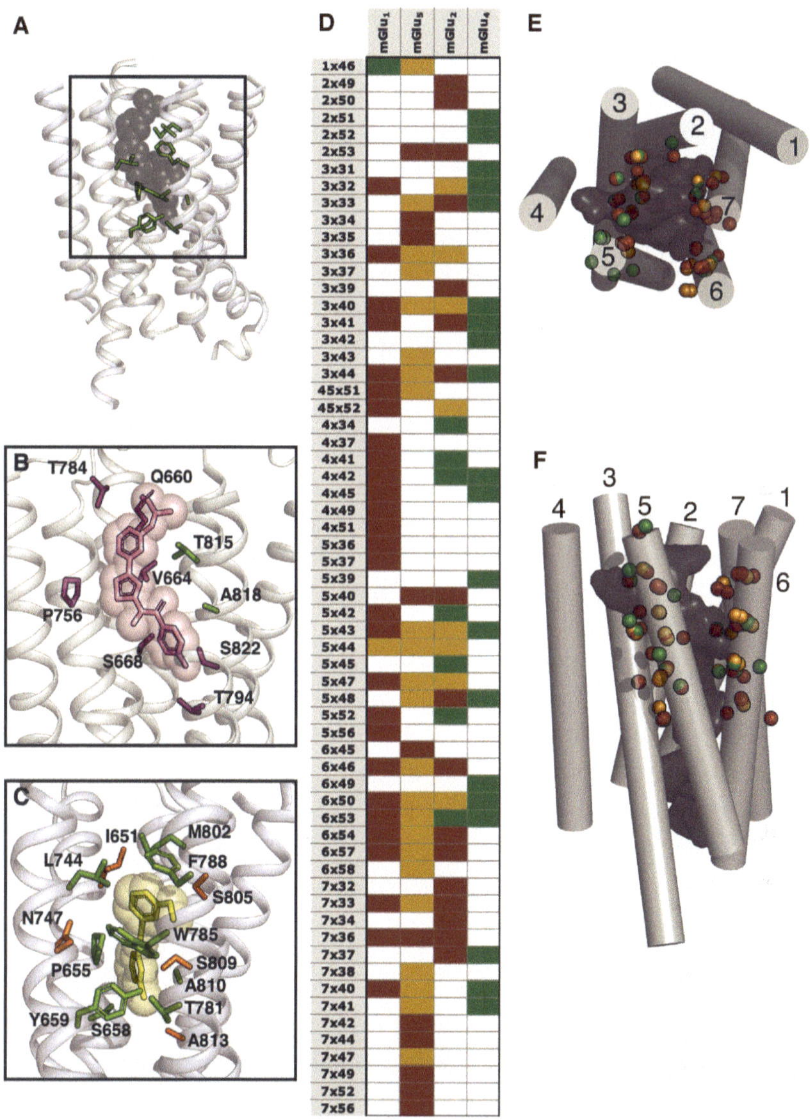

Fig. 6 Combined experiment and modeling to reveal the allosteric binding site. (A) Overlay of the crystal structures of $mGlu_1$ and $mGlu_5$ 7TM domains showing ligands FITM and MMPEP (dark spheres) and amino acids identified from prior SDM studies as being important for their activity (green sticks). (B and C) 7TM domains of $mGlu_1$ and $mGlu_5$ with amino acids affecting NAM activity (green) from Pagano et al. and Litschig et al. ($mGlu_1$) and Malherbe et al. ($mGlu_5$) references that are discussed in the text, and further mutants from the literature (purple and orange). (D) Table summarizing amino acid mutants, identified by their BW numbering, that affect NAM (red), PAM (green) or both NAM and PAM activity (yellow). (E and F) Schematic 7TM domain showing the location of the amino acids affecting NAM (red), PAM (green) or both NAM and PAM activity (yellow).

MPEP (Fig. 4) activity (Malherbe et al., 2003), coinciding with the previous $mGlu_1$ studies (Fig. 6C). Similar reports have been published up to the present day, such as the large scale SDM studies on the $mGlu_2$ (Doornbos et al., 2015; Farinha et al., 2015; Lundström et al., 2011; Pérez-Benito et al., 2017) and $mGlu_5$ receptors (Gregory et al., 2014, 2012). This more recent and substantial body of experimental work was driven by drug discovery groups at F. Hoffmann-La Roche Ltd., Janssen Pharmaceuticals, and Vanderbilt Center for Neuroscience Drug Discovery. It has provided unequivocal information on amino acids relevant for binding, functional activity or glutamate-cooperativity. The current status of mutagenesis studies is summarized in Fig. 6D–F giving a snapshot of the number of amino acids that have been studied and found to affect allosteric modulator activity. As mentioned, much of this work was performed prior to the disclosure of the first mGlu receptor 7TM X-ray crystal structures. At the time there was substantial uncertainty to use these results to generate receptor models and ligand binding modes based only on class A GPCR crystal structures, a concern later confirmed by the diversity of binding modes revealed across GPCR structures, Fig. 3 (Congreve, Oswald, & Marshall, 2017) and differences even within the mGlu family (Christopher et al., 2019). More specifically, despite the apparent convergence of experimental SDM results, hindsight has shown that none of the published modeling attempts of PAM or NAM binding modes at the $mGlu_5$ receptor captured the features, particularly the deeper than expected binding, that was later seen in the first $mGlu_5$ 7TM X-ray structure (Doré et al., 2014).

5. Ligand-based computational modeling of mGlu receptors

With the difficulties to perform structure-based modeling based on distant, low homology X-ray structure templates, computational methods based on the small molecule chemical structure, so-called ligand-based methods, were used to assist drug discovery efforts. For instance, at Janssen these methods were used to identify new $mGlu_2$, $mGlu_5$ and $mGlu_7$ receptor allosteric modulators. For the discovery of $mGlu_2$ receptor PAMs, high-throughput screening delivered a pyridone chemical series that led to the clinical compound JNJ-40411813 (Fig. 4) (Cid et al., 2010; Cid, Duvey, et al., 2012; Cid et al., 2014). Additional chemical scaffolds were needed, and computational methods were used to reveal that the ligands of several different $mGlu_2$ PAM chemotypes shared a common alignment, features and pharmacophore (Tresadern et al., 2010). Pharmacophore models define an ensemble of steric and electronic features necessary for optimal interaction and/or effect with a biological target (Leach, Gillet, Lewis, & Taylor, 2010). They can be calculated from the ligands and bioactivity data alone, by generating, aligning and comparing 3D conformations looking for common features that capture molecular recognition, such as hydrogen bond acceptors or donors, aromatic or lipophilic centers, positively or negatively charged groups, etc. An extension of the pharmacophore method is to compare molecules based on more sophisticated descriptors such as their shape or electrostatic fields (Tresadern & Bemporad, 2010). Thus, for $mGlu_2$ applications a database of chemical fragments was generated and searched using shape and electrostatic similarity to identify alternative scaffolds that shared the overlap and features but with different underlying chemical connectivity. This scaffold-hopping approach led to a novel imidazopyridine scaffold acting as a replacement for the pyridone (Tresadern et al., 2010). Synthesis of close analogues based on the new scaffold resulted in ~100 nM $mGlu_2$ PAMs among the first examples and subsequent optimization led to more potent advanced leads (Cid et al., 2016; Cid, Tresadern, et al., 2012; Doornbos et al., 2017; Trabanco et al., 2012). The scaffold-hopping approach was again used to change from a spirooxindole chemical series to a new benzimidazolone scaffold (de Lucas et al., 2019) as well as to improve the activity of an $mGlu_2$ receptor PAM scaffold fragment (Szabó et al., 2019). In an alternative application, Janssen scientists used the conserved $mGlu_2$ PAM ligand-based alignment to build 3D-quantitative structure–activity relationship (QSAR) and 2D-descriptor machine learning models and predict new potent substituents for a PAM chemical series (Tresadern, Cid, & Trabanco, 2014). Scientists at Merz Pharmaceuticals also used the pharmacophore concept to search for new $mGlu_1$ and $mGlu_5$ NAMs (Mueller et al., 2012; Renner et al., 2007; Vanejevs et al., 2008). Their models identified low micromolar hits for $mGlu_1$ and hits with different chemical substructures for $mGlu_5$. These applications show the value of ligand-based computational modeling for drug discovery in the absence of structure.

The ligand-based modeling of $mGlu_7$ receptor PAMs was more difficult due to the lack of known ligands meaning a pharmacophore model was not possible. An alternative data-driven approach known as proteochemometric (PCM) modeling was used to identify new $mGlu_7$ receptor PAMs (Tresadern et al., 2017). PCM combines multi-target QSAR models into one prediction engine for a target family. Bioactivity data for molecules screened against similar proteins is used as input, and molecular descriptors are used to compare ligands, and amino acid binding site descriptors for receptor similarity. This method made use of the X-ray structures of $mGlu_1$ and $mGlu_5$ 7TM domains to identify the amino acids in the allosteric binding site. Thus, large amounts of Janssen screening data available for mGlu 1, 2 and 5 receptors were used to predict activity versus $mGlu_7$ where little data was available. The PCM model led to new $mGlu_7$ allosteric modulators from several series with one being optimized with further modeling to give a promising series of nanomolar affinity $mGlu_7$ PAMs from computational origins (Cid et al., 2019). In summary, until the first mGlu receptor 7TM structures were published, ligand-based methods were more widespread for computational drug discovery in the mGlu receptor field, afterwards these structures could enable PCM methods and importantly, more accurate structure-based design and analysis.

6. Computational study of $mGlu_2$ receptor allosteric modulators

As mentioned, Janssen is one of many pharmaceutical companies with an interest in the discovery of $mGlu_2$ receptor PAMs and NAMs (Cid et al., 2014, 2016; Doornbos et al., 2015; Trabanco et al., 2012; Van Gool et al., 2017). Experimental mutagenesis studies were performed alongside the medicinal chemistry optimization to determine the ligand binding site. An important aim was to understand functional effect in the context of the ligand-receptor interactions. In the period from 2015 to 2018 several studies were published that confirmed an overlapping binding site and similar interactions among PAMs, and among NAMs, but with some interactions being unique to each set (Cid et al., 2016; Farinha et al., 2015; Pérez-Benito et al., 2017). These studies involved as many as 12 ligands and 39 mutants. Along with binding displacement studies, and deep analysis of structure–activity relationships (SAR), the final analysis making use of computational modeling led to relatively confident predictions of the binding mode of the $mGlu_2$ allosteric modulators. The binding site and mode was later confirmed with the design of a covalent $mGlu_2$ PAM ligand based on the same triazolopyridine scaffold (Doornbos et al., 2019).

In more detail, three PAMs and three NAMs each from different chemical series were studied. Their allosteric functional effect on glutamate activity was confirmed in a $[^{35}S]GTP\gamma S$ assay. Then, all compounds were shown to displace the same tritiated PAM, [^{3}H]JNJ-46281222 (Fig. 4). Mutated receptors were confirmed to express by immunoblotting, showed similar functional glutamate activity, and similar specific binding of a tritiated antagonist suggesting they were well expressed, functional and with an intact orthosteric site. The [^{35}S]GTPγS functional activity was measured for the 6 ligands in 20 mutant receptors. Amino acids $L639^{3.32a.36c}$, $F643^{3.36a.40c}$, $W773^{6.48a.50c}$, and $F776^{6.51a.53c}$ were important for PAM and NAM activity, with $R635^{3.28a.32c}$, $L639^{3.32a.36c}$, and $N735^{5.47a.47c}$ important only for PAMs and $I693^{4.56a.46c}$, $L732^{5.43a.44c}$, $F780^{6.55a.57c}$, and $V798^{7.42a.36c}$ only for NAMs. Thus, allosteric activity was confirmed along with binding at the same site, although with different interactions for PAMs and NAMs. Many analogues from each chemical series were available to develop pharmacophore models for both the PAM and NAM series. This revealed structural features of the ligands essential for activity, for instance a key hydrogen bond acceptor in the central core of the $mGlu_2$ PAMs necessitating a hydrogen bond donor from the binding site.

Active-like and inactive models of the 7TM domain of the $mGlu_2$ receptor were built using the close structural templates from the $mGlu_1$ and $mGlu_5$ X-ray structures. The ligands were docked to identify binding modes that satisfied the mutagenesis and SAR pharmacophore results. In brief, the ligands bound in the expected 7TM site (Fig. 7). All PAMs

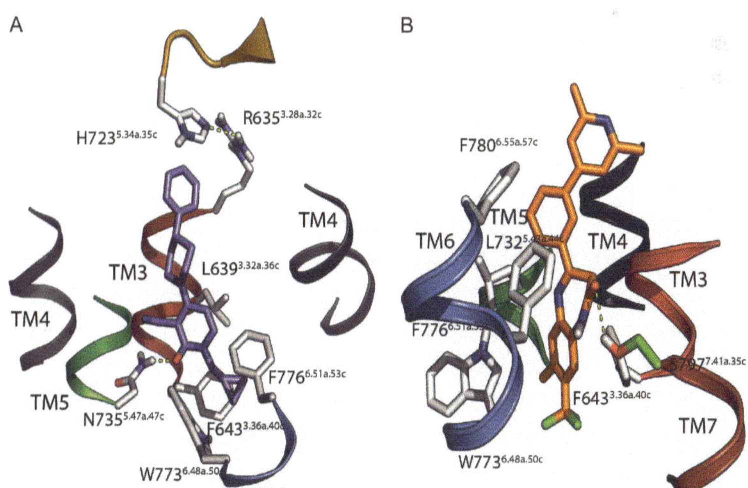

Fig. 7 Proposed binding modes of $mGlu_2$ receptor PAM (A) and NAM (B). *Adapted from Pérez-Benito, L., Doornbos, M. L. J., Cordomí, A., Peeters, L., Lavreysen, H., Pardo, L., et al. (2017). Molecular switches of allosteric modulation of the metabotropic glutamate 2 receptor.* Structure, *25(7), 1153-1162.e1154. https://doi.org/10.1016/j.str.2017.05.021.*

provided a hydrogen bond acceptor to the donor from N735$^{5.47a.47c}$ on TM5, explaining the important pharmacophoric feature and the mutant's effect on activity. The scaffold of the PAMs made aromatic interactions with F643$^{3.36a.40c}$ and F776$^{6.51a.53c}$ while their small hydrophobic substituent bound deepest in the receptor interacting with W773$^{6.48a.50c}$, in agreement with the limited size of this group in the SAR. The PAMs distal tail shows more structural variation and binds toward the extracellular side which is consistent with more varied interactions, in some cases interacting with L639$^{3.32a.36c}$. The NAMs showed a different binding mode in the same site, binding vertically in front of TM6 and making several aromatic interactions with W773$^{6.48a.50c}$, F776$^{6.51a.53c}$, and F780$^{6.55a.57c}$. Their chemical scaffolds were also seen to interact with F643$^{3.36a.40c}$. The interaction of PAMs with the non-conserved N735$^{5.47a.47c}$ provided an explanation for their selectivity versus $mGlu_3$ as this amino acid is Asp in $mGlu_3$. In contrast, $mGlu_2$ NAMs are typically not selective versus $mGlu_3$ and do not interact with this amino acid.

Molecular dynamics (MD) simulations were performed on the PAMs bound in an active-like $mGlu_2$ receptor conformation with G-protein, and the NAMs in an inactive model. The ligands remained stable throughout the simulations providing further confidence in the proposed binding modes (Liu & Kokubo, 2017). The aim of the simulations was to study the effect of the ligands on the amino acids in the vicinity of the binding site. Local structural changes can be reliably studied with microsecond timescale MD simulations, whereas full receptor activation, expected to occur on an approximate 50–100 ms timescale (Hlavackova et al., 2012; Vafabakhsh, Levitz, & Isacoff, 2015), is beyond the scope of current all-atom MD simulations. Analysis identified amino acids with consistent but distinct effects for PAMs compared to NAMs. PAM activation of $mGlu_2$ receptors involved rearrangement of an analogous "transmission switch" in TM3, TM5, and TM6, positions 3.40a, 5.50a, and 6.44a, suggesting consistency with the class A mechanism discussed above. Further structural changes were seen in direct contact with the ligand, one turn above the transmission switch, in an equivalent position to the hydrogen bond between agonist ligand and TM5 S$^{5.46a}$ in class A. These effects were termed a "trigger switch" as they are the initial small local changes provoking the transmission switch movement below. The key hydrogen bond interaction with N735$^{5.47a.47c}$, resembling the interaction between agonists and TM5 in class A, is crucial for the trigger switch action. It causes an inward movement of TM5 (at L738$^{5.50a.50c}$) toward TM3, relocation of Y647$^{3.40a.44c}$ toward

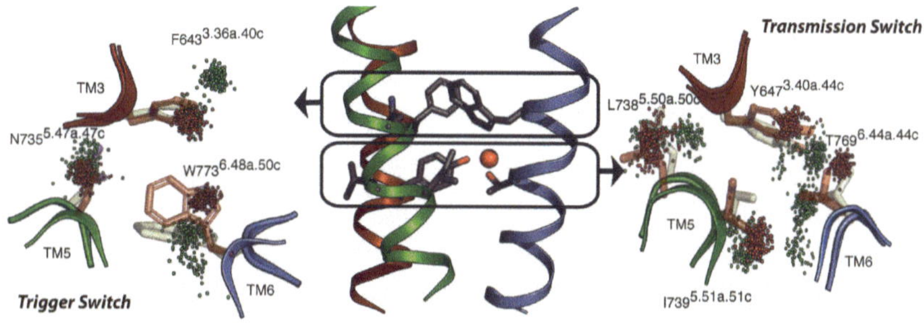

Fig. 8 Comparison of the mechanism of positive and negative allosteric modulation at the mGlu$_2$ receptor. Relative location of the trigger and transmission switch amino acids in the 7TM domain (center). The left and right panels show the position of the amino acids (given as the spheres) in the trigger or transmission switch, respectively, during the MD simulation snapshots, in the presence of either PAM (in green) and NAM (in red). Simulations in presence of PAMs show the hallmark movements of trigger switch induced activation, see text for more details

TM6, and finally repositioning and conformational change of the side chain of T769$^{6.44a.46c}$ from the gauche + to the gauche − or trans conformer (Fig. 8), which was not observed for NAMs. Conformational change of this type in threonine side chains can bend α helices (Ballesteros, Deupi, Olivella, Haaksma, & Pardo, 2000), which in this case would facilitate the outward movement of TM6 for receptor activation. Thus, the similarity with class A activation was revealed, further supported by the understanding that an mGlu receptor 7TM domain can be activated by a PAM alone (El Moustaine et al., 2012).

An interesting aspect of this study was the prospective validation of the hypothesis with new mutants. Mutation of the trigger switch amino acids (F643$^{3.36a.40c}$A, N735$^{5.47a.47c}$D, and W773$^{6.48a.50c}$A) had already been shown to impede PAM allosteric activation despite having no effect on glutamate activity. The new mutations of Y647$^{3.40a.44c}$A and T769$^{6.44a.46c}$A in the transmission switch prevented glutamate activation alone, confirming their role in activation, linking the ECD and intracellular environments. Further mutations such as T769S resulted in lower glutamate activity compared to wild type, while Y647F led to complete loss of activity again, in both cases suggesting an importance of hydrogen bonding and possible water interaction within this switch. It is remarkable that despite studying 40 mutants over many years, various having had no effect (Farinha et al., 2015; Pérez-Benito et al., 2017), the concluding hypothesis was able to pinpoint amino acids relevant for receptor activity.

7. Computational study of $mGlu_5$ receptor allosteric modulators

We performed a similar study for the $mGlu_5$ receptor combining experimental SAR, mutagenesis and computational simulations to investigate the local changes caused by ligand interactions (Llinas del Torrent, Casajuana-Martin, et al., 2019). Interestingly for this receptor, a phenomenon has emerged in which minor changes in ligand chemical structure can result in opposite functional activity (Wood, Hopkins, Brogan, Conn, & Lindsley, 2011). These so-called molecular switches have only been described for the $mGlu_5$ receptor. One example was uncovered in an optimization effort of a $mGlu_5$ partial antagonist (Sharma, Rodriguez, Conn, & Lindsley, 2008). SAR elucidated the changes in ligand chemical structure that caused the change in pharmacological activity, but the origins were not understood. We chose three pairs of NAM PAM analogues to study the origin of the allosteric effect in the $mGlu_5$ receptor, Fig. 9. The ligands present two types of structural change: differing in the position of the substituent methyl group (**1**, **2**) in *meta* giving NAM activity (**1**) or *para* giving a PAM (**2**), or in the type of substituent, ligands **3**, **4**, **5** and **6**. The ligands were structurally similar to MMPEP crystalized in the $mGlu_5$ receptor (Christopher et al., 2019), providing an accurate model for the binding mode, Fig. 9. The ligands were docked into the $mGlu_5$

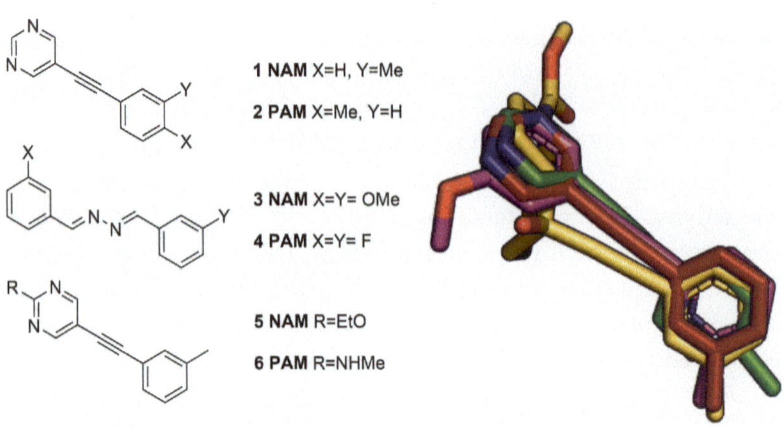

Fig. 9 The three sets of $mGlu_5$ receptor molecular switches. Each pair of molecules have a very similar structure, but opposite allosteric functional activity. The overlay of **1** and **2** (NAM red and PAM green) with crystal structure ligands MMPEP (magenta) and mavoglurant (yellow).

receptor and a series of MD simulations performed. PAMs (**2**, **4**, and **6**) were modeled in an active-like model of the receptor with G-protein while, NAMs (**1**, **3** and **5**) were bound into an inactive model of $mGlu_5$.

Unbiased microsecond timescale MD simulations were used to study how the ligand substituents affected the sidechains in the allosteric site. As a general conclusion, the *meta* substituent of the NAM's phenyl ring in the lower chamber (the *meta* methylphenyl of **1** and **5** or the *meta* methoxyphenyl of **3**) occupies a small cavity between $S658^{3.39a.43c}$ and $Y659^{3.40a.44c}$ as seen also in the X-ray of the NAMs crystalized in $mGlu_5$. This interaction locks the side chains of $S658^{3.39a.43c}$, $Y659^{3.40a.44c}$, and $T781^{6.44a.46c}$ in an "inactive"-like conformation, preventing the movement of amino acids that can be relevant to initiate activation. Analysis of the rotamers of these amino acids showed an important conformational change of $T781^{6.44a.46c}$ when PAMs were bound that was not seen for NAM binding, Fig. 10D and E. As seen in the $mGlu_2$ study, the rotameric change of $T781^{6.44a.46c}$ from gauche+ to gauche− or trans conformer introduces a flexible point in TM6, likely relevant for receptor activation.

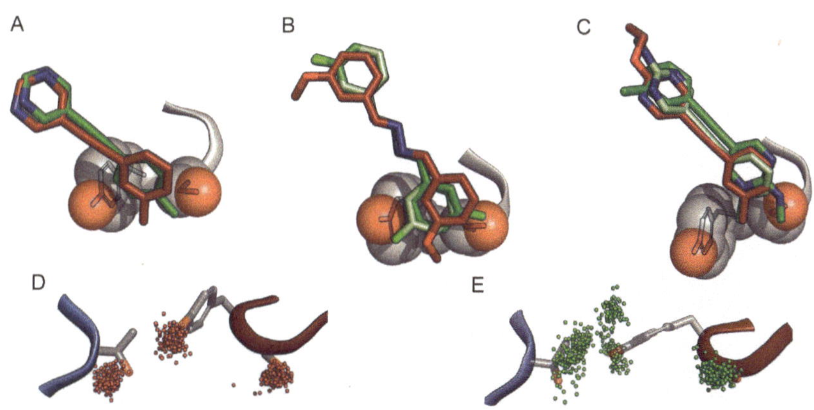

Fig. 10 Blocking interaction of NAMs compared to PAMs. The NAM's *meta* substituent on the aromatic ring in the lower chamber fills a small cavity between $S658^{3.39a.43c}$ and $Y659^{3.40a.44c}$. This prevents the movement of their side chains, and they remain in their stable inactive like conformations. (A) Ligands **1** (red) and **2** (green). (B) Ligands **3** (red) and **4** in the two possible binding modes (green binding mode 1 and light green binding mode 2). (C) Ligands **5** (red) and **6** in the two possible binding modes (green binding mode 1 and light green binding mode 2). (D and E) The movement of $S658^{3.39a.43c}$, $Y659^{3.40a.44c}$, and $T781^{6.44a.46c}$ in the presence of NAMs (red, D) or PAMs (green, E). The spheres show the position of the oxygen side chain atoms at evenly spaced snapshots during the MD simulations in the presence of NAMs or PAMs.

Despite different possible binding modes for the PAMs 4 and 6, Fig. 10B and C, the hypothesis remained consistent.

Control simulations were performed using the *apo* $mGlu_5$ active state bound to the G protein and found to exhibit no rotameric movement of $T781^{6.44a.46c}$. Likewise, repeat simulations of the $mGlu_5$ inactive state with a PAM also showed no movement of the same amino acid. Thus, the observed sidechain movements were not a function of only the ligand, nor only a consequence of the active-state model, but the result of the combination of PAM and active-state receptor. A recent study of two ligands, published following our $mGlu_2$ and $mGlu_5$ reports, also suggested similarity with class A (Cong, Chéron, Golebiowski, Antonczak, & Fiorucci, 2019). They studied one PAM, **4** Fig. 9, and proposed its effect was caused by a shallower binding mode although it is difficult to foresee how the hypothesis could extrapolate to other PAMs. For instance, it does not account for the PAM/NAM switches nor the substantial SAR of both PAMs and NAMs from the same bisarylacetylene scaffold (Emmitte, 2017; Kosuke, Takeshi, & Youichi, 2010). Indeed, the bisarylacetylene is a privileged scaffold for $mGlu_5$ receptor PAMs and NAMs due to its unique narrow linear shape being able to bind deeply by passing the smaller non-conserved amino acids on TMs 3 and 7, $P655^{3.40}$ and $A810^{7.41}$ (larger F and V in group II mGlu receptors for instance) (Doré et al., 2014; Harpsøe et al., 2015). Also, published SAR for bisarylacetylene NAMs was consistent with the *meta* substituent in the lower chamber being crucial for functional activity (Llinas del Torrent, Casajuana-Martin, et al., 2019).

8. Water and mGlu allosteric modulators

For some time, water molecules have been suggested to play an important role in GPCR functional activity (Pardo, Deupi, Dölker, López-Rodríguez, & Campillo, 2007; Venkatakrishnan et al., 2019). Subsequent high-resolution X-ray structures revealed conserved water positions that provided evidence of an unknown function (Miller-Gallacher et al., 2014; Suno et al., 2018; Wang et al., 2017). More recent simulation studies on class A GPCRs have shown that certain water positions create a network of stable water-mediated interactions with differences seen between active and inactive states (Venkatakrishnan et al., 2019). In the study of the $mGlu_2$ receptor, we observed a water molecule entering, forming and stabilizing a network of interactions within the transmission switch during the simulations. We hypothesized that it played an important role on the conformational effects of the adjacent amino acids. The mutation Y647F in the transmission switch, involving only the loss of an OH group, suggested an important hydrogen bond network in this region. In the $mGlu_5$ case the calculation inputs were built starting with the $mGlu_5$ 7TM crystal structure which actually contained a crystallographic water in this position (Doré et al., 2014). Therefore, with more confidence in the position of the water within the transmission switch, we studied its position and interactions throughout the simulations. We observed that it was remarkably more stable for NAMs than PAMs, forming a hydrogen bond bridging interaction between $Y659^{3.40a.44c}$ and $T781^{6.44a.46c}$ 88% of the time in the NAM simulations compared to 29% with the PAMs, Fig. 11. This confirms a role for the water in the functional activity of the receptor, working in tandem with the fixed sidechain conformations, to stabilize the inactive state conformation within the transmission switch.

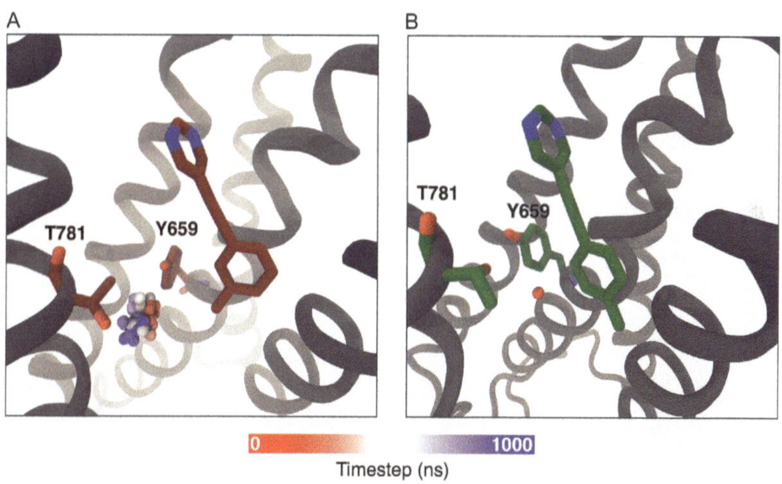

Fig. 11 The importance of water in the inactive state of the mGlu receptor transmission switch. (A) 7TM of $mGlu_5$ receptor bound with NAM **1**. The spheres are water oxygen atom positions extracted from MD simulation snapshots, showing the maintenance of the water within the transmissions switch throughout the simulation duration. (B) Analogous figure showing the $mGlu_5$ 7TM domain binding PAM **2**. Extracting the water sites from MD simulation snapshots reveals the lack of water in the transmission switch during the PAM simulation due to the alternative position of sidechains such as $T781^{6.44a.46c}$.

9. Conclusion

We have discussed a broad scope of computational modeling applied to drug discovery of allosteric modulators of the mGlu receptors. In the absence of high-quality structural templates of the 7TM domain, ligand-based methods such as pharmacophoric overlays, scaffold hopping and PCM models were useful for identifying new hits or lead scaffolds and these approaches remain valuable. Following the breakthroughs in the X-ray structures of the 7TM domains of the $mGlu_1$ and $mGlu_5$ receptors, higher confidence structure-based modeling became possible. In our case, we embarked on detailed studies to reconcile the available experimental information: binding displacement studies, site directed mutagenesis, and SAR with modeled hypotheses of binding modes. With this relatively high-confident starting point, the use of more costly and sophisticated MD simulations revealed the ligand induced conformational changes at atomic resolution. Observing activation of full-length mGlu receptors with such detailed simulations is not possible today, but our work does allow us to inspect the local changes that have been identified in the many breakthrough publications particularly on class A GPCRs as initiating ligand mediated functional activity. In the case of the $mGlu_2$ receptor this was started by a crucial hydrogen bond between PAMs and TM5. We termed these changes a "trigger switch" as they occurred one level above the well-known "transmission switch" and appeared to be the direct conformational changes prompted or stabilized (it is not possible to resolve the difference in this regard) caused by ligand receptor interactions. In the case of $mGlu_5$ receptors, the allosteric modulators bind deeper, therefore bypassing the "trigger switch" and instead interfering directly with the "transmission switch" itself. The NAMs blocked movement and stabilized the inactive conformation, whereas PAMs promoted movement and alternative sidechain conformations. Furthermore, the importance of a water molecule in stabilizing the inactive state of the transmission switch was confirmed. Overall, as well as providing a basic insight into how mGlu receptor allosteric modulators elicit their functional effect, this work could have a large impact on drug design. One could optimize ligands to promote and stabilize the interactions relevant for PAMs and NAMs, for instance, hydrogen bonding interactions of $mGlu_2$ PAMs with TM5, or substituting $mGlu_2$ NAMs in an increasingly linear fashion to promote their blocking interaction in front of TM6, or in the case of $mGlu_5$ considering in detail the role of the *meta* versus *para* substitution of the aromatic ring in the lower chamber. Finally, these studies highlight the value of MD simulations in a drug discovery context.

Acknowledgments

L.P.B. and G.T. thank colleagues at Janssen for continued collaboration and discussions, particularly José-Maria Cid, Andrés A. Trabanco and Hilde Lavreysen the respective chemistry and biology leads on several mGlu programs. We also thank other members of the group of Prof. Pardo who have contributed to the work described in the chapter.

Conflict of interest

L.P.B and G.T. are employees of Janssen Pharmaceutical Research and Development and have been involved in the pre-clinical discovery of small molecule mGlu receptor allosteric modulators. No further conflicts of interest to declare.

References

Alexander, S. P. H., Christopoulos, A., Davenport, A. P., Kelly, E., Marrion, N. V., Peters, J. A., et al. (2017). THE CONCISE GUIDE TO PHARMACOLOGY 2017/18: G protein-coupled receptors. *British Journal of Pharmacology, 174*(S1), S17–S129. https://doi.org/10.1111/bph.13878.

Ballesteros, J. A., Deupi, X., Olivella, M., Haaksma, E. E. J., & Pardo, L. (2000). Serine and threonine residues bend α-helices in the $\chi 1 = g-$ conformation. *Biophysical Journal, 79*(5), 2754–2760. https://doi.org/10.1016/S0006-3495(00)76514-3.

Ballesteros, J. A., & Weinstein, H. (1995). [19] Integrated methods for the construction of three-dimensional models and computational probing of structure-function relations in G protein-coupled receptors. In S. C. Sealfon (Ed.), *Vol. 25. Methods in Neurosciences* (pp. 366–428). Academic Press.

Barnes, S. A., Sheffler, D. J., Semenova, S., Cosford, N. D. P., & Bespalov, A. (2018). Metabotropic glutamate receptor 5 as a target for the treatment of depression and smoking: Robust preclinical data but inconclusive clinical efficacy. *Biological Psychiatry, 83*(11), 955–962. https://doi.org/10.1016/j.biopsych.2018.03.001.

Celli, R., Santolini, I., Van Luijtelaar, G., Ngomba, R. T., Bruno, V., & Nicoletti, F. (2019). Targeting metabotropic glutamate receptors in the treatment of epilepsy: Rationale and current status. *Expert Opinion on Therapeutic Targets, 23*(4), 341–351. https://doi.org/10.1080/14728222.2019.1586885.

Christopher, J. A., Orgován, Z., Congreve, M., Doré, A. S., Errey, J. C., Marshall, F. H., et al. (2019). Structure-based optimization strategies for G protein-coupled receptor (GPCR) allosteric modulators: A case study from analyses of new metabotropic glutamate receptor 5 (mGlu5) X-ray structures. *Journal of Medicinal Chemistry, 62*(1), 207–222. https://doi.org/10.1021/acs.jmedchem.7b01722.

Christopoulos, A. (2014). Advances in G protein-coupled receptor allostery: From function to structure. *Molecular Pharmacology, 86*(5), 463. https://doi.org/10.1124/mol.114.094342.

Cid, J. M., Duvey, G., Cluzeau, P., Nhem, V., Macary, K., Raux, A., et al. (2010). Discovery of 1,5-disubstituted pyridones: A new class of positive allosteric modulators of the metabotropic glutamate 2 receptor. *ACS Chemical Neuroscience, 1*(12), 788–795. https://doi.org/10.1021/cn1000638.

Cid, J. M., Duvey, G., Tresadern, G., Nhem, V., Furnari, R., Cluzeau, P., et al. (2012). Discovery of 1,4-disubstituted 3-cyano-2-pyridones: A new class of positive allosteric modulators of the metabotropic glutamate 2 receptor. *Journal of Medicinal Chemistry*, *55*(5), 2388–2405. https://doi.org/10.1021/jm2016864.

Cid, J. M., Lavreysen, H., Tresadern, G., Pérez-Benito, L., Tovar, F., Fontana, A., et al. (2019). Computationally guided identification of allosteric agonists of the metabotropic glutamate 7 receptor. *ACS Chemical Neuroscience*, *10*(3), 1043–1054. https://doi.org/10.1021/acschemneuro.8b00331.

Cid, J. M., Tresadern, G., Duvey, G., Lütjens, R., Finn, T., Rocher, J.-P., et al. (2014). Discovery of 1-Butyl-3-chloro-4-(4-phenyl-1-piperidinyl)-(1H)-pyridone (JNJ-40411813): A novel positive allosteric modulator of the metabotropic glutamate 2 receptor. *Journal of Medicinal Chemistry*, *57*(15), 6495–6512. https://doi.org/10.1021/jm500496m.

Cid, J. M., Tresadern, G., Vega, J. A., de Lucas, A. I., del Cerro, A., Matesanz, E., et al. (2016). Discovery of 8-trifluoromethyl-3-cyclopropylmethyl-7-[(4-(2,4-difluorophenyl)-1-piperazinyl)methyl]-1,2,4-triazolo[4,3-a]pyridine (JNJ-46356479), a selective and orally bioavailable mGlu2 receptor positive allosteric modulator (PAM). *Journal of Medicinal Chemistry*, *59*(18), 8495–8507. https://doi.org/10.1021/acs.jmedchem.6b00913.

Cid, J. M., Tresadern, G., Vega, J. A., de Lucas, A. I., Matesanz, E., Iturrino, L., et al. (2012). Discovery of 3-Cyclopropylmethyl-7-(4-phenylpiperidin-1-yl)-8-trifluoromethyl [1,2,4]triazolo[4,3-a]pyridine (JNJ-42153605): A positive allosteric modulator of the metabotropic glutamate 2 receptor. *Journal of Medicinal Chemistry*, *55*(20), 8770–8789. https://doi.org/10.1021/jm3010724.

Cong, X., Chéron, J.-B., Golebiowski, J., Antonczak, S., & Fiorucci, S. (2019). Allosteric modulation mechanism of the mGluR5 transmembrane domain. *Journal of Chemical Information and Modeling*, *59*(6), 2871–2878. https://doi.org/10.1021/acs.jcim.9b00045.

Congreve, M., Oswald, C., & Marshall, F. H. (2017). Applying structure-based drug design approaches to allosteric modulators of GPCRs. *Trends in Pharmacological Sciences*, *38*(9), 837–847. https://doi.org/10.1016/j.tips.2017.05.010.

Conn, P. J., Christopoulos, A., & Lindsley, C. W. (2009). Allosteric modulators of GPCRs: A novel approach for the treatment of CNS disorders. *Nature Reviews Drug Discovery*, *8*(1), 41–54. https://doi.org/10.1038/nrd2760.

Conn, P. J., Lindsley, C. W., & Jones, C. K. (2009). Activation of metabotropic glutamate receptors as a novel approach for the treatment of schizophrenia. *Trends in Pharmacological Sciences*, *30*(1), 25–31. https://doi.org/10.1016/j.tips.2008.10.006.

Conn, P. J., & Pin, J.-P. (1997). Pharmacology and functions of metabotropic glutamate receptors. *Annual Review of Pharmacology and Toxicology*, *37*(1), 205–237. https://doi.org/10.1146/annurev.pharmtox.37.1.205.

Cooke, R., & Congreve, M. (2016). Allosteric binding: Structures reveal new ways to tame G protein-coupled receptors. *Future Medicinal Chemistry*, *8*(17), 2005–2007. https://doi.org/10.4155/fmc-2016-0167.

Cordomí, A., Ismail, S., Matsoukas, M.-T., Escrieut, C., Gherardi, M.-J., Pardo, L., et al. (2015). Functional elements of the gastric inhibitory polypeptide receptor: Comparison between secretin- and rhodopsin-like G protein-coupled receptors. *Biochemical Pharmacology*, *96*(3), 237–246. https://doi.org/10.1016/j.bcp.2015.05.015.

Day, P. W., Rasmussen, S. G. F., Parnot, C., Fung, J. J., Masood, A., Kobilka, T. S., et al. (2007). A monoclonal antibody for G protein-coupled receptor crystallography. *Nature Methods*, *4*(11), 927–929. https://doi.org/10.1038/nmeth1112.

de Lucas, A. I., Vega, J. A., Matesanz, E., Linares, M. L., García Molina, A., Tresadern, G., et al. (2019). Spiro-oxindole piperidines and 3-(Azetidin-3-yl)-1H-benzimidazol-2-ones as mGlu2 receptor PAMs. *ACS Medicinal Chemistry Letters*. https://doi.org/10.1021/acsmedchemlett.9b00350.

Doornbos, M. L. J., Cid, J. M., Haubrich, J., Nunes, A., van de Sande, J. W., Vermond, S. C., et al. (2017). Discovery and kinetic profiling of 7-Aryl-1,2,4-triazolo[4,3-a]pyridines: Positive allosteric modulators of the metabotropic glutamate receptor 2. *Journal of Medicinal Chemistry*, *60*(15), 6704–6720. https://doi.org/10.1021/acs.jmedchem.7b00669.

Doornbos, M. L. J., Pérez-Benito, L., Tresadern, G., Mulder-Krieger, T., Biesmans, I., Trabanco, A. A., et al. (2015). Molecular mechanism of positive allosteric modulation of the metabotropic glutamate receptor 2 by JNJ-46281222. *British Journal of Pharmacology*, *173*(3), 588–600. https://doi.org/10.1111/bph.13390.

Doornbos, M. L. J., Wang, X., Vermond, S. C., Peeters, L., Pérez-Benito, L., Trabanco, A. A., et al. (2019). Covalent allosteric probe for the metabotropic glutamate receptor 2: Design, synthesis, and pharmacological characterization. *Journal of Medicinal Chemistry*, *62*(1), 223–233. https://doi.org/10.1021/acs.jmedchem.8b00051.

Doré, A. S., Okrasa, K., Patel, J. C., Serrano-Vega, M., Bennett, K., Cooke, R. M., et al. (2014). Structure of class C GPCR metabotropic glutamate receptor 5 transmembrane domain. *Nature*, *511*, 557. https://doi.org/10.1038/nature13396.

Dror, R. O., Pan, A. C., Arlow, D. H., Borhani, D. W., Maragakis, P., Shan, Y., et al. (2011). Pathway and mechanism of drug binding to G-protein-coupled receptors. *Proceedings of the National Academy of Sciences of the United States of America*, *108*(32), 13118. https://doi.org/10.1073/pnas.1104614108.

El Moustaine, D., Granier, S., Doumazane, E., Scholler, P., Rahmeh, R., Bron, P., et al. (2012). Distinct roles of metabotropic glutamate receptor dimerization in agonist activation and G-protein coupling. *Proceedings of the National Academy of Sciences of the United States of America*, *109*(40), 16342.

Emmitte, K. A. (2017). mGlu5 negative allosteric modulators: A patent review (2013–2016). *Expert Opinion on Therapeutic Patents*, *27*(6), 691–706. https://doi.org/10.1080/13543776.2017.1280466.

Farinha, A., Lavreysen, H., Peeters, L., Russo, B., Masure, S., Trabanco, A. A., et al. (2015). Molecular determinants of positive allosteric modulation of the human metabotropic glutamate receptor 2. *British Journal of Pharmacology*, *172*(9), 2383–2396. https://doi.org/10.1111/bph.13065.

Foster, D. J., & Conn, P. J. (2017). Allosteric modulation of GPCRs: New insights and potential utility for treatment of schizophrenia and other CNS disorders. *Neuron*, *94*(3), 431–446. https://doi.org/10.1016/j.neuron.2017.03.016.

Fredriksson, R., & Schiöth, H. B. (2005). The repertoire of G-protein-coupled receptors in fully sequenced genomes. *Molecular Pharmacology*, *67*(5), 1414. https://doi.org/10.1124/mol.104.009001.

Geng, Y., Bush, M., Mosyak, L., Wang, F., & Fan, Q. R. (2013). Structural mechanism of ligand activation in human GABAB receptor. *Nature*, *504*(7479), 254–259. https://doi.org/10.1038/nature12725.

Gjoni, T., & Urwyler, S. (2008). Receptor activation involving positive allosteric modulation, unlike full agonism, does not result in GABAB receptor desensitization. *Neuropharmacology*, *55*(8), 1293–1299. https://doi.org/10.1016/j.neuropharm.2008.08.008.

González, A., Perez-Acle, T., Pardo, L., & Deupi, X. (2011). Molecular basis of ligand dissociation in β-adrenergic receptors. *PLoS One*, *6*(9), e23815. https://doi.org/10.1371/journal.pone.0023815.

Gregory, K. J., Nguyen, E. D., Malosh, C., Mendenhall, J. L., Zic, J. Z., Bates, B. S., et al. (2014). Identification of specific ligand–receptor interactions that govern binding and cooperativity of diverse modulators to a common metabotropic glutamate receptor 5 allosteric site. *ACS Chemical Neuroscience*, *5*(4), 282–295. https://doi.org/10.1021/cn400225x.

Gregory, K. J., Noetzel, M. J., Rook, J. M., Vinson, P. N., Stauffer, S. R., Rodriguez, A. L., et al. (2012). Investigating metabotropic glutamate receptor 5 allosteric modulator cooperativity, affinity, and agonism: Enriching structure-function studies and structure-activity relationships. *Molecular Pharmacology*, *82*(5), 860. https://doi.org/10.1124/mol.112.080531.

Harpsøe, K., Isberg, V., Tehan, B. G., Weiss, D., Arsova, A., Marshall, F. H., et al. (2015). Selective negative allosteric modulation of metabotropic glutamate receptors—A structural perspective of ligands and mutants. *Scientific Reports*, *5*, 13869. https://doi.org/10.1038/srep13869.

Hauser, A. S., Attwood, M. M., Rask-Andersen, M., Schiöth, H. B., & Gloriam, D. E. (2017). Trends in GPCR drug discovery: New agents, targets and indications. *Nature Reviews Drug Discovery*, *16*, 829. https://doi.org/10.1038/nrd.2017.178.

Hlavackova, V., Zabel, U., Frankova, D., Bätz, J., Hoffmann, C., Prezeau, L., et al. (2012). Sequential inter- and intrasubunit rearrangements during activation of dimeric metabotropic glutamate receptor 1. *Science Signaling*, *5*(237), ra59.

Huang, J., Chen, S., Zhang, J. J., & Huang, X.-Y. (2013). Crystal structure of oligomeric β1-adrenergic G protein-coupled receptors in ligand-free basal state. *Nature Structural & Molecular Biology*, *20*, 419. https://doi.org/10.1038/nsmb.2504.

Huang, W., Manglik, A., Venkatakrishnan, A. J., Laeremans, T., Feinberg, E. N., Sanborn, A. L., et al. (2015). Structural insights into μ-opioid receptor activation. *Nature*, *524*, 315. https://doi.org/10.1038/nature14886.

Isberg, V., de Graaf, C., Bortolato, A., Cherezov, V., Katritch, V., Marshall, F. H., et al. (2015). Generic GPCR residue numbers—Aligning topology maps while minding the gaps. *Trends in Pharmacological Sciences*, *36*(1), 22–31. https://doi.org/10.1016/j.tips.2014.11.001.

Kang, Y., Zhou, X. E., Gao, X., He, Y., Liu, W., Ishchenko, A., et al. (2015). Crystal structure of rhodopsin bound to arrestin by femtosecond X-ray laser. *Nature*, *523*, 561. https://doi.org/10.1038/nature14656.

Koehl, A., Hu, H., Feng, D., Sun, B., Zhang, Y., Robertson, M. J., et al. (2019). Structural insights into the activation of metabotropic glutamate receptors. *Nature*, *566*, 79–84. https://doi.org/10.1038/s41586-019-0881-4.

Komolov, K. E., Du, Y., Duc, N. M., Betz, R. M., Rodrigues, J. P. G. L. M., Leib, R. D., et al. (2017). Structural and functional analysis of a β2-adrenergic receptor complex with GRK5. *Cell*, *169*(3), 407-421.e416. https://doi.org/10.1016/j.cell.2017.03.047.

Kosuke, K., Takeshi, A., & Youichi, S. (2010). Recent patents on positive allosteric modulators of the metabotropic glutamate 5 receptor as a potential treatment for schizophrenia. *Recent Patents on CNS Drug Discovery*, *5*(1), 23–34. https://doi.org/10.2174/157488910789753512.

Krishna Kumar, K., Shalev-Benami, M., Robertson, M. J., Hu, H., Banister, S. D., Hollingsworth, S. A., et al. (2019). Structure of a signaling cannabinoid receptor 1-G protein complex. *Cell*, *176*(3), 448-458.e412. https://doi.org/10.1016/j.cell.2018.11.040.

Kristiansen, K. (2004). Molecular mechanisms of ligand binding, signaling, and regulation within the superfamily of G-protein-coupled receptors: Molecular modeling and mutagenesis approaches to receptor structure and function. *Pharmacology and Therapeutics*, *103*(1), 21–80. https://doi.org/10.1016/j.pharmthera.2004.05.002.

Kruse, A. C., Ring, A. M., Manglik, A., Hu, J., Hu, K., Eitel, K., et al. (2013). Activation and allosteric modulation of a muscarinic acetylcholine receptor. *Nature*, *504*, 101. https://doi.org/10.1038/nature12735.

Kunishima, N., Shimada, Y., Tsuji, Y., Sato, T., Yamamoto, M., Kumasaka, T., et al. (2000). Structural basis of glutamate recognition by a dimeric metabotropic glutamate receptor. *Nature*, *407*, 971. https://doi.org/10.1038/35039564.

Lane, J. R., Sexton, P. M., & Christopoulos, A. (2013). Bridging the gap: Bitopic ligands of G-protein-coupled receptors. *Trends in Pharmacological Sciences*, *34*(1), 59–66. https://doi.org/10.1016/j.tips.2012.10.003.

Leach, A. R., Gillet, V. J., Lewis, R. A., & Taylor, R. (2010). Three-dimensional pharmacophore methods in drug discovery. *Journal of Medicinal Chemistry*, *53*(2), 539–558. https://doi.org/10.1021/jm900817u.

Litschig, S., Gasparini, F., Rueegg, D., Stoehr, N., Flor, P. J., Vranesic, I., et al. (1999). CPCCOEt, a noncompetitive metabotropic glutamate receptor 1 antagonist, inhibits receptor signaling without affecting glutamate binding. *Molecular Pharmacology*, *55*(3), 453.

Liu, K., & Kokubo, H. (2017). Exploring the stability of ligand binding modes to proteins by molecular dynamics simulations: A cross-docking study. *Journal of Chemical Information and Modeling*, *57*(10), 2514–2522. https://doi.org/10.1021/acs.jcim.7b00412.

Liu, X., Masoudi, A., Kahsai, A. W., Huang, L.-Y., Pani, B., Staus, D. P., et al. (2019). Mechanism of β2AR regulation by an intracellular positive allosteric modulator. *Science*, *364*(6447), 1283. https://doi.org/10.1126/science.aaw8981.

Llinas del Torrent, C., Casajuana-Martin, N., Pardo, L., Tresadern, G., & Pérez-Benito, L. (2019). Mechanisms underlying allosteric molecular switches of metabotropic glutamate receptor 5. *Journal of Chemical Information and Modeling*, *59*(5), 2456–2466. https://doi.org/10.1021/acs.jcim.8b00924.

Llinas del Torrent, C., Pérez-Benito, L., & Tresadern, G. (2019). Computational drug design applied to the study of metabotropic glutamate receptors. *Molecules*, *24*(6), 1098. https://doi.org/10.3390/molecules24061098.

Lu, S., & Zhang, J. (2019). Small molecule allosteric modulators of G-protein-coupled receptors: Drug–target interactions. *Journal of Medicinal Chemistry*, *62*(1), 24–45. https://doi.org/10.1021/acs.jmedchem.7b01844.

Lundström, L., Bissantz, C., Beck, J., Wettstein, J. G., Woltering, T. J., Wichmann, J., et al. (2011). Structural determinants of allosteric antagonism at metabotropic glutamate receptor 2: Mechanistic studies with new potent negative allosteric modulators. *British Journal of Pharmacology*, *164*(2b), 521–537. https://doi.org/10.1111/j.1476-5381.2011.01409.x.

Maeda, S., Qu, Q., Robertson, M. J., Skiniotis, G., & Kobilka, B. K. (2019). Structures of the M1 and M2 muscarinic acetylcholine receptor/G-protein complexes. *Science*, *364*(6440), 552. https://doi.org/10.1126/science.aaw5188.

Malherbe, P., Kratochwil, N., Zenner, M.-T., Piussi, J., Diener, C., Kratzeisen, C., et al. (2003). Mutational analysis and molecular modeling of the binding pocket of the metabotropic glutamate 5 receptor negative modulator 2-methyl-6-(phenylethynyl)-pyridine. *Molecular Pharmacology*, *64*(4), 823. https://doi.org/10.1124/mol.64.4.823.

Manglik, A., Kruse, A. C., Kobilka, T. S., Thian, F. S., Mathiesen, J. M., Sunahara, R. K., et al. (2012). Crystal structure of the μ-opioid receptor bound to a morphinan antagonist. *Nature*, *485*(7398), 321–326. https://doi.org/10.1038/nature10954.

Miller-Gallacher, J. L., Nehmé, R., Warne, T., Edwards, P. C., Schertler, G. F. X., Leslie, A. G. W., et al. (2014). The 2.1 Å resolution structure of cyanopindolol-bound β1-adrenoceptor identifies an intramembrane Na+ ion that stabilises the ligand-free receptor. *PloS One*, *9*(3), e92727. https://doi.org/10.1371/journal.pone.0092727.

Monn, J. A., Prieto, L., Taboada, L., Pedregal, C., Hao, J., Reinhard, M. R., et al. (2015). Synthesis and pharmacological characterization of C4-disubstituted analogs of 1S,2S,5R,6S-2-aminobicyclo[3.1.0]hexane-2,6-dicarboxylate: Identification of a potent, selective metabotropic glutamate receptor agonist and determination of agonist-bound human mGlu2 and mGlu3 amino terminal domain structures. *Journal of Medicinal Chemistry*, *58*(4), 1776–1794. https://doi.org/10.1021/jm501612y.

Mueller, R., Dawson, E. S., Meiler, J., Rodriguez, A. L., Chauder, B. A., Bates, B. S., et al. (2012). Discovery of 2-(2-benzoxazoyl amino)-4-aryl-5-cyanopyrimidine as negative allosteric modulators (NAMs) of metabotropic glutamate receptor 5 (mGlu5): From an artificial neural network virtual screen to an in vivo tool compound. *ChemMedChem*, 7(3), 406–414. https://doi.org/10.1002/cmdc.201100510.

Munk, C., Mutt, E., Isberg, V., Nikolajsen, L. F., Bibbe, J. M., Flock, T., et al. (2019). An online resource for GPCR structure determination and analysis. *Nature Methods*, *16*(2), 151–162. https://doi.org/10.1038/s41592-018-0302-x.

Muto, T., Tsuchiya, D., Morikawa, K., & Jingami, H. (2007). Structures of the extracellular regions of the group II/III metabotropic glutamate receptors. *Proceedings of the National Academy of Sciences of the United States of America*, *104*(10), 3759. https://doi.org/10.1073/pnas.0611577104.

Niswender, C. M., & Conn, P. J. (2010). Metabotropic glutamate receptors: Physiology, pharmacology, and disease. *Annual Review of Pharmacology and Toxicology*, *50*(1), 295–322. https://doi.org/10.1146/annurev.pharmtox.011008.145533.

Nygaard, R., Zou, Y., Dror, R. O., Mildorf, T. J., Arlow, D. H., Manglik, A., et al. (2013). The dynamic process of β(2)-adrenergic receptor activation. *Cell*, *152*(3), 532–542. https://doi.org/10.1016/j.cell.2013.01.008.

Pagano, A., Rüegg, D., Litschig, S., Stoehr, N., Stierlin, C., Heinrich, M., et al. (2000). The non-competitive antagonists 2-methyl-6-(phenylethynyl)pyridine and 7-hydroxyiminocyclopropan[b]chromen-1a-carboxylic acid ethyl ester interact with overlapping binding pockets in the transmembrane region of group I metabotropic glutamate receptors. *Journal of Biological Chemistry*, *275*(43), 33750–33758.

Palczewski, K., Kumasaka, T., Hori, T., Behnke, C. A., Motoshima, H., Fox, B. A., et al. (2000). Crystal structure of rhodopsin: A G protein-coupled receptor. *Science*, *289*(5480), 739. https://doi.org/10.1126/science.289.5480.739.

Pándy-Szekeres, G., Munk, C., Tsonkov, T. M., Mordalski, S., Harpsøe, K., Hauser, A. S., et al. (2018). GPCRdb in 2018: Adding GPCR structure models and ligands. *Nucleic Acids Research*, *46*(D1), D440–D446. https://doi.org/10.1093/nar/gkx1109.

Pardo, L., Deupi, X., Dölker, N., López-Rodríguez, M. L., & Campillo, M. (2007). The role of internal water molecules in the structure and function of the rhodopsin family of G protein-coupled receptors. *Chembiochem: A European Journal of Chemical Biology*, *8*(1), 19–24. https://doi.org/10.1002/cbic.200600429.

Pellissier, L. P., Sallander, J., Campillo, M., Gaven, F., Queffeulou, E., Pillot, M., et al. (2009). Conformational toggle switches implicated in basal constitutive and agonist-induced activated states of 5-hydroxytryptamine-4 receptors. *Molecular Pharmacology*, *75*(4), 982. https://doi.org/10.1124/mol.108.053686.

Pérez-Benito, L., Doornbos, M. L. J., Cordomí, A., Peeters, L., Lavreysen, H., Pardo, L., et al. (2017). Molecular switches of allosteric modulation of the metabotropic glutamate 2 receptor. *Structure*, *25*(7), 1153-1162.e1154. https://doi.org/10.1016/j.str.2017.05.021.

Pérez-Benito, L., Henry, A., Matsoukas, M.-T., Lopez, L., Pulido, D., Royo, M., et al. (2018). The size matters? A computational tool to design bivalent ligands. *Bioinformatics*, *34*(22), 3857–3863. https://doi.org/10.1093/bioinformatics/bty422.

Peterlik, D., Flor, P. J., & Uschold-Schmidt, N. (2016). The emerging role of metabotropic glutamate receptors in the pathophysiology of chronic stress-related disorders. *Current Neuropharmacology*, *14*(5), 514–539. https://doi.org/10.2174/1570159X13666150515234920.

Pin, J.-P., & Bettler, B. (2016). Organization and functions of mGlu and GABAB receptor complexes. *Nature*, *540*(7631), 60–68. https://doi.org/10.1038/nature20566.

Pin, J.-P., Galvez, T., & Prézeau, L. (2003). Evolution, structure, and activation mechanism of family 3/C G-protein-coupled receptors. *Pharmacology and Therapeutics*, *98*(3), 325–354. https://doi.org/10.1016/S0163-7258(03)00038-X.

Pin, J.-P., Parmentier, M.-L., & Prézeau, L. (2001). Positive allosteric modulators for γ-aminobutyric acidB receptors open new routes for the development of drugs targeting family 3 G-protein-coupled receptors. *Molecular Pharmacology*, *60*(5), 881. https://doi.org/10.1124/mol.60.5.881.

Pulido, D., Casadó-Anguera, V., Pérez-Benito, L., Moreno, E., Cordomí, A., López, L., et al. (2018). Design of a true bivalent ligand with picomolar binding affinity for a G protein-coupled receptor homodimer. *Journal of Medicinal Chemistry*, *61*(20), 9335–9346. https://doi.org/10.1021/acs.jmedchem.8b01249.

Rasmussen, S. G. F., Choi, H.-J., Rosenbaum, D. M., Kobilka, T. S., Thian, F. S., Edwards, P. C., et al. (2007). Crystal structure of the human β2 adrenergic G-protein-coupled receptor. *Nature*, *450*(7168), 383–387. https://doi.org/10.1038/nature06325.

Rasmussen, S. G. F., DeVree, B. T., Zou, Y., Kruse, A. C., Chung, K. Y., Kobilka, T. S., et al. (2011). Crystal structure of the β2 adrenergic receptor–Gs protein complex. *Nature*, *477*, 549. https://doi.org/10.1038/nature10361.

Renaud, J.-P., Chari, A., Ciferri, C., Liu, W.-T., Rémigy, H.-W., Stark, H., et al. (2018). Cryo-EM in drug discovery: Achievements, limitations and prospects. *Nature Reviews Drug Discovery*, *17*, 471. https://doi.org/10.1038/nrd.2018.77.

Renner, S., Hechenberger, M., Noeske, T., Böcker, A., Jatzke, C., Schmuker, M., et al. (2007). Searching for drug scaffolds with 3D pharmacophores and neural network ensembles. *Angewandte Chemie International Edition*, *46*(28), 5336–5339. https://doi.org/10.1002/anie.200604125.

Romano, C., Yang, W.-L., & O'Malley, K. L. (1996). Metabotropic glutamate receptor 5 is a disulfide-linked dimer. *Journal of Biological Chemistry*, *271*(45), 28612–28616.

Sansuk, K., Deupi, X., Torrecillas, I. R., Jongejan, A., Nijmeijer, S., Bakker, R. A., et al. (2011). A structural insight into the reorientation of transmembrane domains 3 and 5 during family a G protein-coupled receptor activation. *Molecular Pharmacology*, *79*(2), 262.

Serrano-Vega, M. J., Magnani, F., Shibata, Y., & Tate, C. G. (2008). Conformational thermostabilization of the β1-adrenergic receptor in a detergent-resistant form. *Proceedings of the National Academy of Sciences of the United States of America*, *105*(3), 877. https://doi.org/10.1073/pnas.0711253105.

Sharma, S., Rodriguez, A. L., Conn, P. J., & Lindsley, C. W. (2008). Synthesis and SAR of a mGluR5 allosteric partial antagonist lead: Unexpected modulation of pharmacology with slight structural modifications to a 5-(phenylethynyl)pyrimidine scaffold. *Bioorganic & Medicinal Chemistry Letters*, *18*(14), 4098–4101. https://doi.org/10.1016/j.bmcl.2008.05.091.

Sheffler, D. J., Gregory, K. J., Rook, J. M., & Conn, P. J. (2011). Allosteric modulation of metabotropic glutamate receptors. In R. R. Neubig (Ed.), *Vol. 62. Advances in Pharmacology* (pp. 37–77). Academic Press.

Shonberg, J., Kling, R. C., Gmeiner, P., & Löber, S. (2015). GPCR crystal structures: Medicinal chemistry in the pocket. *Bioorganic & Medicinal Chemistry*, *23*(14), 3880–3906. https://doi.org/10.1016/j.bmc.2014.12.034.

Spyridaki, K., Matsoukas, M.-T., Cordomi, A., Gkountelias, K., Papadokostaki, M., Mavromoustakos, T., et al. (2014). Structural-functional analysis of the third transmembrane domain of the corticotropin-releasing factor type 1 receptor: Role in activation and allosteric antagonism. *Journal of Biological Chemistry*, *289*(27), 18966–18977.

Sriram, K., & Insel, P. A. (2018). G protein-coupled receptors as targets for approved drugs: How many targets and how many drugs? *Molecular Pharmacology*, *93*(4), 251. https://doi.org/10.1124/mol.117.111062.

Stansley, B. J., & Conn, P. J. (2018). The therapeutic potential of metabotropic glutamate receptor modulation for schizophrenia. *Current Opinion in Pharmacology*, *38*, 31–36. https://doi.org/10.1016/j.coph.2018.02.003.

Suno, R., Kimura, K. T., Nakane, T., Yamashita, K., Wang, J., Fujiwara, T., et al. (2018). Crystal structures of human orexin 2 receptor bound to the subtype-selective antagonist EMPA. *Structure*, *26*(1), 7-19.e15. https://doi.org/10.1016/j.str.2017.11.005.

Szabó, G., Túrós, G. I., Kolok, S., Vastag, M., Sánta, Z., Dékány, M., et al. (2019). Fragment based optimization of metabotropic glutamate receptor 2 (mGluR2) positive allosteric modulators in the absence of structural information. *Journal of Medicinal Chemistry*, *62*(1), 234–246. https://doi.org/10.1021/acs.jmedchem.8b00161.

Trabanco, A. A., Bartolomé, J. M., & Cid, J. M. (2019). mGluR2 positive allosteric modulators: An updated patent review (2013–2018). *Expert Opinion on Therapeutic Patents*, *29*(7), 497–507. https://doi.org/10.1080/13543776.2019.1637421.

Trabanco, A. A., & Cid, J. M. (2013). mGluR2 positive allosteric modulators: A patent review (2009—Present). *Expert Opinion on Therapeutic Patents*, *23*(5), 629–647. https://doi.org/10.1517/13543776.2013.777043.

Trabanco, A. A., Cid, J. M., Lavreysen, H., Macdonald, G. J., & Tresadern, G. (2011). Progress in the developement of positive allosteric modulators of the metabotropic glutamate receptor 2. *Current Medicinal Chemistry*, *18*(1), 47–68. https://doi.org/10.2174/092986711793979706.

Trabanco, A. A., Tresadern, G., Macdonald, G. J., Vega, J. A., de Lucas, A. I., Matesanz, E., et al. (2012). Imidazo[1,2-a]pyridines: Orally active positive allosteric modulators of the metabotropic glutamate 2 receptor. *Journal of Medicinal Chemistry*, *55*(6), 2688–2701. https://doi.org/10.1021/jm201561r.

Tresadern, G., & Bemporad, D. (2010). Modeling approaches for ligand-based 3D similarity. *Future Medicinal Chemistry*, *2*(10), 1547–1561. https://doi.org/10.4155/fmc.10.244.

Tresadern, G., Cid, J. M., Macdonald, G. J., Vega, J. A., de Lucas, A. I., García, A., et al. (2010). Scaffold hopping from pyridones to imidazo[1,2-a]pyridines. New positive allosteric modulators of metabotropic glutamate 2 receptor. *Bioorganic & Medicinal Chemistry Letters*, *20*(1), 175–179. https://doi.org/10.1016/j.bmcl.2009.11.008.

Tresadern, G., Cid, J.-M., & Trabanco, A. A. (2014). QSAR design of triazolopyridine mGlu2 receptor positive allosteric modulators. *Journal of Molecular Graphics and Modelling*, *53*, 82–91. https://doi.org/10.1016/j.jmgm.2014.07.006.

Tresadern, G., Trabanco, A. A., Pérez-Benito, L., Overington, J. P., van Vlijmen, H. W. T., & van Westen, G. J. P. (2017). Identification of allosteric modulators of metabotropic glutamate 7 receptor using proteochemometric modeling. *Journal of Chemical Information and Modeling*, *57*(12), 2976–2985. https://doi.org/10.1021/acs.jcim.7b00338.

Urwyler, S. (2011). Allosteric modulation of family C G-protein-coupled receptors: From molecular insights to therapeutic perspectives. *Pharmacological Reviews*, *63*(1), 59. https://doi.org/10.1124/pr.109.002501.

Vafabakhsh, R., Levitz, J., & Isacoff, E. Y. (2015). Conformational dynamics of a class C G-protein-coupled receptor. *Nature*, *524*, 497. https://doi.org/10.1038/nature14679.

Van Gool, M., Alonso De Diego, S. A., Delgado, O., Trabanco, A. A., Jourdan, F., Macdonald, G. J., et al. (2017). 1,3,5-Trisubstituted pyrazoles as potent negative allosteric modulators of the mGlu2/3 receptors. *ChemMedChem*, *12*(12), 905–912. https://doi.org/10.1002/cmdc.201700101.

Vanejevs, M., Jatzke, C., Renner, S., Müller, S., Hechenberger, M., Bauer, T., et al. (2008). Positive and negative modulation of group I metabotropic glutamate receptors. *Journal of Medicinal Chemistry*, *51*(3), 634–647. https://doi.org/10.1021/jm0611298.

Venkatakrishnan, A. J., Deupi, X., Lebon, G., Heydenreich, F. M., Flock, T., Miljus, T., et al. (2016). Diverse activation pathways in class A GPCRs converge near the G-protein-coupling region. *Nature*, *536*, 484. https://doi.org/10.1038/nature19107.

Venkatakrishnan, A. J., Deupi, X., Lebon, G., Tate, C. G., Schertler, G. F., & Babu, M. M. (2013). Molecular signatures of G-protein-coupled receptors. *Nature*, *494*, 185. https://doi.org/10.1038/nature11896.

Venkatakrishnan, A. J., Ma, A. K., Fonseca, R., Latorraca, N. R., Kelly, B., Betz, R. M., et al. (2019). Diverse GPCRs exhibit conserved water networks for stabilization and activation. *Proceedings of the National Academy of Sciences of the United States of America, 116*(8), 3288. https://doi.org/10.1073/pnas.1809251116.

Wacker, D., Wang, C., Katritch, V., Han, G. W., Huang, X.-P., Vardy, E., et al. (2013). Structural features for functional selectivity at serotonin receptors. *Science, 340*(6132), 615. https://doi.org/10.1126/science.1232808.

Wang, S., Wacker, D., Levit, A., Che, T., Betz, R. M., McCorvy, J. D., et al. (2017). D4 dopamine receptor high-resolution structures enable the discovery of selective agonists. *Science, 358*(6361), 381. https://doi.org/10.1126/science.aan5468.

Wang, C., Wu, H., Katritch, V., Han, G. W., Huang, X.-P., Liu, W., et al. (2013). Structure of the human smoothened receptor bound to an antitumour agent. *Nature, 497*, 338. https://doi.org/10.1038/nature12167.

Warne, T., Moukhametzianov, R., Baker, J. G., Nehmé, R., Edwards, P. C., Leslie, A. G. W., et al. (2011). The structural basis for agonist and partial agonist action on a β1-adrenergic receptor. *Nature, 469*(7329), 241–244. https://doi.org/10.1038/nature09746.

Weis, W. I., & Kobilka, B. K. (2018). The molecular basis of G protein–coupled receptor activation. *Annual Review of Biochemistry, 87*(1), 897–919. https://doi.org/10.1146/annurev-biochem-060614-033910.

Wise, A., Gearing, K., & Rees, S. (2002). Target validation of G-protein coupled receptors. *Drug Discovery Today*, 7(4), 235–246. https://doi.org/10.1016/S1359-6446(01)02131-6.

Wood, M. R., Hopkins, C. R., Brogan, J. T., Conn, P. J., & Lindsley, C. W. (2011). "Molecular switches" on mGluR allosteric ligands that modulate modes of pharmacology. *Biochemistry, 50*(13), 2403–2410. https://doi.org/10.1021/bi200129s.

Wootten, D., Christopoulos, A., Marti-Solano, M., Babu, M. M., & Sexton, P. M. (2018). Mechanisms of signalling and biased agonism in G protein-coupled receptors. *Nature Reviews Molecular Cell Biology, 19*(10), 638–653. https://doi.org/10.1038/s41580-018-0049-3.

Wu, H., Wang, C., Gregory, K. J., Han, G. W., Cho, H. P., Xia, Y., et al. (2014). Structure of a class C GPCR metabotropic glutamate receptor 1 bound to an allosteric modulator. *Science, 344*(6179), 58.

Xu, F., Wu, H., Katritch, V., Han, G. W., Jacobson, K. A., Gao, Z.-G., et al. (2011). Structure of an agonist-bound human A2A adenosine receptor. *Science, 332*(6027), 322. https://doi.org/10.1126/science.1202793.

Xue, L., Rovira, X., Scholler, P., Zhao, H., Liu, J., Pin, J.-P., et al. (2015). Major ligand-induced rearrangement of the heptahelical domain interface in a GPCR dimer. *Nature Chemical Biology, 11*(2), 134–140. https://doi.org/10.1038/nchembio.1711.

Zhang, H., Qiao, A., Yang, D., Yang, L., Dai, A., de Graaf, C., et al. (2017). Structure of the full-length glucagon class B G-protein-coupled receptor. *Nature, 546*, 259. https://doi.org/10.1038/nature22363.

CHAPTER TWO

Structure-based discovery and development of metabotropic glutamate receptor 5 negative allosteric modulators

Kirstie A. Bennett[a,*], John A. Christopher[a], Benjamin G. Tehan[b]
[a]Sosei Heptares, Cambridge, United Kingdom
[b]OMass Therapeutics, Oxford, United Kingdom
[*]Corresponding author: e-mail address: kirstie.bennett@soseiheptares.com

Contents

Abstract

The metabotropic glutamate (mGlu) receptors are a family of eight class C G protein-coupled receptors (GPCRs) which modulate cell signaling and synaptic transmission to the major excitatory neurotransmitter L-glutamate (L-glutamic acid). Due to their role in modulating glutamate response, their widespread distribution in the central nervous system (CNS) and some evidence of dysregulation in disease, the mGlu receptors have become attractive pharmacological targets. As the orthosteric (glutamate) binding site is highly conserved across the eight mGlu receptors, it is difficult not only to generate ligands with subtype selectivity but, due to the nature of the binding site, with suitable

Advances in Pharmacology, Volume 88
ISSN 1054-3589
https://doi.org/10.1016/bs.apha.2020.03.001

drug-like properties to allow oral bioavailability and CNS penetration. Selective pharmacological targeting of a single receptor subtype can be achieved by targeting alternative (allosteric) binding sites. The nature of the allosteric binding pockets allows ligands to be developed that have good physical chemical properties as evidenced by several allosteric modulators of mGlu receptors entering clinical trials. The first negative allosteric modulators of the metabotropic glutamate 5 ($mGlu_5$) receptor were discovered from high throughput screening activities. An alternative approach to drug discovery is to use structural knowledge to enable structure-based drug design (SBDD), which allows the design of molecules in a more rational, rather than empirical, fashion. Here we will describe the process of SBDD in the discovery of the $mGlu_5$ negative allosteric modulator HTL0014242 and describe how knowledge of receptor structure can also be used to gain insights into the receptor activation mechanisms.

Abbreviations

7TM	seven transmembrane
CDPPB	3-cyano-*N*-(1,3-diphenyl-1*H*-pyrazol-5-yl)benzamide
CPPHA	*N*-[4-chloro-2-[(1,3-dihydro-1,3-dioxo-2*H*-isoindol-2-yl)methyl]phenyl]-2-hydroxybenzamide
CRD	cysteine-rich domain
Cryo-EM	cryogenic electron microscopy
HTL0014242	3-chloro-5-[6-(5-fluoropyridin-2-yl)pyrimidin-4-yl]benzonitrile
mGlu	metabotropic glutamate
MPEP	2-methyl-6-(phenylethynyl)-pyridine
M-MPEP	2-methyl-6-((3-methoxyphenyl)ethynyl)-pyridine
NAL	neutral allosteric ligand
PAM	positive allosteric modulator
SAR	structure activity relationship
SBDD	structure-based drug design
VFT	venus flytrap domain

1. Introduction

Structure-based drug design (SBDD) is a powerful and well established approach for the discovery and optimization of hit compounds to lead series and candidate molecules (Ronald, 2020; van Montfort & Workman, 2017; Wang, Song, Li, & Chen, 2018). The approach leverages experimental information of a ligand bound to the protein of interest, typically from an X-ray structure, to allow medicinal and computational chemists to target molecule designs in a rational, rather than empirical, fashion. Such guidance in design processes allows molecules for synthesis to be targeted based on structural hypotheses. This guides effort toward regions of exploration where profitable interactions with the protein target may be made or enhanced, and molecular properties of the molecule optimized, rather than relying on approaches where synthetically available vectors from a molecule are explored empirically. Empirical approaches unguided by structural data may result in larger numbers of compounds needing to be synthesized in an optimization campaign to reach a candidate molecule and frequently a bias toward areas of chemistry that are readily accessible synthetically will be apparent. In addition to X-ray structural information, data from nuclear magnetic resonance (NMR) (Sugiki, Furuita, Fujiwara, & Kojima, 2018) or cryogenic electron microscopy (cryo-EM) (Scapin, Potter, & Carragher, 2018) structures can be used to guide SBDD. SBDD approaches can help overcome issues of 'flat' or poorly developable structure activity relationships (SAR) by guiding the exploration of areas of a chemical series to better fit into the binding pocket of the target.

Characterization of regions within a binding pocket, for example, in terms of hydrophobicity/hydrophilicity and amenability to specifically designed molecular interactions including hydrogen bonding, π-π stacking and electrostatic interactions, is also key to SBDD (Bissantz, Kuhn, & Stahl, 2010). These considerations allow a molecule to be tailored to the characteristics of a binding site to optimize affinity for the target, but also give the opportunity for the properties of a molecule to be optimized toward the desired 'drug-like' characteristics required for the intended route of administration and duration of action at the target.

To date, application of SBDD to enzyme targets, for which the protein can be readily purified and crystallized, has yielded the greatest success, with many molecules derived from SBDD principles now on the market (Alex & Millan, 2011). Protein classes including HIV protease inhibitors and kinase inhibitors and more recently very challenging protein-protein interaction targets such as Bcl-x_L, and MDM2-p53, have yielded success through SBDD (Jubb, Higueruelo, Winter, & Blundell, 2012). Due to their conformational flexibility and instability outside of the cell membrane, GPCRs and other membrane proteins have until the last decade been poorly tractable to structural biology approaches. Technological and scientific advances in the GPCR arena in particular have opened up the potential for this highly valuable target class to be leveraged by SBDD (Congreve, Dias, & Marshall, 2014; Katritch, Cherezov, & Stevens, 2012) and in particular mGlu receptor 5 (mGlu$_5$), as detailed in this chapter, has been one of the early success stories for the application of fragment-based, and structure-based, drug discovery.

2. Interest in targeting the $mGlu_5$ receptor in CNS disorders

The $mGlu_5$ receptor is widely expressed throughout the central nervous system (CNS). The receptor is predominantly located post-synaptically, regulating and fine-tuning neuronal excitability and synaptic transmission, through its modulation of various signal transduction pathways and interactions with other transmitter systems (Bach, Isaac, & Slassi, 2007). Across mammalian species high $mGlu_5$ receptor expression is observed in the cortex, striatum and hippocampus with moderate levels in the thalamus and low levels in the cerebellum (Patel et al., 2007). There is a wealth of pre-clinical and clinical evidence suggesting the potential of antagonists of $mGlu_5$ to have therapeutic potential in several CNS disorders, for example, anxiety, treatment-resistant depression, fragile X syndrome, levodopa-induced dyskinesias in Parkinson's disease, gastroesophageal reflux disease and addiction (for a review see Slassi et al., 2005; also see Table 1). Indeed, several ligands which reduce $mGlu_5$ activity have been developed and progressed into clinical trials.

3. $mGlu_5$ receptor negative allosteric modulator clinical trials

A negative allosteric modulator (NAM) is a ligand that reduces the action of an orthosteric agonist, endogenous activator or antagonist by combining with an allosteric site of the receptor macromolecule (Christopoulos et al., 2014). All compounds which have entered clinical trials that reduce glutamate (L-glutamate, **1**, Fig. 2) responses via the $mGlu_5$ receptor as the primary target are captured in Table 1. All these compounds act at an allosteric site (i.e., act as NAMs) rather than acting at the glutamate (orthosteric) binding site. Note the breadth of diseases in which $mGlu_5$ NAMs have been tested.

To date no ligand which targets the $mGlu_5$ receptor has made it to market. The reasoning behind this may be choice of disease and study design (for example, see the review on Fragile X trials by Berry-Kravis et al., 2018) or dose-limiting adverse events (adverse psychiatric disorders such as hallucinations or psychotomimetic effects) which have been observed in some clinical trials (for an example see Youssef et al., 2018).

Table 1 Details of $mGlu_5$ ligands tested in clinical trials.

Identifier	Originator	Structure	Disease(s)	Key references
Fenobam	McNeil Laboratories	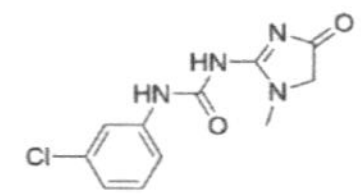	Anxiety	Pecknold, McClure, Appeltauer, Wrzesinski, and Allan (1982)
Dipraglurant	Addex Pharma	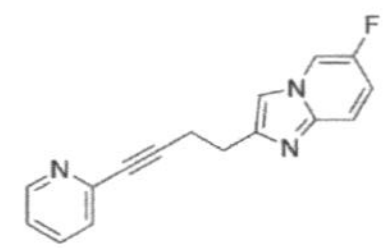	PD-LID, dystonia	Sciamanna et al. (2014) and Tison et al. (2016)
Raseglurant	Addex Pharma	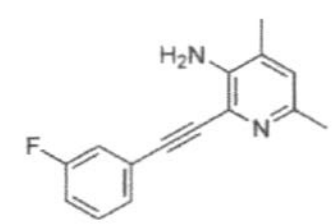	GERD, episodic migraine, dental anxiety	Marin and Goadsby (2010) and Zerbib et al. (2011)
Mavoglurant	Novartis	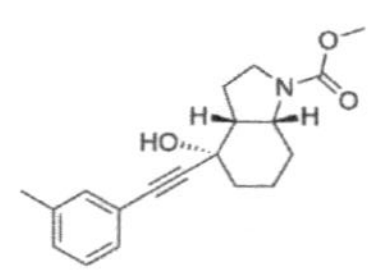	PD-LID, HD, FXS, OCD, addiction	Berg et al. (2011), Jacquemont et al. (2011), Reilmann et al. (2015), and Rutrick et al. (2017)
Basimglurant	Roche	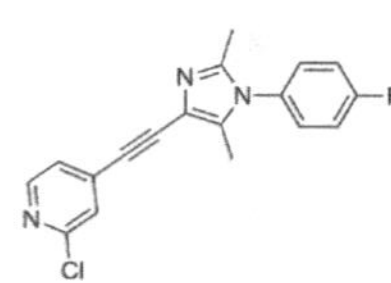	MDD, FXS	Fuxe and Borroto-Escuela (2015) and Youssef et al. (2018)

Continued

Table 1 Details of $mGlu_5$ ligands tested in clinical trials.—cont'd

Identifier	Originator	Structure	Disease(s)	Key references
AZD9272	AstraZeneca	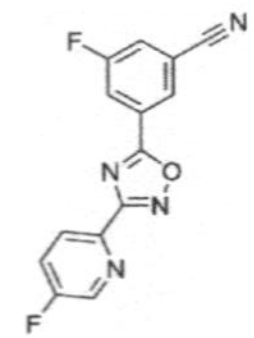	Pain	Kalliomäki, Huizar, Kågedal, Hägglöf, and Schmelz (2013)
AZD2066	AstraZeneca	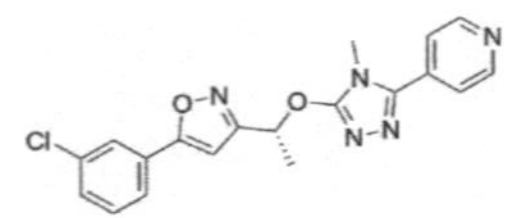	MDD, neuropathic pain, GERD	Jaso et al. (2016) and Rohof et al. (2012); NCT00857623
AZD2516	AstraZeneca	Undisclosed	Neuropathic pain, GERD	Ståhle, Karlsten, Jonzon, Eriksson, and Kågedal (2012)
STX-107	Seaside Therapeutics	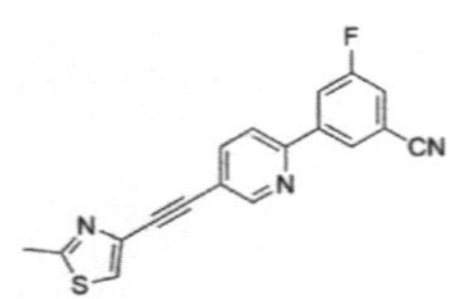	FXS	NCT01325740
HTL0014242	Sosei Heptares	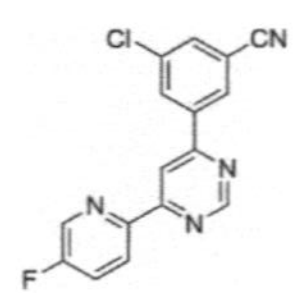	Neurology indications	Christopher et al. (2015)

PD-LID: Parkinson's disease levodopa-induced dyskinesias; GERD: gastroesophageal reflux disease; HD: Huntingdon's disease; FXS: fragile X syndrome; MDD: major depressive disorder; OCD: obsessive compulsive disorder.
The name, structure and indication of $mGlu_5$ NAMs which have entered clinical trials.

4. Overview of the general mGlu receptor architecture

There are eight metabotropic glutamate receptors ($mGlu_{1-8}$) which are subdivided into three groups based on sequence similarity, coupling to G protein pathways and pharmacology; Group I ($mGlu_1$ and $mGlu_5$) Group II ($mGlu_2$ & $mGlu_3$) and III ($mGlu_4$, $mGlu_6$, $mGlu_7$ and $mGlu_8$). To gain subtype selectivity, drug discovery campaigns at $mGlu_5$ have targeted the allosteric sites rather than the orthosteric (i.e., glutamate binding) site.

All mGlu receptors share a common molecular architecture, comprising of a Venus Flytrap (VFT) domain linked via a cysteine-rich domain (CRD) to a hepta-helical transmembrane domain (7TM) with a large disordered C-terminus (Seebahn, Sticht, & Enz, 2013) which contains multiple interaction sites for proteins such as calmodulin (Choi, Chung, & Roche, 2011) (Fig. 1).

The VFT domain compromises the orthosteric binding site to which the endogenous ligand, glutamate binds. X-ray crystal structures of $mGlu_1$ VFT have been solved which reveals the VFT remains in a resting 'open' state, which closes upon glutamate binding whereas antagonists stabilize the resting state by essentially wedging the protomer in the open confirmation (Tsuchiya, Kunishima, Kamiya, Jingami, & Morikawa, 2002). The mGlu receptors form obligatory dimers through disulfide bonds linking the

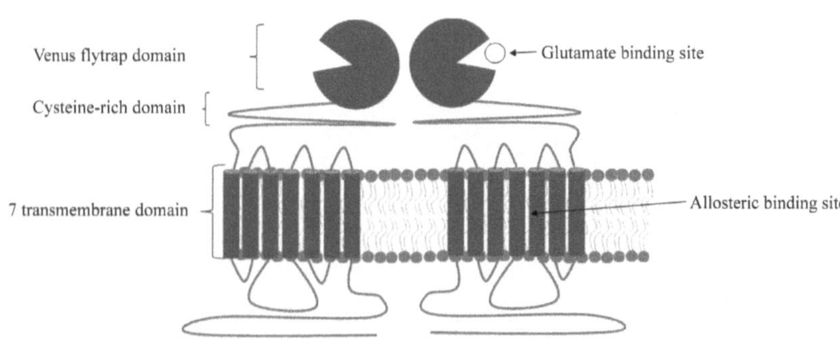

Fig. 1 Cartoon of the general architecture of the mGlu receptors. The mGlu receptors exit as homodimers. The Venus flytrap domain (VFT) contains the orthosteric (glutamate) binding site. The VFT is linked to the 7 transmembrane domain (7TM) via the cysteine-rich domain (CRD). The CRD helps transmit structural changes upon glutamate binding into a structural change in the 7TM region to activate G protein signaling. The 7TM domain contains the allosteric binding site. For $mGlu_5$ two allosteric binding sites have been described.

VFT domains (Kunishima et al., 2000; Muto, Tsuchiya, Morikawa, & Jingami, 2007; Romano et al., 2001; Romano, Yang, & O'Malley, 1996).

The CRD is a semi-rigid domain which contains nine critical cysteine residues, eight of which are linked by disulfide bridges (Muto et al., 2007). The CRD interacts with two regions of the second extracellular loop in the 7TM region, acting a rigid fulcrum to aid propagation of agonist-induced conformational changes at the VFT to structural changes in the 7TM region which results in G protein activation (Koehl et al., 2019). It is within the 7TM domain that the allosteric binding sites are located.

5. Rationale for targeting the allosteric sites of the $mGlu_5$ receptor

Ligands have been developed which target the orthosteric site of $mGlu_5$ resulting in class I selective agonists such as L-quisqualate (**2**, Fig. 2) which is the most potent group I agonist and antagonists such

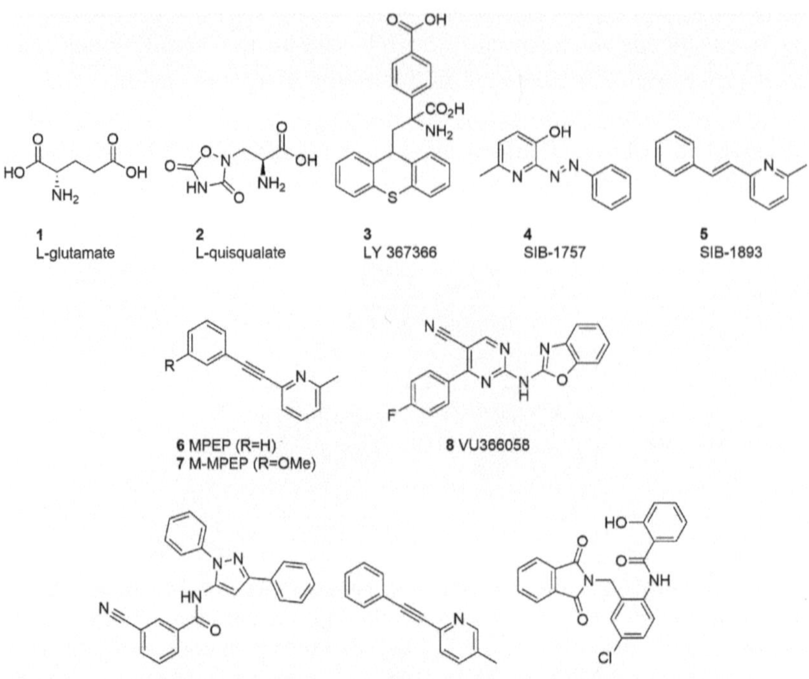

Fig. 2 Chemical structures of L-glutamate 1, L-glutamic acid 2, LY 367366 3, SIB-1757 4, SIB-1893 5, MPEP 6, M-MPEP 7, VU366058 8, CDPPB 9, 5-MPEP 10 and CPPHA 11.

as LY 367366 (**3**, Fig. 2) (Schoepp, Jane, & Monn, 1999). However, orthosteric ligands are glutamate derived acidic molecules which have failed to achieve appropriate profiles for clinical progression, exhibiting challenges such as poor pharmacokinetics, low CNS penetration, and poor selectivity. For example, L-quisqualate is also known to activate AMPA receptors and LY 367366 can also antagonize group II & III mGlu receptors. There are no known selective $mGlu_5$ orthosteric antagonist ligands developed to date. To overcome these challenges, drug discovery efforts have targeted the more tractable allosteric binding site in the 7TM domain.

Allosteric modulators may potentiate or inhibit the affinity and/or the efficacy of an orthosteric ligand, a property described as 'co-operativity.' As well as negative allosteric modulators (NAMs), ligands which act to increase efficacy of an orthosteric ligand, so called positive allosteric modulators (PAMs) and ligands which display neutral effect on orthosteric ligand but are known to bind in the allosteric sites (neutral allosteric ligands or NALs) have been described.

6. Allosteric sites on the $mGlu_5$ receptor: Pharmacological and mutagenesis studies

Fenobam (McN-3377) (Table 1) was the first $mGlu_5$ negative allosteric modulator discovered, an imidazole developed by McNeill labs in the late 1970s (Porter et al., 2005) which acted as an anxiolytic but at the time the target was unknown. It took until 2005 until the target of fenobam was discovered with studies showing fenobam to act as a potent $mGlu_5$ negative allosteric modulator of glutamate signaling (Porter et al., 2005). Thus, the first described $mGlu_5$ negative allosteric modulators were SIB-1757 and SIB-1893 (**4**, **5**, Fig. 2) which were discovered in a high throughput screening campaign through a collaborative effort between SIBIA Neurosciences Inc., and Novartis (Varney et al., 1999). SIB-1757 and SIB-1893 were demonstrated to exhibit non-competitive antagonism of glutamate signaling in Schild analysis. SIB-1893 was developed further by increasing $mGlu_5$ selectivity (100-fold) yielding 2-methyl-6-(phenylethynyl)-pyridine (MPEP, **6**, Fig. 2) (Gasparini et al., 1999) Using a series of chimeric receptors and point mutations the binding site of MPEP was shown to be in the 7TM domain located in TM 3, 6, and 7 (Gregory, Dong, Meiler, & Conn, 2011; Kuhn et al., 2002). While MPEP has negative allosteric modulation of glutamate function (Gasparini et al., 1999) studies have shown that L-quisqualate and glutamate occupancy of the orthosteric binding site has no effect on the affinity of [^{3}H]MPEP in rat cortical membranes of astrocytes, i.e., L-quisqualate and glutamate display neutral affinity co-operativity with MPEP (Bradley, Langmead, Watson, & Challiss, 2011). The negative allosteric modulation of glutamate efficacy and the neutral affinity co-operativity with glutamate mean that $mGlu_5$ NAM activity should be unaffected by high concentrations of glutamate that may be present in disease states which is an advantage over orthosteric ligands which would be competitive with glutamate. Methylation of MPEP led to the higher affinity analogue 2-methyl-6-((3-methoxyphenyl)ethynyl)-pyridine (M-MPEP, **7**, Fig. 2) (Gasparini et al., 2002).

The majority of $mGlu_5$ NAMs originated from the $mGlu_5$ tool compound MPEP and feature the same 1,2-diarylalkyne architecture but concerns over a structural link between the alkyne moiety and hepatotoxicity via glutathione conjugation (Zhang et al., 2014) yielded a broadening of the landscape to include non-alkyne $mGlu_5$ NAMs.

One strategy that has been used to generate novel chemotypes without the alkyne moiety is virtual screening. Mueller et al., 2012 trained an Artificial Neural Network (ANN) model that was using data generated from a published HTS screen (Rodriguez et al., 2010). Using the ANN model, a virtual screen of a commercially available compound library lead to the identification of two 2-(2-benzoxazolylamino)-4-phenylpyrimidines which represented a novel chemotype. Optimization revealed the series to have flat SAR but did allow the identification of the tool compound VU366058 (**8**, Fig. 2) (Mueller et al., 2012).

3-Cyano-*N*-(1,3-diphenyl-1*H*-pyrazol-5-yl)benzamide (CDPPB, **9**, Fig. 2) (Lindsley et al., 2004) was the first $mGlu_5$ PAM discovered through optimizing NAM hits in a traditional high throughput screening method. CDPPB is a positive allosteric modulator of glutamate increasing the potency of glutamate in a concentration-dependent manner (positive efficacy modulation) and has been described to increase the affinity of L-quisqualate in a radioligand binding assay in rat astrocytes and cortical membranes (positive affinity modulation) (Bradley et al., 2011). In radioligand binding experiments CDPPB competitively competes with [^{3}H] MPEP binding (Chen et al., 2007) and so can be classed as binding to the same site as MPEP.

As well as PAMs and NAMs neutral allosteric ligands (NALs) have been identified such as 5-MPEP (**10**, Fig. 2) which blocks CPPHA-induced potentiation of $mGlu_5$ responses and binds to the MPEP allosteric site (Chen et al., 2007)

The 7TM domains of mGlu receptors can act like a prototypical family A (or rhodopsin like-receptor) GPCR whereby truncation of the N-terminal domain (VFT & CRD) results in a receptor that is fully functional, albeit which cannot be activated by orthosteric ligands (Goudet et al., 2004). Evidence that ligands such as MPEP acted at an allosteric site was confirmed by demonstrating this truncated receptor could be directly activated by PAMs and blocked by NAMs (Goudet et al., 2004).

A second structurally distinct site to the MPEP site has been described, this is the binding site of the PAM *N*-[4-chloro-2-[(1,3-dihydro-1,3-dioxo-2*H*-isoindol-2-yl)methyl]phenyl]-2-hydroxybenzamide (CPPHA, **11**, Fig. 2). CPPHA does not displace binding of [^{3}H]MPEP nor [^{3}H]L-quisqualate (O'Brien et al., 2004) but does act as a PAM to increase the potency of L-quisqualate and glutamate signaling. Mutagenesis studies show that a A809$^{7.39}$V mutation (numbering following Class C nomenclature as described in Pin, Galvez, and Prézeau, 2003) reduces binding of ligands to the MPEP site has no effect on the response to CPPHA but F585$^{1.45}$I in TM1 eliminated CPPHA-mediated potentiation of glutamate responses without affecting MPEP's NAM properties. To date no NAM ligands have been described to bind to this site (Chen, Goudet, Pin, & Conn, 2008).

7. Allosteric sites on the mGlu$_5$ receptor: X-ray crystal structure of the 7TM region

The first crystal structure of the mGlu$_5$ 7TM was published in 2014 (Doré et al., 2014) and was solved in complex with the negative allosteric modulator (NAM) mavoglurant (Table 1). The mGlu$_5$ crystallographic structure at 2.6 Å unambiguously shows the binding of the mavoglurant in the mGlu$_5$ allosteric pocket. The allosteric pocket is located ~8 Å from the extracellular side and is comprised of an upper and lower chamber connected by a narrow linker region. The allosteric pocket has a slight tilt relative to the axis of the TM bundle, and is defined by residues from TM2, TM3, TM5, TM6 and TM7. The upper chamber, in which the saturated bicyclic ring system of mavoglurant sits, is predominately hydrophobic, defined by Val806$^{7.36}$, Met802$^{7.32}$, Phe788$^{6.53}$, Trp785$^{6.50}$, Leu744$^{5.44}$, Ile651$^{3.36}$, Pro655$^{3.40}$ and Asn747$^{5.47}$. The Asn747$^{5.47}$ nitrogen hydrogen bonds to the carbonyl oxygens of Gly652$^{3.37}$ and the carbamate tail of mavoglurant, with the methoxy terminal portion of the carbamate sitting in a cavity defined by Leu744$^{5.44}$, Pro743$^{5.43}$ and Ile651$^{3.36}$. The importance of many of these residues in allosteric ligand binding to mGlu$_5$ had been suggested previously in mutagenesis studies (Gregory et al., 2013; Malherbe et al., 2006, 2003; Pagano et al., 2000). This structure provided a significant step forward in the prosecution and understanding of $mGlu_5$ ligands, in addition to clearly highlighting how selectivity was obtained over the related Group 1 glutamate receptor, $mGlu_1$ via comparison to the $mGlu_1$ 7TM crystal structure also solved in 2014 (Wu et al., 2014).

8. Structure-based drug design at $mGlu_5$: Discovery of HTL0014242

Identification of the $mGlu_5$ NAM HTL0014242 (Fig. 3; Table 1) using fragment- and structure-based drug discovery approaches was reported in 2015 as the first example of SBDD for the target (Christopher et al., 2015). A thermostabilized form of the $mGlu_5$ receptor (StaR® protein) demonstrated increased tolerance of high DMSO concentrations compared to wild-type receptor and enabled fragment screening in a high-concentration radioligand binding format. The radioligand used was $[^3H]$-M-MPEP, itself a NAM ligand, thus allowing identification of fragment hits competitive with the radioligand that functioned as NAMs.

The highly ligand efficient fragment **12** (Fig. 3) was one of a number of hits from the screen and was initially progressed through exploration of phenyl group replacements for the upper pyrazole ring, supported by the identification of a similar hit from the fragment screen with a substituted phenyl in place of the pyrazole (Christopher et al., 2015). In addition, a strategy employed to progress the hits sought to identify common motifs within high affinity $mGlu_5$ NAMs reported in the literature and hybridize these into the chemotype identified from fragment screening. The initial hit expansion chemistry was guided by the use of an advanced homology model that

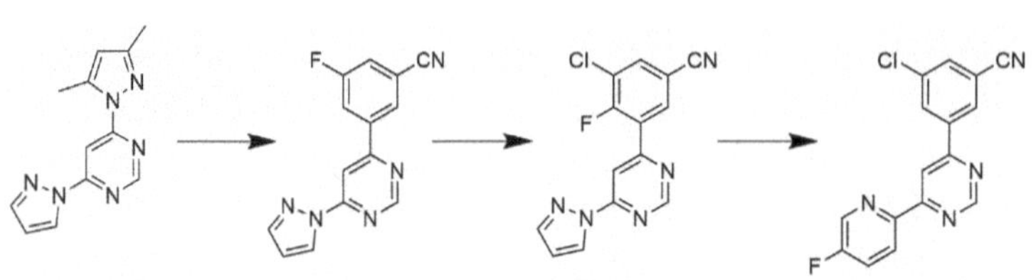

12 $mGlu_5$ pK_i 5.2 LE 0.40

13 $mGlu_5$ pK_i 7.2 LE 0.49

14 $mGlu_5$ pK_i 9.3 LE 0.60

HTL0014242 $mGlu_5$ pK_i 9.3 LE 0.57

Fig. 3 Structure-based drug discovery progression of fragment screening hit **12** to clinical candidate NAM HTL0014242.

had been refined by receptor mutagenesis information from the literature and from a significant dataset originating from the mutagenesis process that had resulted in the StaR® protein used for the fragment screen.

Computational modeling and selection for synthesis, focused in large part on hybridization as noted above, allowed rapid progression of the hit to a series of pyrazoles exemplified by **12** (Fig. 3), which demonstrated significantly enhanced affinity, ligand efficiency and lipophilic ligand efficiency over the initial fragment **12**. Key to the identification of **13** was the incorporation of a substituted 3-cyanophenyl motif in the upper portion of the molecule from the literature molecule hybridization approach.

By this time in the medicinal chemistry campaign the first X-ray structure of $mGlu_5$, in complex with the NAM, mavoglurant, had been solved in our laboratories (Doré et al., 2014). The crystallography construct was subsequently used to generate structures of molecules within the series, including **14** and the molecule ultimately selected as the clinical candidate from the series, HTL0014242. The X-ray structure of **14** revealed a hydrogen bond from $Ser809^{7.39}$ accepted by the pyrazole ring nitrogen, an observation which coupled with a need for improved metabolic stability in the series led to an exploration of alternative heterocyclic groups. Pyridine substitution was particularly effective in yielding an appropriate balance between activity and metabolic stability and ultimately the candidate molecule resulted from a thorough exploration of this region of the chemotype. In the context of the top ring, the X-ray structural information concurred with our initial SAR observations that hydrophobicity was required to drive high affinity. Evaluation of halogen and methyl substitution to complement the electronic character between this region of the chemotype and the receptor binding site allowed the affinity to be optimized into the nanomolar region. Furthermore, the structures of **14** and HTL0014242 rationalized the observed critical SAR requirement for nitrile substitution in the 3-position of the phenyl ring, revealing a water-mediated hydrogen bonding interaction with the backbone carbonyl of $Val740^{5.40}$. Any efforts to modify or remove this moiety had resulted in significantly diminished activity. SAR options in the central pyrimidine ring were minimal, as changing this to a pyridine or other diazine heterocycles resulted in a significant drop in affinity.

Comparison of the X-ray structures of **14** and HTL0014242 with that of mavoglurant revealed an outward movement in the side chain of $Val806^{7.36}$ by approximately 1 Å to accommodate the pyrimidine linker in the narrow channel linking the upper and lower regions of the binding site occupied by the rings of each chemotype.

HTL0014242 emerged from the structure-based drug discovery campaign detailed above as the molecule in the series with the best balance of affinity, potency and in-vitro metabolic stability and upon further profiling was demonstrated to have excellent selectivity within the $mGlu_{1-8}$ family of receptors and across a broader panel of selectivity targets (Christopher et al., 2015). An excellent pre-clinical PK profile in rat and dog supported progression into rat ex vivo autoradiography receptor occupancy, in-vivo efficacy and repeat dose rat toxicology studies ahead of candidate nomination, and the molecule is currently in Phase I clinical trials (NCT03785054).

During the drug discovery campaign that led to HTL0014242, further crystal structures of literature molecules were solved in our laboratories to broaden the information base from which our SBDD efforts could draw upon. Structures of fenobam and M-MPEP were subsequently published (Christopher et al., 2018), together with retrospective analyses of the published SAR of these chemotypes in the context of the new structural information, with a particular emphasis on how the use of structural information in tandem with Group Efficiency calculations and thorough evaluation of the energetics of water molecules can facilitate a detailed understanding of the SAR. Although further examples of $mGlu_5$ SBDD have not yet emerged the availability of multiple crystal structures in the public domain of diverse ligands and the retrospective analyses of historic SAR datasets provide the tools for further advances in the area.

The protein backbone of the two structures are in close agreement with the mavoglurant structure (4OO9) with Cα root-mean-square deviation values of 0.23 and 0.26 Å between compound **14** and HTL0014242 (Christopher et al., 2015) structures, respectively. Surprisingly, however, in the studies of **14** the side chain of $Trp785^{6.50}$ is now found in a $\chi 1$ trans orientation, placing the indole ring system toward the center of the helical bundle where the NH of the indole moiety forms a hydrogen bond with $Ser809^{7.39}$. This differing rotamer drastically alters the shape and electrostatics of the allosteric site, resulting in a much smaller pocket with significantly different properties. The rearrangement of residues within the allosteric pocket would occlude binding of mavoglurant from the 4OO9 structure, due to a severe clash from the side chain of $Trp785^{6.50}$ with the previously observed position of the saturated bicyclic ring system. In addition to this significant rearrangement there is a subtle movement of TM7 around the position $Val806^{7.36}$. This subtle movement out of ~0.5 Å is caused by the interaction between the pyrimidine core of the compounds and residue $Val806^{7.36}$. The movement allows for the much larger linking pyrimidine-core group within the narrow linker region, whereas previously it was thought that only narrow alkyne or alkene groups could be tolerated in this area. This subtle movement has opened up completely different possibilities within medicinal chemistry for the further prosecution of this target.

Like mavoglurant, the pyrimidine ligands are found in the allosteric pocket, comprised of an upper and lower chamber connected by a narrow linker region, ~8 Å from the receptor surface. The, $mGlu_5$ selective, lower chamber accommodates the pyrazole and pyridyl ring systems of **13** and HTL0014242, respectively, it is defined by $Ala810^{7.40}$ and $Pro655^{3.40}$, bordered on one side by $Ile625^{2.46}$, $Gly628^{2.49}$, $Ser654^{3.39}$, and $Ser658^{3.43}$ and on the other by $Tyr659^{3.44}$ and $Ser809^{7.39}$. In both structures the $Ser809^{7.39}$ is within hydrogen bonding distance to the nitrogen atoms within the respective pyrazole and pyridyl ring systems. The crystallographic water seen between $Tyr659^{3.44}$ and $Ser809^{7.39}$ is also seen in the pyrimidine complexes. This water molecule and disruption of its hydrogen bonding network, which had been linked to observed changes in ligand pharmacology, did not exhibit these pharmacological changes within this series of compounds analyzed.

The narrow linker region, which is perturbed by ~1 Å, as mentioned previously can accommodate a pyrimidine linker which traverses the narrow channel in the allosteric pocket formed between $Tyr659^{3.44}$, $Ser809^{7.39}$, $Val806^{7.36}$ and $Pro655^{3.40}$.

The upper chamber of the pyrimidine complexes defined primarily by $Trp785^{6.50}$, to the bottom, and $Phe788^{6.53}$ and $Met802^{7.32}$, to the top, with $Ser805^{7.35}$, $Val806^{7.36}$, and $Leu744^{5.44}$ forming the sides have significantly different properties to the upper chamber of the $mGlu_5$ mavoglurant complex, while remaining mostly hydrophobic in nature, they now exhibit a greater proportion of aromatic character fitting with the SAR of the series and highlighting the significance of utilizing a top ring system with its correct electronic character (Christopher et al., 2015). Additionally, the meta cyano substituent of the upper half of the compounds with the pyrimidine core can be seen to form a water-mediated hydrogen bond with the backbone carbonyl of $Val740^{5.40}$.

In the fenobam and M-MPEP structures (Christopher et al., 2018) a similar overall organization for the seven transmembrane helices is observed as in previously reported $mGlu_5$ pyrimidine structures. For both complexes, the upper chamber $Trp785^{6.50}$ adopts $\chi1$ *trans*-rotameric state, with its indole ring nitrogen hydrogen bonding to the $Tyr659^{3.44}$ and $Ser809^{7.39}$ side chains. This conformation was first observed in the $mGlu_5$ complex structures with **14** and HTL0014242.

9. Further learnings from structural information: Selectivity between $mGlu_5$ and $mGlu_1$

Comparison of the allosteric binding sites in the $mGlu_5$ 7TM structure (Doré et al., 2014) with that of the $mGlu_1$ 7TM structure (Wu et al., 2014) highlighted how selectivity could be gained between the Group 1 glutamate receptors. In the $mGlu_5$ structure the alkyne linker of mavoglurant traverses a narrow channel between $Tyr659^{3.44}$, $Ser809^{7.39}$, $Val806^{7.36}$ and $Pro655^{3.40}$, with the hydroxyl substituent at the upper end sitting almost equidistant between, and within hydrogen bonding distance of, the hydroxyl oxygens from $Ser809^{7.39}$ and $Ser805^{7.35}$. In the $mGlu_1$ structure the $Pro655^{3.40}$ is replaced by $Ser668^{3.53}$ in a $\chi 1$ trans orientation, this orientation of $Ser668^{3.53}$ blocks the narrow binding pocket and access to the lower chamber for $mGlu_1$ ligands. Notably, however, the $Trp798^{6.50}$ ($mGlu_1$) is in a similar gauche −ve $\chi 1$ orientation as is seen in the $mGlu_5$ ($Trp785^{6.50}$) structure with mavoglurant. This occlusion of the narrow traversing region from the upper to the lower chamber of the $mGlu_5$ allosteric binding site leads to the exceptional selectivity seen for $mGlu_5$ modulators occupying both regions (Fig. 4).

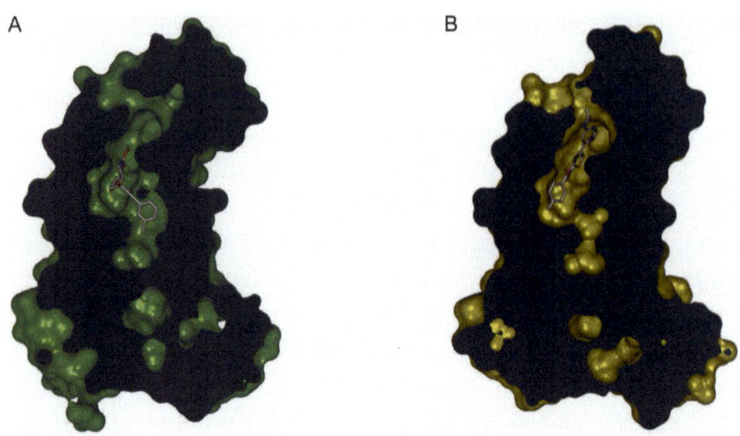

Fig. 4 Comparison of the $mGlu_1$ and $mGlu_5$ allosteric binding sites. Panel (A) shows a slabbed version of the $mGlu_5$ structure (4OO9) with mavoglurant bound. The larger cavity in the center of the structure enables the 3-methylphenyl ring of mavoglurant to sit lower in the pocket, this pocket is not accessible in the $mGlu_1$ structure (B). Panel (B) shows a slabbed depiction of the $mGlu_1$ structure (4or2), the narrow base of the central pocket is not accessible by the ligand FM9 and hence, relative to $mGlu_5$, it sits much higher in the pocket.

10. Further learnings from structural information: Mode switching

The field of mGlu NAM and PAM drug discovery has long been confounded by mode switching of modulators, the phenomenon has also been reported for numerous mavoglurant-related alkyne linker series (Sams, Mikkelsen, Brodbeck, Pu, & Ritzén, 2011; Sharma, Rodriguez, Conn, & Lindsley, 2008; Vanejevs et al., 2008; Wood, Hopkins, Brogan, Conn, & Lindsley, 2011). This makes $mGlu_5$-mavoglurant structure an ideal template in which to further investigate this observation. Predominately the ligand structural changes implicated in the NAM/PAM switch mechanism of mavoglurant-related compounds seems to be on the part of the ligand that occupies the lower chamber. The 3-methylphenyl ring of mavoglurant which occupies the lower chamber of the $mGlu_5$ allosteric site sits between Ala810$^{7.40}$ and Pro655$^{3.40}$, bordered on one side by Ile625$^{2.46}$, Gly628$^{2.49}$, Ser654$^{3.39}$, Ser658$^{3.43}$ and on the other by Tyr659$^{3.44}$. This lower part of mavoglurant is within 4 Å of a network of hydrogen bonds involving the side chains of Tyr659$^{3.44}$, Thr781$^{6.46}$, the main-chain carbonyl of Ser809$^{7.39}$ and a water molecule at the bottom of the allosteric pocket (Fig. 5). Varying the

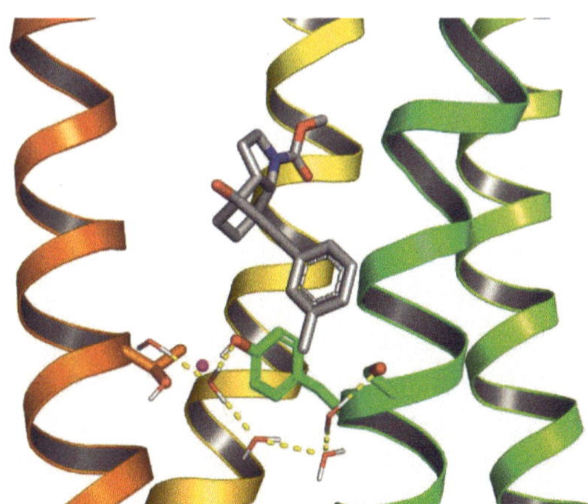

Fig. 5 The structural basis of NAM/PAM molecular switches. A crystallographic water molecule in the $mGlu_5$ mavoglurant binding site (mavoglurant in gray, water molecule in magenta) hydrogen bonds to Tyr659$^{3.44}$, Thr781$^{6.46}$, and the main-chain of Ser809$^{7.39}$. A predicted network of waters is shown overlaid with H-bonds (yellow). This network of water molecules is proposed to facilitate activation. Subtle changes to allosteric modulators influence the stability of this water network and may lead to molecular switching within closely related series of molecules.

3-methyl substituent on the phenyl ring in related compounds from methoxy to chloro to fluoro switches the ligand from a NAM to NAL to a PAM, respectively (O'Brien et al., 2003). Furthermore, mutation of Thr781$^{6.46}$ (Thr780rat) and Ser809$^{7.39}$ (Ser808rat) to alanine also switches the pharmacology of alkyne type PAMs (Gregory et al., 2013). The unusual changes in ligand pharmacology resulting from perturbation of the network around the water point to a potential activation switch holding TM7, TM3 and TM6 together at the base of the pocket, and a structural basis for modulation of the conformational spectra of the receptor.

In the mGlu$_5$ crystal structure the interactions in mGlu$_5$ selective sub-pocket are primarily mediated by Ile625$^{2.46}$, Ser658$^{3.43}$, Tyr659$^{3.44}$, Ser809$^{7.39}$, Ala810$^{7.40}$. A water molecule coordinated to Tyr659$^{3.44}$, Thr781$^{6.46}$, and the main-chain of Ser809$^{7.39}$ is located directly adjacent to the 3-methyl substituent of mavoglurant (Fig. 5). The crystallographic water adjacent to mavoglurant is calculated to be very stable using WaterFLAP software and further prediction of water molecules in the apo-mGlu$_5$ cavity places a water molecule 0.5 Å from the position observed in the crystal structure Fig. 5. This predicted network of water molecules could move to fill voids, and create different hydrogen bonding networks, therefore lowering the energy required to reach the active state. Variations in mavoglurant-like ligands, and other mode switching series, could change the environment the water network feels, thereby stabilizing or destabilizing the water molecules and lowering or raising the barrier to activation. These changes in the stabilization of the water network can also be borne out by changes in the hydrophobicity of this region, e.g., mutation of Thr781$^{6.46}$ and Ser809$^{7.39}$ to alanine switches the pharmacology of alkyne PAMs to NAMs (Gregory et al., 2014, 2013; Mühlemann et al., 2006).

Taking this initial step of analyzing the energetics of water molecules alone one step further, a group comprised of researchers from Jannsen Research and the University of Barcelona were able to show, by utilizing molecular dynamics (MD) of related pairs of mGlu$_5$ NAM/PAM compounds, that there were indeed statistically significant different orientations of residues in the binding site that could distinguish the two scenarios (del Torrent, Casajuana-Martin, Pardo, Tresadern, & Pérez-Benito, 2019). Docking followed by MD calculations for three sets of PAM and NAM pairs consistently showed the role of specific interactions formed between ligand substituents and amino acid side chains that block or promote local movements associated with receptor activation. The work highlighted the value added by applying MD to understand functional activity in drug design programs, in addition to providing valuable insight into the mechanisms of class C GPCR allosteric activation.

11. Further learnings from structural information: Full receptor activation process

Multiple cryo-EM and crystallographic structures in conjunction with signaling studies from Koehl et al. (2019) give a fascinating insight into the possible structural changes that are occurring in the activation of the mGlu receptors enabling a macroscopic view of the full activation process from an orthosteric agonist. This was briefly summarized on the section discussing the mGlu architecture but worth mentioning further here. The authors show that the activation profile of mGlu receptors requires inter and intra-subunit conformational changes. This was demonstrated by concentration-dependently challenging a constitutively active $mGlu_5$ construct with the 7TM negative allosteric modulator, MPEP. This fascinating paper highlights how an orthosteric agonist stabilizes a compact conformation of the VFT domain, which in turn interacts with the adjacent CRD. Work by Koehl et al. (2019) revealed that the CRD domain propagates further conformational changes through to the 7TM region via interactions with the extracellular loop 2 (ECL2). Thus the ECL2-CRD interaction is the structural basis of the allostery between the 7TM region and the extracellular domains. These exceptional studies highlight new possible regions for the allosteric modulation of mGlu proteins.

12. Conclusion

Targeting the allosteric site of the $mGlu_5$ receptor offers several advantages over targeting the orthosteric site, namely, improved subtype selectivity, better physico-chemical properties, improved CNS penetration and, as neutral affinity co-operativity with glutamate. Use of SBDD aided design of the novel $mGlu_5$ NAM HTL0014242. While structures are powerful tools for SBDD they can also give a further glimpse into activation mechanisms.

Conflict of interest

K.A.B., J.A.C. are current, and B.G.T. former, employees of Sosei Heptares, a biopharmaceutical company that specializes in GPCR SBDD and have a $mGlu_5$ NAM in clinical trials.

References

Alex, A. A., & Millan, D. S. (2011). *Contribution of structure-based drug design to the discovery of marketed drugs*. https://doi.org/10.1039/9781849733410-00108.

Bach, P., Isaac, M., & Slassi, A. (2007). Metabotropic glutamate receptor 5 modulators and their potential therapeutic applications. *Expert Opinion on Therapeutic Patents*, *17*, 371–384.

Berg, D., Godau, J., Trenkwalder, C., Eggert, K., Csoti, I., Storch, A., et al. (2011). AFQ056 treatment of levodopa-induced dyskinesias: Results of 2 randomized controlled trials. *Movement Disorders*, *26*, 1243–1250.

Berry-Kravis, E. M., Lindemann, L., Jønch, A. E., Apostol, G., Bear, M. F., Carpenter, R. L., et al. (2018). Drug development for neurodevelopmental disorders: Lessons learned from fragile X syndrome. *Nature Reviews. Drug Discovery*, *17*, 280–299.

Bissantz, C., Kuhn, B., & Stahl, M. (2010). A medicinal chemist's guide to molecular interactions. *Journal of Medicinal Chemistry*, *53*, 5061–5084.

Bradley, S. J., Langmead, C. J., Watson, J. M., & Challiss, J. R. (2011). Quantitative analysis reveals multiple mechanisms of allosteric modulation of the mGlu5 receptor in rat Astroglia. *Molecular Pharmacology*, *79*, 874–885.

Chen, Y., Goudet, C., Pin, J.-P., & Conn, J. P. (2008). N-{4-chloro-2-[(1,3-dioxo-1,3-dihydro-2H-isoindol-2-yl)methyl]phenyl}-2-hydroxybenzamide (CPPHA) acts through a novel site as a positive allosteric modulator of group 1 metabotropic glutamate receptors. *Molecular Pharmacology*, *73*, 909–918.

Chen, Y., Nong, Y., Goudet, C., Hemstapat, K., de Paulis, T., Pin, J.-P., et al. (2007). Interaction of novel positive allosteric modulators of metabotropic glutamate receptor 5 with the negative allosteric antagonist site is required for potentiation of receptor responses. *Molecular Pharmacology*, *71*, 1389–1398.

Choi, K., Chung, S., & Roche, K. W. (2011). Differential binding of calmodulin to Group I metabotropic glutamate receptors regulates receptor trafficking and signaling. *The Journal of Neuroscience*, *31*, 5921–5930.

Christopher, J. A., Aves, S. J., Bennett, K. A., Doré, A. S., Errey, J. C., Jazayeri, A., et al. (2015). Fragment and structure-based drug discovery for a class C GPCR: Discovery of the mGlu5 negative allosteric modulator HTL14242 (3-chloro-5-[6-(5-fluoropyridin-2-yl)pyrimidin-4-yl]benzonitrile). *Journal of Medicinal Chemistry*, *58*, 6653–6664.

Christopher, J. A., Orgován, Z., Congreve, M., Doré, A. S., Errey, J. C., Marshall, F. H., et al. (2018). Structure-based optimization strategies for G protein-coupled receptor (GPCR) allosteric modulators: A case study from analyses of new metabotropic glutamate receptor 5 (mGlu 5) X-ray structures. *Journal of Medicinal Chemistry*, *62*, 207–222.

Christopoulos, A., Changeux, J.-P., Catterall, W. A., Fabbro, D., Burris, T. P., Cidlowski, J. A., et al. (2014). International union of basic and clinical pharmacology. XC. Multisite pharmacology: Recommendations for the nomenclature of receptor allosterism and allosteric ligands. *Pharmacological Reviews*, *66*, 918–947.

Congreve, M., Dias, J. M., & Marshall, F. H. (2014). Structure-based drug design for G protein-coupled receptors. *Progress in Medicinal Chemistry*, *53*, 1–63, (chapter 1).

del Torrent, C., Casajuana-Martin, N., Pardo, L., Tresadern, G., & Pérez-Benito, L. (2019). Mechanisms underlying allosteric molecular switches of metabotropic glutamate receptor 5. *Journal of Chemical Information and Modeling*, *59*, 2456–2466.

Doré, A. S., Okrasa, K., Patel, J. C., Serrano-Vega, M., Bennett, K., Cooke, R. M., et al. (2014). Structure of class C GPCR metabotropic glutamate receptor 5 transmembrane domain. *Nature*, *511*, 557–562.

Fuxe, K., & Borroto-Escuela, D. O. (2015). Basimglurant for treatment of major depressive disorder: A novel negative allosteric modulator of metabotropic glutamate receptor 5. *Expert Opinion on Investigational Drugs*, *24*, 1247–1260.

Gasparini, F., Andres, H., Flor, P., Heinrich, M., Inderbitzin, W., Lingenhöhl, K., et al. (2002). [3H]-M-MPEP, a potent, subtype-selective radioligand for the metabotropic glutamate receptor subtype 5. *Bioorganic & Medicinal Chemistry Letters*, *12*, 407–409.

Gasparini, F., Lingenhöhl, K., Stoehr, N., Flor, P. J., Heinrich, M., Vranesic, I., et al. (1999). 2-Methyl-6-(phenylethynyl)-pyridine (MPEP), a potent, selective and systemically active mGlu5 receptor antagonist. *Neuropharmacology*, *38*, 1493–1503.

Goudet, C., Gaven, F., Kniazeff, J., Vol, C., Liu, J., Cohen-Gonsaud, M., et al. (2004). Heptahelical domain of metabotropic glutamate receptor 5 behaves like rhodopsin-like receptors. *Proceedings of the National Academy of Sciences of the United States of America*, *101*, 378–383.

Gregory, K. J., Dong, E. N., Meiler, J., & Conn, J. P. (2011). Allosteric modulation of metabotropic glutamate receptors: Structural insights and therapeutic potential. *Neuropharmacology*, *60*, 66–81.

Gregory, K. J., Nguyen, E. D., Malosh, C., Mendenhall, J. L., Zic, J. Z., Bates, B. S., et al. (2014). Identification of specific ligand–receptor interactions that govern binding and cooperativity of diverse modulators to a common metabotropic glutamate receptor 5 allosteric site. *ACS Chemical Neuroscience*, *5*, 282–295.

Gregory, K. J., Nguyen, E. D., Reiff, S. D., Squire, E. F., Stauffer, S. R., Lindsley, C. W., et al. (2013). Probing the metabotropic glutamate receptor 5 (mGlu5) positive allosteric modulator (PAM) binding pocket: Discovery of point mutations that engender a "molecular switch" in PAM pharmacology. *Molecular Pharmacology*, *83*, 991–1006.

Jacquemont, S., Curie, A., des Portes, V., Torrioli, M., Berry-Kravis, E., Hagerman, R. J., et al. (2011). Epigenetic modification of the FMR1 gene in fragile X syndrome is associated with differential response to the mGluR5 antagonist AFQ056. *Science Translational Medicine*, *3*, 64ra1.

Jaso, B. A., Niciu, M. J., Iadarola, N. D., Lally, N., Richards, E. M., Park, M., et al. (2016). Therapeutic modulation of glutamate receptors in major depressive disorder. *Current Neuropharmacology*, *15*, 57–70.

Jubb, H., Higueruelo, A. P., Winter, A., & Blundell, T. L. (2012). Structural biology and drug discovery for protein–protein interactions. *Trends in Pharmacological Sciences*, *33*, 241–248.

Kalliomäki, J., Huizar, K., Kågedal, M., Hägglöf, B., & Schmelz, M. (2013). Evaluation of the effects of a metabotropic glutamate receptor 5-antagonist on electrically induced pain and central sensitization in healthy human volunteers. *European Journal of Pain*, *17*, 1465–1471.

Katritch, V., Cherezov, V., & Stevens, R. C. (2012). Diversity and modularity of G protein-coupled receptor structures. *Trends in Pharmacological Sciences*, *33*, 17–27.

Koehl, A., Hu, H., Feng, D., Sun, B., Zhang, Y., Robertson, M. J., et al. (2019). Structural insights into the activation of metabotropic glutamate receptors. *Nature*, *566*, 79–84.

Kuhn, R., Pagano, A., Stoehr, N., Vranesic, I., Flor, P., Lingenhöhl, K., et al. (2002). In vitro and in vivo characterization of MPEP, an allosteric modulator of the metabotropic glutamate receptor subtype 5: Review article. *Amino Acids*, *23*, 207–211.

Kunishima, N., Shimada, Y., Tsuji, Y., Sato, T., Yamamoto, M., Kumasaka, T., et al. (2000). Structural basis of glutamate recognition by a dimeric metabotropic glutamate receptor. *Nature*, *407*, 971–977.

Lindsley, C. W., Wisnoski, D. D., Leister, W. H., O'brien, J. A., Lemaire, W., Williams, D. L., et al. (2004). Discovery of positive allosteric modulators for the metabotropic glutamate receptor subtype 5 from a series of N-(1,3-diphenyl-1H-pyrazol-5-yl)benzamides that potentiate receptor function in vivo. *Journal of Medicinal Chemistry*, *47*, 5825–5828.

Malherbe, P., Kratochwil, N., Mühlemann, A., Zenner, M., Fischer, C., Stahl, M., et al. (2006). Comparison of the binding pockets of two chemically unrelated allosteric antagonists of the mGlu5 receptor and identification of crucial residues involved in the inverse agonism of MPEP. *Journal of Neurochemistry*, *98*, 601–615.

Malherbe, P., Kratochwil, N., Zenner, M.-T., Piussi, J., Diener, C., Kratzeisen, C., et al. (2003). Mutational analysis and molecular modeling of the binding pocket of the metabotropic glutamate 5 receptor negative modulator 2-methyl-6-(phenylethynyl)-pyridine. *Molecular Pharmacology*, *64*, 823–832.

Marin, J. C., & Goadsby, P. J. (2010). Glutamatergic fine tuning with ADX-10059: A novel therapeutic approach for migraine? *Expert Opinion on Investigational Drugs*, *19*, 555–561.

Mueller, R., Dawson, E., Meiler, J., Rodriguez, A., Chauder, B., Bates, B., et al. (2012). Discovery of 2-(2-benzoxazoyl amino)-4-aryl-5-cyanopyrimidine as negative allosteric modulators (NAMs) of metabotropic glutamate receptor 5 (mGlu5): From an artificial neural network virtual screen to an in vivo tool compound. *ChemMedChem*, 7, 406–414.

Mühlemann, A., Ward, N. A., Kratochwil, N., Diener, C., Fischer, C., Stucki, A., et al. (2006). Determination of key amino acids implicated in the actions of allosteric modulation by 3,3′-difluorobenzaldazine on rat mGlu5 receptors. *European Journal of Pharmacology*, *529*, 95–104.

Muto, T., Tsuchiya, D., Morikawa, K., & Jingami, H. (2007). Structures of the extracellular regions of the group II/III metabotropic glutamate receptors. *Proceedings of the National Academy of Sciences of the United States of America*, *104*, 3759–3764.

O'Brien, J. A., Lemaire, W., Chen, T.-B., Chang, R. S., Jacobson, M. A., Ha, S. N., et al. (2003). A family of highly selective allosteric modulators of the metabotropic glutamate receptor subtype 5. *Molecular Pharmacology*, *64*, 731–740.

O'Brien, J. A., Lemaire, W., Wittmann, M., Jacobson, M. A., Ha, S. N., Wisnoski, D. D., et al. (2004). A novel selective allosteric modulator potentiates the activity of native metabotropic glutamate receptor subtype 5 in rat forebrain. *Journal of Pharmacology and Experimental Therapeutics*, *309*, 568–577.

Pagano, A., Ruegg, D., Litschig, S., Stoehr, N., Stierlin, C., Heinrich, M., et al. (2000). The non-competitive antagonists MPEP and CPCCOEt interact with overlapping binding pockets in the transmembrane region of group-I metabotropic glutamate receptors. *Journal of Biological Chemistry*, *275*, 33750–33758.

Patel, S., Hamill, T. G., Connolly, B., Jagoda, E., Li, W., & Gibson, R. E. (2007). Species differences in mGluR5 binding sites in mammalian central nervous system determined using in vitro binding with [18F]F-PEB. *Nuclear Medicine and Biology*, *34*, 1009–1017.

Pecknold, J. C., McClure, D., Appeltauer, L., Wrzesinski, L., & Allan, T. (1982). Treatment of anxiety using fenobam (a nonbenzodiazepine) in a double-blind standard (diazepam) placebo-controlled study. *Journal of Clinical Psychopharmacology*, *2*, 129–132.

Pin, J.-P., Galvez, T., & Prézeau, L. (2003). Evolution, structure, and activation mechanism of family 3/C G-protein-coupled receptors. *Pharmacology & Therapeutics*, *98*, 325–354.

Porter, R. H., Jaeschke, G., Spooren, W., Ballard, T. M., Büttelmann, B., Kolczewski, S., et al. (2005). Fenobam: A clinically validated nonbenzodiazepine anxiolytic is a potent, selective, and noncompetitive mGlu5 receptor antagonist with inverse agonist activity. *Journal of Pharmacology and Experimental Therapeutics*, *315*, 711–721.

Reilmann, R., Rouzade-Dominguez, M., Saft, C., Süssmuth, S. D., Priller, J., Rosser, A., et al. (2015). A randomized, placebo-controlled trial of AFQ056 for the treatment of chorea in Huntington's disease. *Movement Disorders*, *30*, 427–431.

Rodriguez, M., Grier, C., Jones, E., Herman, A., Kane, R., Smith, R., et al. (2010). Discovery of novel allosteric modulators of metabotropic glutamate receptor subtype 5 reveals chemical and functional diversity and in vivo activity in rat behavioural models of anxiolytic and antipsychotic activity. *Molecular Pharmacology*, *78*, 1105–1123.

Rohof, W., Lei, A., Hirsch, D., Ny, L., Astrand, M., Hansen, M., et al. (2012). The effects of a novel metabotropic glutamate receptor 5 antagonist (AZD2066) on transient lower oesophageal sphincter relaxations and reflux episodes in healthy volunteers. *Alimentary Pharmacology & Therapeutics*, *35*, 1231–1242.

Romano, C., Miller, J., Hyrc, K., Dikranian, S., Mennerick, S., Takeuchi, Y., et al. (2001). Covalent and noncovalent interactions mediate metabotropic glutamate receptor mGlu5 dimerization. *Molecular Pharmacology*, *59*, 46–53.

Romano, C., Yang, W.-L., & O'Malley, K. L. (1996). Metabotropic glutamate receptor 5 is a disulfide-linked dimer. *Journal of Biological Chemistry*, *271*, 28612–28616.

Ronald, J.-P. (2020). *Structural biology in drug discovery* (1st ed.). Wiley & Sons Ltd.

Rutrick, D., Stein, D. J., Subramanian, G., Smith, B., Fava, M., Hasler, G., et al. (2017). Mavoglurant augmentation in OCD patients resistant to selective serotonin reuptake inhibitors: A proof-of-concept, randomized, placebo-controlled, phase 2 study. *Advances in Therapy*, *34*, 524–541.

Sams, A., Mikkelsen, G., Brodbeck, R. M., Pu, X., & Ritzén, A. (2011). Efficacy switching SAR of mGluR5 allosteric modulators: Highly potent positive and negative modulators from one chemotype. *Bioorganic & Medicinal Chemistry Letters*, *21*, 3407–3410.

Scapin, G., Potter, C. S., & Carragher, B. (2018). Cryo-EM for small molecules discovery, design, understanding, and application. *Cell Chemical Biology*, *25*, 1318–1325.

Schoepp, D. D., Jane, D. E., & Monn, J. A. (1999). Pharmacological agents acting at subtypes of metabotropic glutamate receptors. *Neuropharmacology*, *38*, 1431–1476.

Sciamanna, G., Ponterio, G., Tassone, A., Maltese, M., Madeo, G., Martella, G., et al. (2014). Negative allosteric modulation of mGlu5 receptor rescues striatal D2 dopamine receptor dysfunction in rodent models of DYT1 dystonia. *Neuropharmacology*, *85*, 440–450.

Seebahn, A., Sticht, H., & Enz, R. (2013). Expression, purification, and structural analysis of intracellular C-termini from metabotropic glutamate receptors. *Methods in Enzymology*, *520*, 257–279, (chapter 12).

Sharma, S., Rodriguez, A. L., Conn, J. P., & Lindsley, C. W. (2008). Synthesis and SAR of a mGluR5 allosteric partial antagonist lead: Unexpected modulation of pharmacology with slight structural modifications to a 5-(phenylethynyl)pyrimidine scaffold. *Bioorganic & Medicinal Chemistry Letters*, *18*, 4098–4101.

Slassi, A., Isaac, M., Edwards, L., Minidis, A., Wensbo, D., Mattsson, J., et al. (2005). Recent advances in non-competitive mGlu5 receptor antagonists and their potential therapeutic applications. *Current Topics in Medicinal Chemistry*, *5*, 897–911.

Ståhle, L., Karlsten, R., Jonzon, B., Eriksson, B., & Kågedal, M. (2012). Safety evaluation of the mGluR5 antagonists AZD9272, AZD2066 and AZD2516 in healthy volunteers and patients with neuropathic pain or major depressive disorder. In *14th World congress on pain Aug 27–31;* Milan, Italy.

Sugiki, T., Furuita, K., Fujiwara, T., & Kojima, C. (2018). Current NMR techniques for structure-based drug discovery. *Molecules*, *23*, 148.

Tison, F., Keywood, C., Wakefield, M., Durif, F., Corvol, J., Eggert, K., et al. (2016). A phase 2A trial of the novel mGluR5-negative allosteric modulator dipraglurant for levodopa-induced dyskinesia in Parkinson's disease. *Movement Disorders*, *31*, 1373–1380.

Tsuchiya, D., Kunishima, N., Kamiya, N., Jingami, H., & Morikawa, K. (2002). Structural views of the ligand-binding cores of a metabotropic glutamate receptor complexed with an antagonist and both glutamate and Gd3+. *Proceedings of the National Academy of Sciences of the United States of America*, *99*, 2660–2665.

van Montfort, R. L., & Workman, P. (2017). Structure-based drug design: Aiming for a perfect fit. *Essays in Biochemistry*, *61*, 431–437.

Vanejevs, M., Jatzke, C., Renner, S., Müller, S., Hechenberger, M., Bauer, T., et al. (2008). Positive and negative modulation of group I metabotropic glutamate receptors. *Journal of Medicinal Chemistry*, *51*, 634–647.

Varney, M., Cosford, N., Jachec, C., Rao, S., Sacaan, A., Lin, F., et al. (1999). SIB-1757 and SIB-1893: Selective, noncompetitive antagonists of metabotropic glutamate receptor type 5. *The Journal of Pharmacology and Experimental Therapeutics*, *290*, 170–181.
Wang, X., Song, K., Li, L., & Chen, L. (2018). Structure-based drug design strategies and challenges. *Current Topics in Medicinal Chemistry*, *18*, 998–1006.
Wood, M. R., Hopkins, C. R., Brogan, J. T., Conn, J. P., & Lindsley, C. W. (2011). "Molecular switches" on mGluR allosteric ligands that modulate modes of pharmacology. *Biochemistry*, *50*, 2403–2410.
Wu, H., Wang, C., Gregory, K. J., Han, G., Cho, H. P., Xia, Y., et al. (2014). Structure of a class C GPCR metabotropic glutamate receptor 1 bound to an allosteric modulator. *Science*, *344*, 58–64.
Youssef, E. A., Berry-Kravis, E., Czech, C., Hagerman, R. J., Hessl, D., Wong, C. Y., et al. (2018). Effect of the mGluR5-NAM basimglurant on behavior in adolescents and adults with fragile X syndrome in a randomized, double-blind, placebo-controlled trial: FragXis phase 2 results. *Neuropsychopharmacology*, *43*, 503–512.
Zerbib, F., des Varannes, B. S., Roman, S., Tutuian, R., Galmiche, J.-P., Mion, F., et al. (2011). Randomised clinical trial: Effects of monotherapy with ADX10059, a mGluR5 inhibitor, on symptoms and reflux events in patients with gastro-oesophageal reflux disease. *Alimentary Pharmacology & Therapeutics*, *33*, 911–921.
Zhang, L., Balan, G., Barreiro, G., Boscoe, B. P., Chenard, L. K., Cianfrogna, J., et al. (2014). Discovery and preclinical characterization of 1-methyl-3-(4-methylpyridin-3-yl)-6-(pyridin-2-ylmethoxy)-1H-pyrazolo-[3,4-b]pyrazine (PF470): A highly potent, selective, and efficacious metabotropic glutamate receptor 5 (mGluR5) negative allosteric modulator. *Journal of Medicinal Chemistry*, *57*, 861–877.

Further reading

Niswender, C. M., & Conn, J. P. (2010). Metabotropic glutamate receptors: Physiology, pharmacology, and disease. *Annual Review of Pharmacology and Toxicology*, *50*, 295–322.

CHAPTER THREE

The function and allosteric control of the human sweet taste receptor

Guy Servant[a,*], Terry Kenakin[b], Lan Zhang[a], Mark Williams[a], Nicole Servant[c]

[a]Firmenich Inc., San Diego, CA, United States
[b]Department of Pharmacology, University of North Carolina School of Medicine, Chapel Hill, NC, United States
[c]Eurofins DiscoverX, San Diego, CA, United States
[*]Corresponding author: e-mail address: guy.servant@firmenich.com

Contents

Abstract

Humans perceive sweet taste via activation of a specific taste receptor expressed at the surface of taste receptor cells located on the tongue and soft palate papillae. The sweet taste receptor functions as an obligate heterodimer, comprising two different class C GPCR subunits. This receptor is unique in that it is activated or modulated by a plethora of ligands from highly diverse chemical classes, from small molecules to peptides and proteins and interacting with topologically distinct sites on each of its subunits. Modulators acting at separate functional domains of the sweet taste receptor can behave as full agonists. However, contrary to observations made with other class C GPCRs such as the metabotropic glutamate receptors and the γ-aminobutyric acid type B receptor ($GABA_B$) receptor, modulators interacting within the allosteric sites in the transmembrane domains of the sweet taste receptor only exert a relatively small effect on the affinity and efficacy of the agonist interacting at the orthosteric binding site located within the Venus fly trap domain (VFD). Newly identified potent and efficacious positive allosteric modulators (PAM)s of the sweet taste receptor rather interact at a site in close proximity to the agonist, within the VFD, display significant probe dependence, and markedly increase the affinity of the orthosteric ligand. Several sweet taste

Advances in Pharmacology, Volume 88
ISSN 1054-3589
https://doi.org/10.1016/bs.apha.2020.01.002

receptor inhibitors have also been characterized. Functional studies reveal a complex relationship between different ligands. Whether the antagonist will be surmountable or insurmountable and will act competitively or non-competitively largely depends on the agonist being studied and the location of its interaction site on the receptor.

Abbreviations

CRD cysteine-rich domain
GABA γ-aminobutyric acid
GPCR G protein-coupled receptor
mGluRs metabotropic glutamate receptors
MSG monosodium glutamate
NAM negative allosteric modulator
NHDC neohesperidin dihydrochalcone
PAM positive allosteric modulator
TMD transmembrane domain
VFD Venus fly trap domain

1. Introduction

Remarkably similar to the case of receptors for the senses for vision and smell (Schou, Pedersen, & Christensen, 2015), receptors for three of the five primary tastes also consist of several G protein-coupled receptors (GPCRs) (Chandrashekar, Hoon, Ryba, & Zuker, 2006; Meyerhof, Behrens, Brockhoff, Bufe, & Kuhn, 2005). Bitter taste is mediated by a group of 25 class A GPCRs in humans whereas sweet and savory (also called umami) taste are mediated by two related obligatory heterodimeric class C GPCRs: T1R2/T1R3 for sweet taste and T1R1/T1R3 for umami taste (Chandrashekar et al., 2006). A channel selective for protons, OTOP1, expressed in a subpopulation of taste receptor cells makes up the primary receptor for the detection of protons or sourness (Teng et al., 2019; Tu et al., 2018; Zhang et al., 2019). The primary salt receptors in rodent consists of the epithelial sodium channel ENaC and other receptors or channels with a lower sensitivity to salt (Chandrashekar et al., 2010; Oka, Butnaru, von Buchholtz, Ryba, & Zuker, 2013). However ENaC plays only a minor role, at best, for salt detection in human and, as a result, the search for other primary salt receptor(s) still goes on.

The bitter taste receptor family, thought to be the result of several gene duplication events, has been studied extensively over the last ~20 years (Jaggupilli, Howard, Upadhyaya, Bhullar, & Chelikani, 2016). It is now known that each receptor can be activated by numerous different ligands and that, conversely, bitter ligands can activate numerous bitter receptors

(Meyerhof et al., 2010). In addition, several haplotypes have been identified explaining our different detection thresholds or sensitivity to bitter compounds (Bufe et al., 2005; Pronin et al., 2007). Bitter taste GPCRs can also be modulated by allosteric ligands (Behrens & Meyerhof, 2013; Slack et al., 2010). However, this review will focus on functional allosteric interactions between the different domains of the human sweet taste receptor. This large protein contains multiple ligand binding sites making it ideal to study allosteric interaction (Fig. 1). Properties of these different domains, how they interact with each other and their ligands will be presented and analyzed in the broader context of family C GPCRs, such as the metabotropic glutamate receptor family and the $GABA_B$ receptor where receptor domains function, structure and allosteric interactions are now understood at the molecular level (Kim, Chen, Abrol, Goddard, & Guthrie, 2017; Koehl et al., 2019; Pin & Bettler, 2016; Pin, Kniazeff, Prezeau, Liu, & Rondard, 2019).

2. The human sweet taste receptor and its ligands

Humans can detect dozens of different sweetener molecules. These include sugars such as glucose, fructose, sucrose, lactose, maltose, galactose and trehalose, sugar alcohols such as sorbitol, xylitol, mannitol, maltitol, erythritol, isomalt, lactitol and glycerol, artificial non-caloric sweeteners such as aspartame, neotame, advantame, sucralose, saccharin, acesulfame K, cyclamate, P-4000, perillartine, neohesperidin dihydrochalcone (NHDC), guanidinium sweeteners and dulcin, natural non-caloric sweeteners such as steviol glycosides, mogrosides, phyllodulcin, monatin, polypodoside A and osladin and finally natural non-caloric sweet proteins such as monellin, thaumatin, miraculin, brazzein, mabinlin, pentadin, lysozyme, neoculin and curculin (DuBois, 2016). Representative molecules from these different chemical classes do not show much structural similarity, ranging from low molecular weight small molecules (acesulfame K; 201 g/mol) to large proteins of several kDa (Fig. 1). Furthermore, the sweetness detection threshold for these different sweeteners varies by more than five orders of magnitudes (Li & Servant, 2008). These observations had led early taste physiologists and neuroscientists to postulate that there had to be more than one sweet taste receptor to account for such chemical diversity and range in relative potency (DuBois, 2016). In late 1990s and early 2000s sequencing of subtracted cDNA libraries from lingual tissue and clever analysis of sequences in close proximity to the *Sac* locus in mice led to the identification of three genes, TAS1R1, TAS1R2 and TAS1R3 (Hoon et al.,

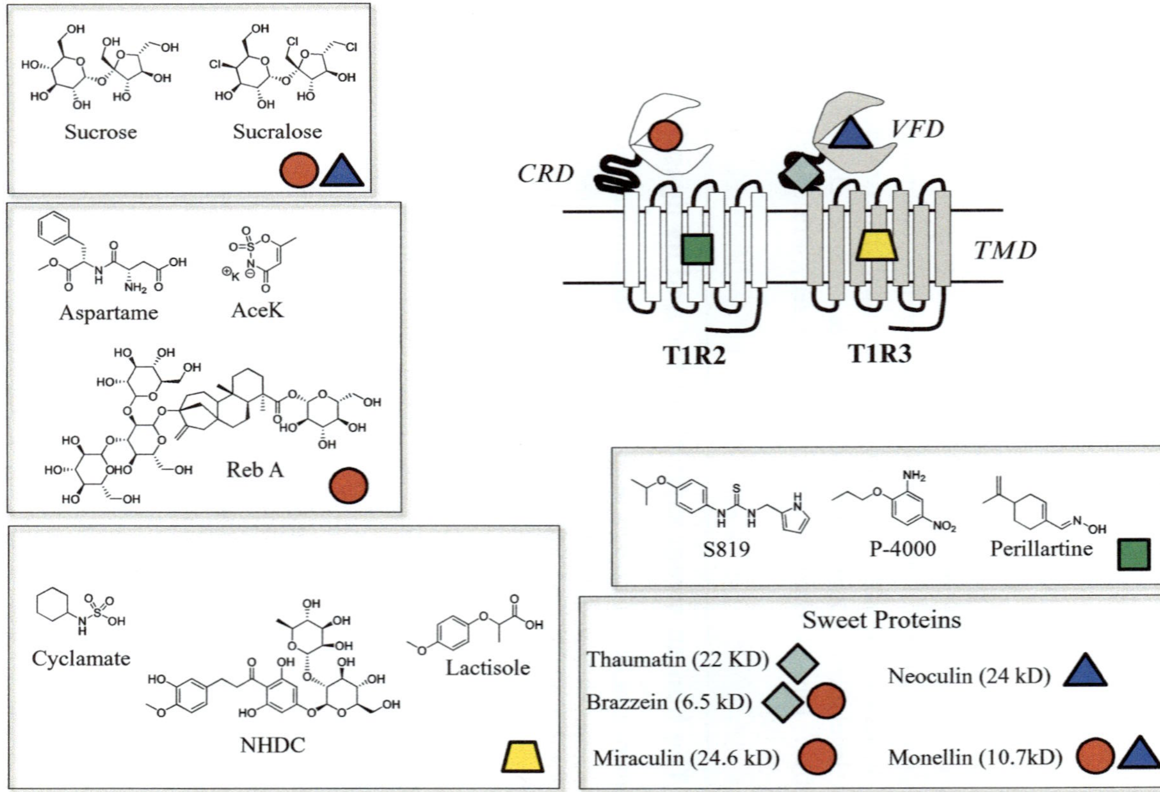

Fig. 1 Location of interaction between agonists, sweeteners and the human sweet taste receptor. The human sweet taste receptor comprises two subunits, T1R2 and T1R3. Each of the subunit is a family C GPCR made up of three distinct functional domains, the Venus fly trap domain (VFD) the cysteine rich domain (CRD) and the transmembrane domain (TMD). The VFD of T1R2 contains the binding site for natural carbohydrates and is therefore considered the orthosteric binding site. The CRDs of T1R2 and T1R3 also play a role in ligand binding but most probably help propagate signal from the VFD to the TMD involved in signal transduction, G protein coupling and signal termination. The TMDs of T1R2 and T1R3 also behave as typical class A GPCRs. These domains contain allosteric ligand binding sites for several agonists and sweeteners and binding at these loci leads to receptor activation.

1999; Kitagawa, Kusakabe, Miura, Ninomiya, & Hino, 2001; Max et al., 2001; Montmayeur, Liberles, Matsunami, & Buck, 2001; Sainz, Korley, Battey, & Sullivan, 2001), coding for family C GPCRs, that were later found to associate into heterodimers to form the sweet taste receptor and the umami taste receptor (Fig. 1) (Li et al., 2002; Nelson et al., 2002, 2001). Knock out studies in mice confirmed that sweet and umami taste are mediated through these receptors (Zhao et al., 2003). Yet, additional receptors and channels have been proposed to contribute to the detection of sweet and umami tasting substances in rodents (Chaudhari, Landin, & Roper, 2000; Damak et al., 2003; Maruyama, Pereira, Margolskee, Chaudhari, & Roper, 2006; Ohkuri et al., 2009; Yasumatsu et al., 2012; Yee, Sukumaran, Kotha, Gilbertson, & Margolskee, 2011). However, we now know, using cell-based assays, that co-expression of T1R2/T1R3 and T1R1/T1R3 is sufficient to recapitulate the basic human taste experience. Every sweeteners ever evaluated in T1R2/T1R3 assays not only activate the receptor but do so with the predicted rank order of potency (Li & Servant, 2008). Similarly, activation of human T1R1/T1R3 by glutamate happens at concentration known to elicit a savory taste and, importantly, ribonucleotides such as IMP and GMP, known to impart a strong enhancement of the glutamate savory note, behave as efficacious positive allosteric modulators (PAMs) of T1R1/T1R3 (Li et al., 2002; Nelson et al., 2002).

3. Human sweet taste receptor binding sites and signal transmission within the heterodimer

If there is only one sweet taste receptor then how can such a diverse set of ligands accommodate a single binding pocket? They do not. In fact, the human sweet taste receptor encompasses at least five distinct domains required for activation by ligands (Fig. 1). Rodents are less sensitive or not at all responsive to certain sweeteners such as aspartame, neotame, cyclamate, NHDC, monellin and others (Xu et al., 2004). It turns out that mouse or rat T1R2 and T1R3 coding sequences differ from their human counterparts in specific regions required for binding of these sweeteners. Receptors chimera, made up of human and rat domains (i.e., a VFD coming from the human subunit linked to a transmembrane domain (TMD) subunit coming from the rat subunit or vice versa) were evaluated in cell-based assays and responses to different ligands were monitored. Using this approach, complemented with site directed mutagenesis and modeling, a rather complex and surprising sweetener binding map has emerged. Sucrose (and probably other carbohydrates), sucralose, aspartame, neotame, saccharin, AceK and

D-tryptophan interact within the VFT of T1R2 whereas cyclamate and NHDC interact within the TMD of T1R3 (Fig. 1) (DuBois, 2016; Jiang et al., 2005; Maillet et al., 2015; Masuda et al., 2012; Winnig, Bufe, Kratochwil, Slack, & Meyerhof, 2007; Winnig, Bufe, & Meyerhof, 2005; Xu et al., 2004). Other functional sites are found within the TMD of T1R2 for perillartine, P-4000 and new sweetener called S819 (Fig. 1) (DuBois, 2016; Servant & Servant, 2019; Slack, 2012; Xu et al., 2004). Larger sweeteners such as sweet proteins interact with domains comprising the cysteine-rich domain (CRD) of T1R3 and probably outside surfaces of the T1R2 and T1R3 VFDs (Fig. 1) (Assadi-Porter et al., 2010; DuBois, 2016; Jiang et al., 2004; Koizumi et al., 2007; Koizumi et al., 2011; Masuda et al., 2013; Nakajima et al., 2008; Sanematsu et al., 2016; Walters & Hellekant, 2006). In biochemical studies sucrose, sucralose and even glucose bind to the isolated and purified VFD of not only mouse T1R2 on but also mouse T1R3, as measured by changes in intrinsic tryptophan fluorescence suggesting yet another potential binding site for carbohydrate sweeteners (Fig. 1) (Nie, Vigues, Hobbs, Conn, & Munger, 2005).

How the sweet taste receptor subunits work together to ultimately transmit the signal to the G protein and to elicit intracellular signaling is still unclear as a crystal structure of the human sweet taste receptor bound to different ligands has been elusive. However, assumptions can be drawn or hypotheses can be formulated from work conducted on mGluRs and the $GABA_B$ receptor. First, it is important to identify which receptor subunit propagates the signal to the G protein. In family C GPCRs, within a heterodimer ($GABA_B$ receptor) or even homodimers such as metabotropic glutamate receptors (mGluRs), only one GPCR subunit of the dimer binds to and activates the G protein (Pin & Bettler, 2016; Pin et al., 2019). In the sweet receptor, three independent observations suggest that G protein binding and activation most likely occurs at the intracellular face of the T1R2 subunit (Fig. 2). First, the use of human-rodent receptor chimera points to T1R2 as critical for G protein activation. While the human sweet taste receptors couples efficiently to $G\alpha_{15}$ in vitro, the rat receptor fails to do so. Replacement of the rat T1R2-TDM sequence by its human counterpart, in the presence of a wild-type rat T1R3, rescues signaling. Conversely, replacement of the human T1R2-TMD sequence by its rat counter-part abolishes signaling (Xu et al., 2004). Second, purified G proteins of the $G\alpha_{i/o}$ family get activated in vitro by applications of membranes containing hT1R2 but not hT1R3 (Sainz et al., 2007). Lastly, cells expressing hT1R2 on its own or even exclusively expressing the TMD of hT1R2 show G protein activation by allosteric ligands (Servant & Servant, 2019; Slack, 2012).

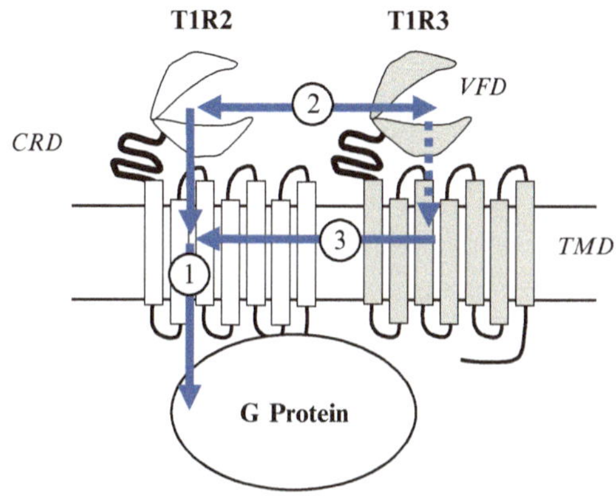

Fig. 2 Potential signal transmission mechanisms within the human sweet taste receptor subunits. In path 1, allosteric ligands interacting at the T1R2-TMD stabilize its active conformation and lead to G protein activation. In path 2, orthosteric ligands interacting at the VFD domains activate the TMDs via the CRD ultimately leading to G protein activation. It is still not clear if VFD activation of the T1R3-TMD is necessary to achieve full receptor activation or if signal transmission occurs entirely through the T1R2-TMD. In path 3, allosteric ligands interacting at the T1R3-TMD directly stabilize an active conformation leading to transactivation of the T1R2-TMD and subsequent G protein activation.

Therefore, allosteric agonists interacting within T1R2-TMD can stabilize an activated conformation of the domain, leading to G protein activation, even in the absence of T1R3 (path 1, Fig. 2). Conversely, orthosteric agonists interacting within the T1R2-VFD fail to activate the T1R2-TMD, and ultimately the G protein in the absence of T1R3 (Li et al., 2002). Recent breakthroughs in the glutamate receptor family and modeling studies provide clues to the sweet receptor activation mechanism and highlight the crucial role played by the heterodimer VFD lobes interface for activation by orthosteric agonists. In brief, closure of the VFDs by orthosteric ligands is thought to stabilize a conformation which decreases the distance between the VFD lower lobes and the respective CRDs of the two subunits. This change is transmitted by the rigid CRD to the TMD resulting in a significant re-orientation between the transmembrane helices interfaces, from a TM4–5/TM4–5 inter-subunit interface to a TM6/TM6 inter-subunit interface, and a compaction of the transmembrane helical bundle subsequently leading to G protein activation (Kim et al., 2017; Koehl et al., 2019). So, it is very likely that orthosteric agonist-induced activation requires the participation and interaction of both sweet receptor VFDs in order to propagate signal transmission to the T1R2-TMD (path 2, Fig. 2). Similarly to signaling mechanisms elucidated for mGluRs and $GABA_B$ (Pin & Bettler, 2016; Pin et al., 2019), it is also likely that signal transmission from the allosteric site located within the T1R3-TMD occurs through trans-activation of the adjacent T1R2-TDM (path 3, Fig. 2). In this scenario, agonist-bound T1R3-TMD stabilizes the active conformation of the T1R2-TMD which then relays signaling to the G protein. This mechanism would need to be experimentally confirmed in the context of the sweet taste receptor. For example, a headless hT1R2 subunit, devoid of its VFD should still be able to transmit signal from an allosteric agonist-bound T1R3-TMD. Also, the effect of a negative allosteric modulator interacting within the T1R3-TMD points to a functional interaction between the two TMDs (see Section 6). Direct signal transmission from an activated VFD to an adjacent but different TMD subunit (trans-activation) has not been noted so far and is unlikely, due to the strict requirement of the CRD to transmit signal between the two domains (Pin & Bettler, 2016). It is, however, conceivable that stabilization of a T1R3-VFD closed conformation could lead to activation of the T1R2-TMD subunit through interaction with the adjacent T1R2-VFD (Path 2, Fig. 2). In agreement, in a $GABA_B$ receptor mutant where the $GABA_{B1}$-TMD has been reduced to one TMD (the seventh helix), GABA is still able to activate the receptor by transactivation of the $GABA_{B2}$-VFD (Monnier et al., 2011). In mGluRs, closure of the two VFDs is necessary for full receptor activation while in the $GABA_B$ receptor closure of the $GABA_{B1}$ VFD is sufficient to confer full activity (Pin & Bettler, 2016; Pin et al., 2019). No such studies have been conducted so far on the sweet taste receptor so the relative contribution of each VFD orthosteric binding sites to the sweet receptor activation level is currently unknown.

4. Evaluation of sweetener synergy at the human sweet taste receptor

Taste studies in human volunteers suggest potential synergy between sweeteners. Evaluation of binary or more complex sweetener mixtures with human volunteers reveal combinations where the sweetness intensity of the mixture is apparently greater than the sum of the sweetness intensity level of each sweetener component (Reyes, Gravina, & Hayes, 2019; Schiffman et al., 1995; Schiffman, Sattely-Miller, Graham, Booth, & Gibes, 2000). However, in most cases apparent sweetness synergy can only be achieved at low sweetener levels or, conversely, sweetness suppression has actually been observed at higher sweetener levels (Schiffman et al., 1995). Moreover, several undesired properties of sweeteners, mostly noted in both artificial and natural non-caloric sweeteners, such as delayed sweet onset, lingering sweetness, bitterness or a licorice off-note make interpretation of taste data (aimed at detecting sweetness synergy) much more challenging (Servant, Tachdjian, Li, & Karanewsky, 2011). For example, components of a sweetener blend, saccharin and cyclamate, reported to act synergistically in taste tests (Schiffman et al., 1995; Vincent, Lynch, Pohley, Helgren, & Kirchmeyer, 1955) are now known to actually inhibit each other bitter taste receptors therefore minimizing the effect of bitterness on sweetness suppression (Keast, Bournazel, & Breslin, 2003) and, explaining, in part, the increase in apparent sweetness for the blend (Behrens, Blank, & Meyerhof, 2017). With the identification of the sweet taste receptor and the development of robust cell-based assays (Li & Servant, 2008; Servant et al., 2010), synergy between different combinations of sweeteners, acting at different domains of the heterodimer, can be precisely measured without the inherent complexities and limitations of human taste tests.

Binding of sweeteners to the TMDs of hT1R3 and hT1R2 only minimally influence the affinity of sweeteners interacting within the VFD of T1R2. NHDC and cyclamate are prototypical sweeteners interacting at overlapping binding sites within the TMD of T1R3 (Winnig et al., 2007) (Fig. 1). Evaluation of the effect of increasing concentrations of either sweetener on the potency and efficacy of sucrose, binding at the orthosteric site, yields the dose-response curves depicted in Fig. 3B and C. At 25 μM, NHDC causes a 1.7-fold leftward shift (EC_{50} ratio or $EC_{50}R$) in the sucrose dose-response (Table 1). Similarly, at its highest dose cyclamate only produces an $EC_{50}R$ of 1.5 and a slight increase in efficacy (Table 1). Note that in both experiments, increasing concentrations of allosteric ligands results in concomitant elevation of the sucrose curve's bottom asymptote, as expected since the sweeteners are allosteric agonists at the human sweet taste receptor (Fig. 3A). To precisely analyze the cooperative nature of the different sweeteners, dose-response data can be fitted to an operational model of allosterism:

$$Effect = \frac{E_m(\tau_A[A](K_B+\alpha\beta[B])+\tau_B[B]K_A)^n}{([A]K_B+K_AK_B+K_A[B]+\alpha[A][B])^n+(\tau_A[A](K_B+\alpha\beta[_B]+\tau_B[B]K_A)^n}$$

This model includes parameters describing and quantifying the effect of the modulator on the affinity (α) and efficacy (β) of the orthosteric ligand. Values of α and β greater than 1.0 indicate positive cooperativity on affinity

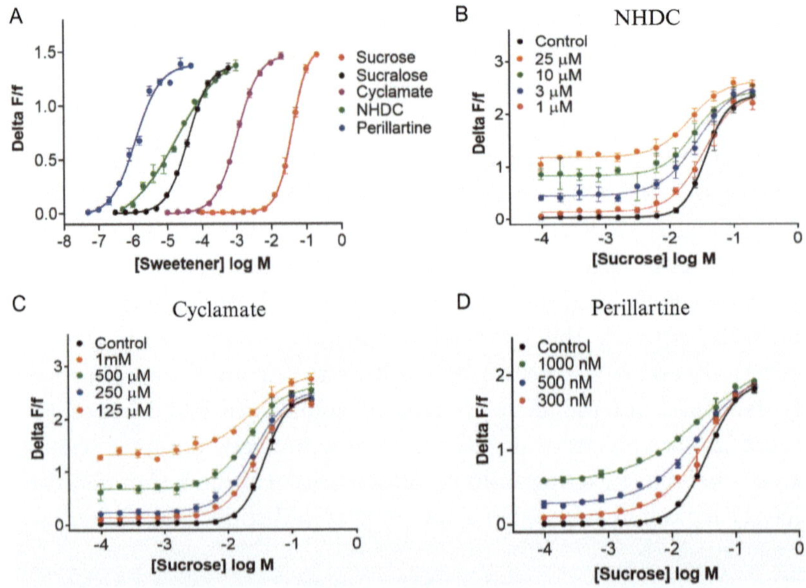

Fig. 3 Evaluation of allosteric agonist effects on orthosteric sweetener activity in a cell-based assay for the human sweet taste receptor. An assay was developed in U2OS cells, stably expressing hT1R2, hT1R3, and allowing detection of receptor activity by calcium mobilization. (A) Dose-response curves of orthosteric agonists (sucrose and sucralose) and allosteric agonists used in the study are shown. Panels (B) through (F), effect of increasing concentrations of the depicted allosteric agonists on the sucrose dose-response in the receptor assay. Each data point corresponds to a triplicate or quadruplicate determinations and each experiment is representative of at least three separate experiments.

and efficacy, respectively, and should be constant for a given set of ligands and GPCR across different assay systems (Ehlert, 2005; Kenakin, 2005; Price et al., 2005). The α values produced for NHDC and cyclamate are 0.3 and 1, respectively, (Table 1), suggesting little to no impact of these sweeteners binding on sucrose affinity and a loose structural coupling between the VFD of T1R2 and the TMD of T1R3. On the other hand, β values of 20 would suggest positive cooperativity on efficacy, suggesting facilitation of signaling upon activation of the sweet receptor by these two topologically distinct sites (Table 1). This could explain, in part, the low level of synergy detected in taste tests between cyclamate-sucrose and NHDC-sucrose sweetener pairs (Schiffman et al., 1995). An earlier study reported an apparent synergy between NHDC-sucrose and cyclamate-sucrose combinations using a sweet taste receptor cell-based assay (Fujiwara et al., 2012). However, the relatively poor sucrose effect in the assay, on its own, made it

Table 1 Summary of cell-based assay data from Figs. 3 and 4 and allosteric model fitting results for detection of synergy.

1	2	3	4	6	7	8	9	10	11
Allosteric modulator	**Orthosteric agonist**	K_A	τ_A	K_B	τ_B	n	$EC_{50}R$	α	β
SE-1	Sucralose	75 μM	1.85	60 μM	0	2.0	18	26	1.4
FEMA 4774	Sucrose	1.3 M	30	100 μM	0	1.4	12	30	1
NHDC	Sucrose	1.5 M	30	50 μM	3	1.8	1.7	0.3	20
Cyclamate	Sucrose	1.5 M	30	12 mM	12	1.8	1.5	1	20
Perillartine	Sucrose	1.2 M	30	4 μM	3.5	1.8	1.4	1	3

Cell-based assay data was fitted to the operational model of allosterism described as followed:

$$Effect = \frac{E_m(\tau_A[A](K_B+\alpha\beta[B])+\tau_B[B]K_A)^n}{([A]K_B+K_AK_B+K_A[B]+\alpha[A][B])^n+(\tau_A[A](K_B+\alpha\beta[B])+\tau_B[B]K_A)^n}$$

where $[A]$ = agonist concentration, E_m = system maximal response, n = slope of the curve, $[B]$ = modulator concentration, K_A = equilibrium-dissociation constant of agonist-receptor complex, K_B = equilibrium-dissociation constant of modulator-receptor complex, τ_A = efficacy of agonist, τ_B = efficacy of modulator, $EC_{50}R$ = leftward shift magnitude of the agonist EC_{50} in the presence of the modulator, α = effect of modulator on agonist affinity, β = effect of modulator on agonist efficacy.

difficult to quantify enhancement. In addition NHDC effect as a sweet taste enhancer has been historically difficult to reproduce (Kroeze, 2000). Similarly, interaction of perillartine with the TMD of hT1R2 only minimally influences binding of sucrose to its orthosteric binding site. At 1 μM, perillartine produces an $EC_{50}R$ of 1.4 (Fig. 3D) and operational model fitting of the data produces an α value of 1 and a β value of 3 pointing to overall low cooperativity on sucrose affinity and efficacy (Table 1).

5. Identification of potent and efficacious PAMs for the human sweet taste receptor

The obesity crisis in America and other parts of the world has forced food and beverages companies to reformulate some of their products with lower levels of sugar (Servant et al., 2011). While the use of non-caloric sweeteners such as aspartame, sucralose, AceK, Rebaudioside A and others has allowed reduction of the caloric load in products, their adoption by consumers has relatively been limited due to the overall poor taste of these sweeteners (Tan, Wee, Tomic, & Forde, 2019). In fact even after the identification or the development of more than 100 different sweeteners over the last century, none of them can fully replace the taste of sugar (DuBois, 2016; DuBois & Prakash, 2012). Furthemore, since combination of sweeteners have also proven of limited utility to boost overall sweetness intensity (see above); more tools are necessary to improve the taste quality of consumer products with reduced sugar content. The establishment of sweet taste receptor cell-based assays in the early 2000s has allowed screening of vast collections of synthetic and natural compounds to identify novel modulators and as a result of this discovery effort five novel PAMs for the human sweet taste receptors have been developed and commercialized.

The first PAM for the human sweet taste receptor was identified following a high throughput screening campaign conducted with sucralose, a sucrose analogue with a ~1000 improved potency compared to the natural sugar (Figs. 1 and 3A) (Servant et al., 2010). In a sweet taste receptor assay, SE-1, a pyrimidine-thione somewhat related to saccharin, causes a drastic leftward shift in the sucralose dose-response by 18-folds without elevating the sucralose's curve bottom asymptote, the signature of a pure PAM (Fig. 4A) (Servant et al., 2010). In agreement, SE-1 does not activate the sweet taste receptor on its own but synergizes considerably with sucralose in a dose-dependent fashion (Fig. 4B) (Servant et al., 2010). In clear contrast to other allosteric sweeteners, SE-1 displays a significant positive cooperativity on the affinity of the orthosteric agonist, sucralose, with an α value of 26 (Table 1). SE-1 (and its analogues) exhibits a clear probe dependence, that is, it selectively enhances the activity of sucralose and to a lower extent sucrose and neotame while exhibiting no effect on other sweeteners (Fig. 4C) (Servant et al., 2010). Similarly, probe dependence has been observed for other for mGluR family members where allosteric modulators selectively affect the affinity and efficacy of different orthosteric ligands (Gregory & Conn, 2015). A simple modification on SE-1, replacing the thiol by a ketone on the pyrimidine ring to improve its stability, produced SE-2 (also called FEMA 4669), a selective sucralose modifier which received regulatory approval in 2008 (Fig. 4D) (Servant et al., 2010). In sensory tests with human trained panelists SE-2 (FEMA 4669) allows for greater than 75% reduction in sucralose levels while preserving sweetness intensity (Fig. 4D) (Servant et al., 2010). Additional screening campaigns and/or further optimization of the earlier lead series SE-1 have so far produced four other PAMs for the sweet taste receptors: FEMA 4701, FEMA 4774, FEMA 4802 and FEMA 4899, each exhibiting selective enhancement of either sucrose, sucralose or fructose activity (Arthur, Karanewsky, Liu, Chi, & Markison, 2015; Arthur, Karanewsky, Luksic, Goodfellow, & Daniels, 2015; Karanewsky

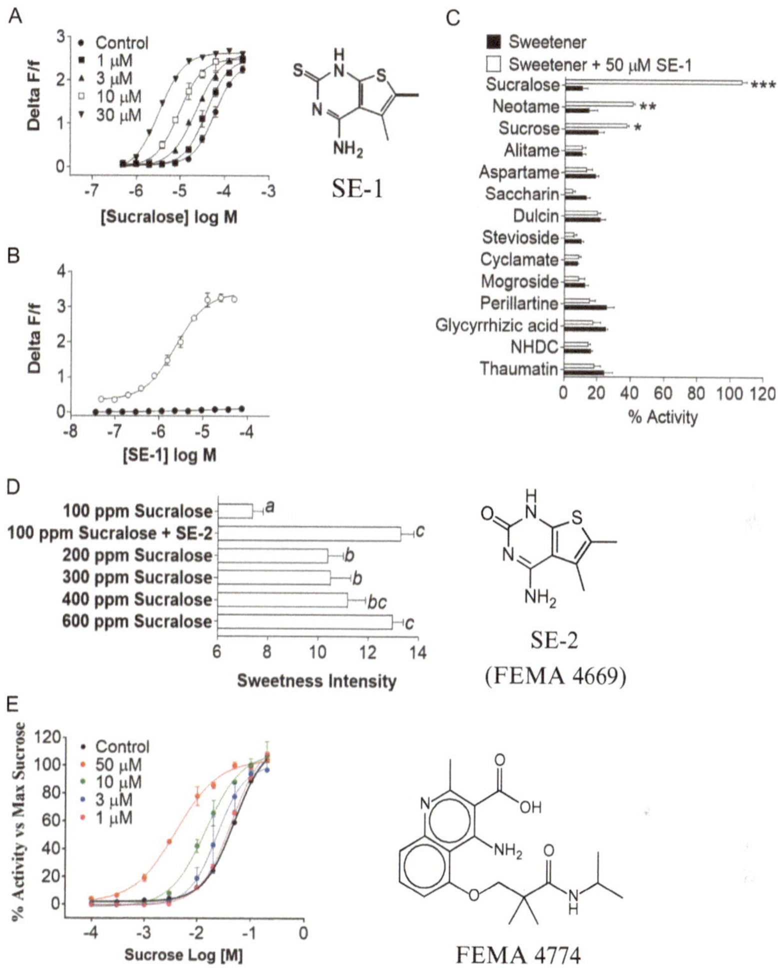

Fig. 4 Identification of potent and efficacious PAMs for the human sweet taste receptors. (A) SE-1 induces a dose-dependent decrease in sucralose EC_{50} in the human sweet receptor cell-based assay. (B) SE-1 lacks agonist activity on its own. Increasing concentrations of SE-1, in the presence (open circles) and absence (closed circles) of a sup-optimal concentration of sucralose, indicate that it behaves as a pure PAM on the human sweet taste receptor. (C) SE-1 displays marked probe dependency in the cell-based assay, selectively enhancing the activity of only a few sweeteners including sucralose, sucrose and neotame. (D) SE-2, a closely related stable analogue of SE-1, enhances the sweetness levels of a 100 ppm sucralose solution to that of a 600 ppm sucralose solution in human trained taste panelists. (E) FEMA 4774 corresponds to another pure PAM of the sweet taste receptor with improved effect on sucrose enhancement. As shown on the graph, FEMA 4774 induces a dose-dependent decrease in sucrose EC_{50} in the human sweet receptor cell-based assay. *Data depicted in panels (A) through (D) were reproduced from Servant, G., Tachdjian, C., Tang, X. Q., Werner, S., Zhang, F., Li, X., et al. (2010). Positive allosteric modulators of the human sweet taste receptor enhance sweet taste.* Proceedings of the National Academy of Sciences of the United States of America, 107*(10), 4746–4751.*

et al., 2017). For comparison with experiments shown in Fig. 3, where allosteric sweeteners are evaluated on their effect on sucrose activity, example of synergy achieved with a potent sucrose enhancer, FEMA 4774, is shown in Fig. 4E. Just like FEMA 4669, it behaves as a pure PAM of the sweet taste receptor and significantly enhances the affinity of sucrose for its binding site, with a α value of 30 (Table 1).

The higher level of synergy achieved with these new PAMs, relative to any other allosteric sweeteners combined with a clear probe dependence are highly suggestive of a unique mechanism of action, different than the ones described for other family C GPCR allosteric modulators which typically interact within the TMD to increase the potency and sometimes the efficacy of the orthosteric ligand interacting within the VFD (Conn, Christopoulos, & Lindsley, 2009; Gregory, Dong, Meiler, & Conn, 2011). Mutagenesis and modeling studies suggest that these novel PAMs indeed interact within the VFD of T1R2 in close proximity to the orthosteric binding site located near the hinge region (Zhang et al., 2010). Sweetener binding is thought to stabilize a closed confirmation of the VFD, leading to receptor activation (Pin & Bettler, 2016; Pin et al., 2019). Closure of the VFD creates an additional binding pocket located anteriorly, opposite to the hinge region, where modulator binding, mostly achieved through hydrophobic interactions, is thought to further stabilize sweetener binding (Zhang et al., 2010). This mechanism of action explains, at least in part, the observed probe dependence or why only T1R2 VFD interacting orthosteric ligands can synergize with this class of allosteric modulators. Further selectivity is also probably achieved by steric hindrance. It is likely that larger sweeteners interacting within the T1R2 VFD such as steviosides and rebaudiosides occupy the same binding pocket as SE-1 and its derivatives therefor precluding their function (Zhang et al., 2010). Interestingly, the mechanism of action for these newly isolated sweet taste receptor PAMs is very similar to the effect of 5′ ribonucleotides on the umami taste receptor (Zhang et al., 2008).

Among the sweet taste receptor allosteric modulators evaluated, the VFD-interacting modulator SE-1 and its analogues stand out in terms of the magnitude of synergy achieved with orthosteric ligands. In that respect, the human sweet taste receptor is somewhat of an oddity within the class C GPCR family. Indeed, every potent and efficacious PAMs identified or developed for the metabotropic glutamate receptors and the $GABA_B$ receptor interact within the TMD of the receptor subunits (Conn et al., 2009; Gregory et al., 2011). PAMs for group III mGluRs have been reported to exhibit more than 100-fold shits in EC_{50} potentiation for glutamate in a cell-based assay (Le Poul et al., 2012) while group I and II PAMs also display robust potentiation of 20- to 30-fold (Gregory et al., 2013; O'Brien et al., 2018). So, why are the modulator-induced changes in conformation within the TMD of the sweet taste receptor not more significantly affecting binding or activity of the orthosteric ligands at the VFD? At least with respect to the cell-based assay, each functional domain of the sweet receptor seem to be able to function almost independently and while there has to be a tight "inward" functional coupling between the VFD and the TMD, to link binding of the agonist at the VFD to G protein activation by the TMD (Fig. 2), the effect of "outward" coupling of the TMD on VFD function seems much less evident, at least up to now. Perhaps the low affinity VFD binding pocket for carbohydrate sweeteners is harder to stabilize in a significantly higher affinity state, by the activated TMD, due to the inability of the low affinity orthosteric ligands to engage more residues within the VFD. In that regard it is worth mentioning that glutamate and GABA have affinities in the high nM to low μM range for their respective receptors (Gregory et al., 2013; Malherbe et al., 2008; O'Brien et al., 2018). In support of this hypothesis, Ca^{2+} displays an EC_{50} of 2 mM for the CaSR and its prototypical TMD-interacting PAM, Cinacalcet, only induces a twofold shift in a cell-based assay (Nemeth et al., 2004). We have yet to identify or optimize TMD-interacting positive allosteric modulators as efficient as their VFD-interacting counterparts. Screening on higher affinity VFD interacting sweeteners could potentially lead to the identification of other classes of efficacious PAMs for the sweet taste receptor, including some interacting at the TMDs of either hT1R2 or hT1R3. Alternatively, the high level of constitutive activity of the human sweet taste receptor (Galindo-Cuspinera, Winnig, Bufe, Meyerhof, & Breslin, 2006) (Servant, unpublished) could possibly limit the impact of TMD conformational change on VFD function, if the latter is, most of the time, in a partially activated and higher affinity state on its own or as a result of a functional interaction with an activated TMD.

6. Human sweet taste receptor inhibitors

Several sweetness inhibitors and human sweet taste receptor blockers have been identified over the years. These include lactisole, gymnemic acid, amiloride, phenoxy herbicides and fibrates such as chlofibric and bezafibric acids (Sigoillot, Brockhoff, Meyerhof, & Briand, 2012). Monosodium glutamate (MSG), the canonical orthosteric ligand of the umami taste receptor also inhibits the human sweet taste receptor most likely by competing at the orthosteric T1R2-VFD binding site (Shim et al., 2015). Even sweeteners including saccharin and AceK, typical orthosteric agonists (Fig. 1), have been shown to inhibit sweet taste and the human sweet taste receptor when utilized at higher concentrations, suggesting the presence of a second and lower affinity inhibitory binding site probably located within the T1R3-TMD (Galindo-Cuspinera et al., 2006; Masuda et al., 2012; Sigoillot et al., 2012). Lactisole, or the sodium salt of ±2-(4-methoxyphenoxy) propanoic acid (Fig. 1) is by far the best characterized sweetness inhibitor. In taste tests, lactisole inhibits the sweetness of several carbohydrate and non-caloric sweeteners but has also been shown to exhibit a certain level of selectivity in taste tests (Johnson, Birch, & MacDougall, 1994; Schiffman, Booth, Sattely-Miller, Graham, & Gibes, 1999) suggesting that distinct classes of sweeteners may potentially compete with lactisole at the receptor level. With the use of receptor chimeras, site directed mutagenesis and modeling, the lactisole binding site was located within the extracellular side of the T1R3-TMD between helices 3, 5 and 6 (Jiang et al., 2005; Nakagita et al., 2019; Winnig et al., 2007; Xu et al., 2004). In vitro lactisole acts has an insurmountable non-competitive antagonist with sweeteners interacting within the T1R2-VFD, including aspartame, AceK (Winnig et al., 2007) and saccharin (Fig. 5A). The effect on lactisole on saccharin function on the sweet taste receptor and modeling of the dose-responses data is consistent with an allosteric antagonism ($\alpha = 0.8$, $\beta = 0.015$). On the other hand, lactisole behaves as an apparent competitive antagonist vis-à-vis sweeteners interacting within the T1R3-TMD such as cyclamate and NHDC, suggesting that these molecules share at least overlapping binding pockets (Winnig et al., 2007). In the receptor assay lactisole also shows what appears to look like a typical behavior of a genuine competitive antagonist with monellin (Fig. 5B), who's binding region has been mapped mostly within the extracellular domains of the heterodimer (Fig. 1 and section on binding sites above). The shifted monellin dose-response curves are parallel and analysis with equidistant and the slope of the Schild regression is close to unity (Fig. 5C). However, this pattern of effect could also be consistent with allosteric antagonism with these allosteric parameters ($\alpha = 0.07$, $\beta = 0.9$). Molecules of low α values leaves open the possibility that lactisole, in fact, still allosterically blocks the effects of these sweeteners. In addition to its properties as a classical insurmountable non-competitive antagonist (Fig. 5A), lactisole behaves as a negative allosteric modulator (NAM) with sweeteners interacting within the T1R2-TMD such as perillartine (Fig. 5D). In this case, the shifted dose-response curves appear to approach

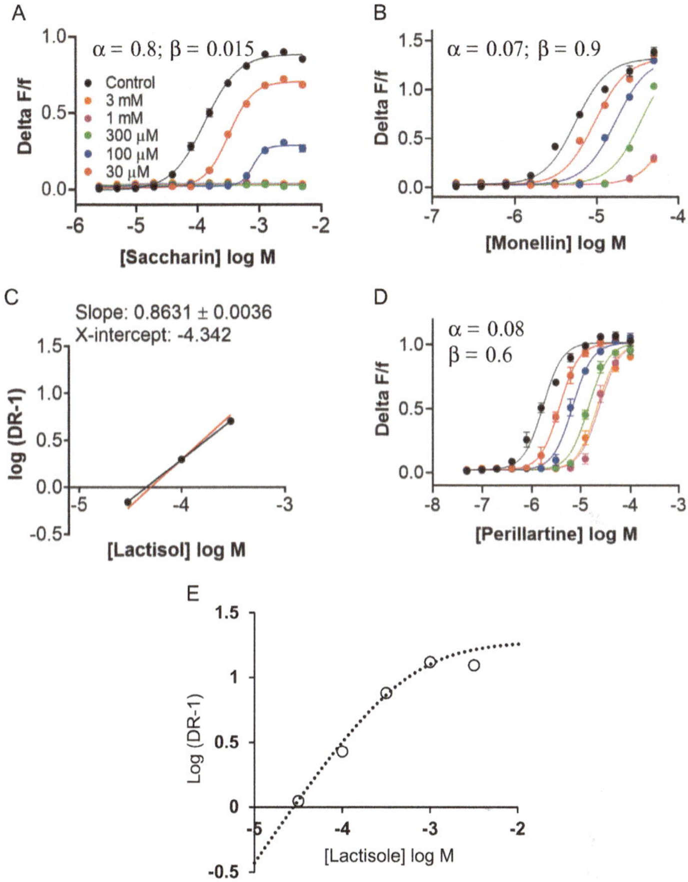

Fig. 5 Effect of the sweet receptor antagonist lactisole of sweetener activity in the human sweet receptor cell-based assay. An assay was developed in U2OS cells, stably expressing hT1R2, hT1R3, and allowing detection of receptor activity by calcium mobilization. (A) Lactisole behaves as an insurmountable non-competitive antagonist with saccharin. (B) Lactisole behaves as an apparent competitive antagonist with monellin. (C) Schild's regression analysis of the monellin data set (black line) produces a slope close to unity (red line). (D) Lactisole behaves as a NAM on perillartine. (E) Schild's regression analysis of the perillartine data produces a curvilinear slope instead of a linear slope. α and β values were obtained after fitting the data to the operational model of allosterism described in the main body of the manuscript. Each data point corresponds to a quadruplicate determinations and each experiment is representative of at least three separate experiments.

saturation at higher concentrations. Analysis with the functional allosteric model yields a prediction of a curvilinear Schild's regression that fits the antagonist data points (Fig. 5E) with values of $\alpha = 0.08$ and $\beta = 0.6$. So the sweet receptor assay exposes three clear and distinct effects for lactisole, competitive, insurmountable non-competitive antagonism and NAM, depending on the sweetener being studied, revealing a functional selectivity vis-a-vis different agonists and the complex allosteric nature of the sweet taste receptor. Lactisole's mechanism of action is still not fully understood at the molecular level. One possibility is that upon binding, lactisole stabilizes an inactive conformation of the T1R3-TMD which then stabilizes the inactive conformation of the T1R2-TMD, precluding G protein activation. Sweeteners interacting with the orthosteric site on T1R2-VFD, such as saccharin (Masuda et al., 2012), cannot overcome this inhibition, either because the VFDs cannot adopt a closed conformation in the presence of lactisole and/or because the closed and active form of the VFDs cannot stimulate the lactisole-bound and inactivated T1R3/T1R2-TMDs. On the other hand, sweeteners that can functionally compete with lactisole in the assay are either competitive or non-competitive binders. Ligands such as NHDC and cyclamate (Winnig et al., 2007), competitively compete with lactisole and, at high concentrations, prevent its binding to the receptor as suggested by the Schild's regression analysis. Monellin, a relatively large sweetener, is made of 2 polypeptides of 45 and 50 amino acid residues and that are linked via non-covalent interactions (Kant, 2005). Monellin's behavior implies that, if indeed it is a competitive binder with lactisole, at least a portion of the polypeptide lies in close proximity to the lactisole binding site within the TMD of hT1R3. Sweeteners binding and directly activating the T1R2-TMD (and the associated G protein) such as perillartine (Fig. 3) can overcome the effect of lactisole's stabilization of the T1R3-TMD in an inactive conformation however at a cost of a drop of more than 10-fold in its apparent affinity (Fig. 5). It will be of interest of determine the effects of some other sweet taste receptor antagonists with different properties and pharmacology. For example the binding site of amiloride was recently mapped on the T1R2-TMD (Zhao, Xu, Meng, & Liu, 2018). Testing the dominance of T1R2-TMD inhibition over activation of the whole sweet taste receptor by sweeteners interacting at different domains could provide additional clues on how these sites functionally interact.

7. Conclusion

Two fundamental breakthroughs are still missing to better understand how the different domains of the sweet taste receptor interact and influence each other. First, a structure of the heterodimer bound to orthosteric and allosteric sweeteners and novel PAMs (SE-2 or others). This would provide crucial information on location of binding sites, could confirm or further refine the mechanism of action of the new PAMs and even potentially allow for rational design of new modulators with perhaps even greater potency, efficacy and with altered selectivity. Second, the development of robust binding assays to precisely measure the extent of PAM or NAM's influence on affinity vs efficacy. Classical binding assay approaches have been a challenge with the sweet taste receptor since the ligand affinities (in the high mM range for carbohydrate sweeteners) are low relative to other GPCR ligands. The development of homogeneous assays measuring receptor subunits conformational changes as a measure of ligand binding (Doumazane et al., 2013) could also help in further refining our understanding of ligand interactions at the sweet taste receptor. High throughput screening of synthetic chemical libraries have yielded potent and efficacious new PAMs but these are of limited chemical diversity and are afflicted with significant sweetener selectivity. Screening of larger commercially available synthetic chemical library on one sweetener may not produce many more active pharmacophores. Rather, diverse sets of compounds could be screened using several representative and commercially relevant sweeteners, even binding at different domains of the sweet taste receptor. In addition, exploring the more complex chemical diversity present in plant and microbial extracts may provide new lead series. Family C GPCR modulators have been shown to behave as molecular switches, whereby small chemical modifications can significantly alter the pharmacology of the modulator, changing its properties from a PAM to a NAM or even a neutral allosteric binder (Gregory & Conn, 2015). Perhaps modifications of lactisole, amiloride, or other reported bitter taste receptor NAMs could lead to the identification of novel PAMs with utility in the flavor industry.

Conflict of interest

G.S., M.W. and L.Z. are employed at Firmenich Inc., a corporation that specializes in the development and commercialization of flavors and fragrances. T.K. and N.S. have no conflicts of interest to declare.

References

Arthur, A. J., Karanewsky, D. S., Liu, H., Chi, B., & Markison, S. (2015). Toxicological evaluation of the flavour ingredient 4-amino-5-(3-(isopropylamino)-2,2-dimethyl-3-oxopropoxy)-2-methylquinoline-3-carboxylic acid. *Toxicology Reports*, *2*, 1255–1264.

Arthur, A. J., Karanewsky, D. S., Luksic, M., Goodfellow, G., & Daniels, J. (2015). Toxicological evaluation of two flavors with modifying properties: 3-((4-amino-2,2-dioxido-1H-benzo[c][1,2,6]thiadiazin-5-yl)oxy)-2,2-dimethyl-N-pro pylpropanamide and (S)-1-(3-(((4-amino-2,2-dioxido-1H-benzo[c][1,2,6]thiadiazin-5-yl)oxy)methyl) pipe ridin-1-yl)-3-methylbutan-1-one. *Food and Chemical Toxicology*, *76*, 33–45.

Assadi-Porter, F. M., Maillet, E. L., Radek, J. T., Quijada, J., Markley, J. L., & Max, M. (2010). Key amino acid residues involved in multi-point binding interactions between brazzein, a sweet protein, and the T1R2-T1R3 human sweet receptor. *Journal of Molecular Biology, 398*(4), 584–599.

Behrens, M., Blank, K., & Meyerhof, W. (2017). Blends of non-caloric sweeteners saccharin and cyclamate show reduced off-taste due to TAS2R bitter receptor inhibition. *Cell Chemical Biology, 24*(10), 1199–1204.

Behrens, M., & Meyerhof, W. (2013). Bitter taste receptor research comes of age: From characterization to modulation of TAS2Rs. *Seminars in Cell & Developmental Biology, 24*(3), 215–221.

Bufe, B., Breslin, P. A., Kuhn, C., Reed, D. R., Tharp, C. D., Slack, J. P., et al. (2005). The molecular basis of individual differences in phenylthiocarbamide and propylthiouracil bitterness perception. *Current Biology, 15*(4), 322–327.

Chandrashekar, J., Hoon, M. A., Ryba, N. J., & Zuker, C. S. (2006). The receptors and cells for mammalian taste. *Nature, 444*(7117), 288–294.

Chandrashekar, J., Kuhn, C., Oka, Y., Yarmolinsky, D. A., Hummler, E., Ryba, N. J., et al. (2010). The cells and peripheral representation of sodium taste in mice. *Nature, 464*(7286), 297–301.

Chaudhari, N., Landin, A. M., & Roper, S. D. (2000). A metabotropic glutamate receptor variant functions as a taste receptor. *Nature Neuroscience, 3*(2), 113–119.

Conn, P. J., Christopoulos, A., & Lindsley, C. W. (2009). Allosteric modulators of GPCRs: A novel approach for the treatment of CNS disorders. *Nature Reviews. Drug Discovery, 8*(1), 41–54.

Damak, S., Rong, M., Yasumatsu, K., Kokrashvili, Z., Varadarajan, V., Zou, S., et al. (2003). Detection of sweet and umami taste in the absence of taste receptor T1r3. *Science, 301*(5634), 850–853.

Doumazane, E., Scholler, P., Fabre, L., Zwier, J. M., Trinquet, E., Pin, J. P., et al. (2013). Illuminating the activation mechanisms and allosteric properties of metabotropic glutamate receptors. *Proceedings of the National Academy of Sciences of the United States of America, 110*(15), E1416–E1425.

DuBois, G. E. (2016). Molecular mechanism of sweetness sensation. *Physiology & Behavior, 164*(Pt. B), 453–463.

DuBois, G. E., & Prakash, I. (2012). Non-caloric sweeteners, sweetness modulators, and sweetener enhancers. *Annual Review of Food Science and Technology, 3*, 353–380.

Ehlert, F. J. (2005). Analysis of allosterism in functional assays. *The Journal of Pharmacology and Experimental Therapeutics, 315*(2), 740–754.

Fujiwara, S., Imada, T., Nakagita, T., Okada, S., Nammoku, T., Abe, K., et al. (2012). Sweeteners interacting with the transmembrane domain of the human sweet-taste receptor induce sweet-taste synergisms in binary mixtures. *Food Chemistry, 130*(3), 561–568.

Galindo-Cuspinera, V., Winnig, M., Bufe, B., Meyerhof, W., & Breslin, P. A. (2006). A TAS1R receptor-based explanation of sweet 'water-taste'. *Nature, 441*(7091), 354–357.

Gregory, K. J., & Conn, P. J. (2015). Molecular insights into metabotropic glutamate receptor allosteric modulation. *Molecular Pharmacology, 88*(1), 188–202.

Gregory, K. J., Dong, E. N., Meiler, J., & Conn, P. J. (2011). Allosteric modulation of metabotropic glutamate receptors: Structural insights and therapeutic potential. *Neuropharmacology, 60*(1), 66–81.

Gregory, K. J., Herman, E. J., Ramsey, A. J., Hammond, A. S., Byun, N. E., Stauffer, S. R., et al. (2013). N-aryl piperazine metabotropic glutamate receptor 5 positive allosteric modulators possess efficacy in preclinical models of NMDA hypofunction and cognitive enhancement. *The Journal of Pharmacology and Experimental Therapeutics, 347*(2), 438–457.

Hoon, M. A., Adler, E., Lindemeier, J., Battey, J. F., Ryba, N. J., & Zuker, C. S. (1999). Putative mammalian taste receptors: A class of taste-specific GPCRs with distinct topographic selectivity. *Cell, 96*(4), 541–551.

Jaggupilli, A., Howard, R., Upadhyaya, J. D., Bhullar, R. P., & Chelikani, P. (2016). Bitter taste receptors: Novel insights into the biochemistry and pharmacology. *The International Journal of Biochemistry & Cell Biology*, 77(Pt. B), 184–196.

Jiang, P., Cui, M., Zhao, B., Liu, Z., Snyder, L. A., Benard, L. M., et al. (2005). Lactisole interacts with the transmembrane domains of human T1R3 to inhibit sweet taste. *The Journal of Biological Chemistry, 280*(15), 15238–15246.

Jiang, P., Cui, M., Zhao, B., Snyder, L. A., Benard, L. M., Osman, R., et al. (2005). Identification of the cyclamate interaction site within the transmembrane domain of the human sweet taste receptor subunit T1R3. *The Journal of Biological Chemistry, 280*(40), 34296–34305.

Jiang, P., Ji, Q., Liu, Z., Snyder, L. A., Benard, L. M., Margolskee, R. F., et al. (2004). The cysteine-rich region of T1R3 determines responses to intensely sweet proteins. *The Journal of Biological Chemistry, 279*(43), 45068–45075.

Johnson, C., Birch, G. G., & MacDougall, D. B. (1994). The effect of the sweetness inhibitor 2(-4-methoxyphenoxy)propanoic acid (sodium salt) (Na-PMP) on the taste of bitter-sweet stimuli. *Chemical Senses, 19*(4), 349–358.

Kant, R. (2005). Sweet proteins—Potential replacement for artificial low calorie sweeteners. *Nutrition Journal, 4*, 5.

Karanewsky, D. S., Servant, G., Liu, H., Chi, B., Ida, L., Saganich, M., et al. (2017). Toxicological evaluation of the flavour ingredient N-(1-((4-amino-2,2-dioxido-1H-benzo[c][1,2,6]thiadiazin-5-yl)oxy)-2-methylpropan- 2-yl)-2,6-dimethylisonicotinamide (S2218). *Toxicology Reports, 4*, 507–520.

Keast, R. S., Bournazel, M. M., & Breslin, P. A. (2003). A psychophysical investigation of binary bitter-compound interactions. *Chemical Senses, 28*(4), 301–313.

Kenakin, T. (2005). New concepts in drug discovery: Collateral efficacy and permissive antagonism. *Nature Reviews. Drug Discovery, 4*(11), 919–927.

Kim, S. K., Chen, Y., Abrol, R., Goddard, W. A., 3rd, & Guthrie, B. (2017). Activation mechanism of the G protein-coupled sweet receptor heterodimer with sweeteners and allosteric agonists. *Proceedings of the National Academy of Sciences of the United States of America, 114*(10), 2568–2573.

Kitagawa, M., Kusakabe, Y., Miura, H., Ninomiya, Y., & Hino, A. (2001). Molecular genetic identification of a candidate receptor gene for sweet taste. *Biochemical and Biophysical Research Communications, 283*(1), 236–242.

Koehl, A., Hu, H., Feng, D., Sun, B., Zhang, Y., Robertson, M. J., et al. (2019). Structural insights into the activation of metabotropic glutamate receptors. *Nature, 566*(7742), 79–84.

Koizumi, A., Nakajima, K., Asakura, T., Morita, Y., Ito, K., Shmizu-Ibuka, A., et al. (2007). Taste-modifying sweet protein, neoculin, is received at human T1R3 amino terminal domain. *Biochemical and Biophysical Research Communications, 358*(2), 585–589. https://doi.org/10.1016/j.bbrc.2007.04.171.

Koizumi, A., Tsuchiya, A., Nakajima, K., Ito, K., Terada, T., Shimizu-Ibuka, A., et al. (2011). Human sweet taste receptor mediates acid-induced sweetness of miraculin. *Proceedings of the National Academy of Sciences of the United States of America, 108*(40), 16819–16824.

Kroeze, J. H. (2000). Neohesperidin dihydrochalcone is not a taste enhancer in aqueous sucrose solutions. *Chemical Senses, 25*(5), 555–559.

Le Poul, E., Bolea, C., Girard, F., Poli, S., Charvin, D., Campo, B., et al. (2012). A potent and selective metabotropic glutamate receptor 4 positive allosteric modulator improves movement in rodent models of Parkinson's disease. *The Journal of Pharmacology and Experimental Therapeutics, 343*(1), 167–177.

Li, X., & Servant, G. (2008). Functional characterization of the human sweet taste receptor: High-throughput screening assay development and structural function relation. *ACS Symposium Series*, *979*, 368–385.

Li, X., Staszewski, L., Xu, H., Durick, K., Zoller, M., & Adler, E. (2002). Human receptors for sweet and umami taste. *Proceedings of the National Academy of Sciences of the United States of America*, *99*(7), 4692–4696.

Maillet, E. L., Cui, M., Jiang, P., Mezei, M., Hecht, E., Quijada, J., et al. (2015). Characterization of the binding site of aspartame in the human sweet taste receptor. *Chemical Senses*, *40*(8), 577–586.

Malherbe, P., Masciadri, R., Norcross, R. D., Knoflach, F., Kratzeisen, C., Zenner, M. T., et al. (2008). Characterization of (R,S)-5,7-di-tert-butyl-3-hydroxy-3-trifluoromethyl-3H-benzofuran-2-one as a positive allosteric modulator of GABAB receptors. *British Journal of Pharmacology*, *154*(4), 797–811.

Maruyama, Y., Pereira, E., Margolskee, R. F., Chaudhari, N., & Roper, S. D. (2006). Umami responses in mouse taste cells indicate more than one receptor. *The Journal of Neuroscience*, *26*(8), 2227–2234.

Masuda, K., Koizumi, A., Nakajima, K., Tanaka, T., Abe, K., Misaka, T., et al. (2012). Characterization of the modes of binding between human sweet taste receptor and low-molecular-weight sweet compounds. *PLoS One*, 7(4), e35380.

Masuda, T., Taguchi, W., Sano, A., Ohta, K., Kitabatake, N., & Tani, F. (2013). Five amino acid residues in cysteine-rich domain of human T1R3 were involved in the response for sweet-tasting protein, thaumatin. *Biochimie*, *95*(7), 1502–1505.

Max, M., Shanker, Y. G., Huang, L., Rong, M., Liu, Z., Campagne, F., et al. (2001). Tas1r3, encoding a new candidate taste receptor, is allelic to the sweet responsiveness locus Sac. *Nature Genetics*, *28*(1), 58–63.

Meyerhof, W., Batram, C., Kuhn, C., Brockhoff, A., Chudoba, E., Bufe, B., et al. (2010). The molecular receptive ranges of human TAS2R bitter taste receptors. *Chemical Senses*, *35*(2), 157–170.

Meyerhof, W., Behrens, M., Brockhoff, A., Bufe, B., & Kuhn, C. (2005). Human bitter taste perception. *Chemical Senses*, *30*(Suppl. 1), i14–i15.

Monnier, C., Tu, H., Bourrier, E., Vol, C., Lamarque, L., Trinquet, E., et al. (2011). Trans-activation between 7TM domains: Implication in heterodimeric GABAB receptor activation. *The EMBO Journal*, *30*(1), 32–42.

Montmayeur, J. P., Liberles, S. D., Matsunami, H., & Buck, L. B. (2001). A candidate taste receptor gene near a sweet taste locus. *Nature Neuroscience*, *4*(5), 492–498.

Nakagita, T., Ishida, A., Matsuya, T., Kobayashi, T., Narukawa, M., Hirokawa, T., et al. (2019). Structural insights into the differences among lactisole derivatives in inhibitory mechanisms against the human sweet taste receptor. *PLoS One*, *14*(3), e0213552.

Nakajima, K., Morita, Y., Koizumi, A., Asakura, T., Terada, T., Ito, K., et al. (2008). Acid-induced sweetness of neoculin is ascribed to its pH-dependent agonistic-antagonistic interaction with human sweet taste receptor. *FASEB Journal*, *22*(7), 2323–2330.

Nelson, G., Chandrashekar, J., Hoon, M. A., Feng, L., Zhao, G., Ryba, N. J., et al. (2002). An amino-acid taste receptor. *Nature*, *416*(6877), 199–202.

Nelson, G., Hoon, M. A., Chandrashekar, J., Zhang, Y., Ryba, N. J., & Zuker, C. S. (2001). Mammalian sweet taste receptors. *Cell*, *106*(3), 381–390.

Nemeth, E. F., Heaton, W. H., Miller, M., Fox, J., Balandrin, M. F., Van Wagenen, B. C., et al. (2004). Pharmacodynamics of the type II calcimimetic compound cinacalcet HCl. *The Journal of Pharmacology and Experimental Therapeutics*, *308*(2), 627–635.

Nie, Y., Vigues, S., Hobbs, J. R., Conn, G. L., & Munger, S. D. (2005). Distinct contributions of T1R2 and T1R3 taste receptor subunits to the detection of sweet stimuli. *Current Biology: CB*, *15*(21), 1948–1952.

O'Brien, D. E., Shaw, D. M., Cho, H. P., Cross, A. J., Wesolowski, S. S., Felts, A. S., et al. (2018). Differential pharmacology and binding of mGlu2 receptor allosteric modulators. *Molecular Pharmacology*, *93*(5), 526–540.

Ohkuri, T., Yasumatsu, K., Horio, N., Jyotaki, M., Margolskee, R. F., & Ninomiya, Y. (2009). Multiple sweet receptors and transduction pathways revealed in knockout mice by temperature dependence and gurmarin sensitivity. *American Journal of Physiology*, *296*(4), R960–R971.

Oka, Y., Butnaru, M., von Buchholtz, L., Ryba, N. J., & Zuker, C. S. (2013). High salt recruits aversive taste pathways. *Nature*, *494*(7438), 472–475.

Pin, J. P., & Bettler, B. (2016). Organization and functions of mGlu and GABAB receptor complexes. *Nature*, *540*(7631), 60–68.

Pin, J. P., Kniazeff, J., Prezeau, L., Liu, J. F., & Rondard, P. (2019). GPCR interaction as a possible way for allosteric control between receptors. *Molecular and Cellular Endocrinology*, *486*, 89–95.

Price, M. R., Baillie, G. L., Thomas, A., Stevenson, L. A., Easson, M., Goodwin, R., et al. (2005). Allosteric modulation of the cannabinoid CB1 receptor. *Molecular Pharmacology*, *68*(5), 1484–1495.

Pronin, A. N., Xu, H., Tang, H., Zhang, L., Li, Q., & Li, X. (2007). Specific alleles of bitter receptor genes influence human sensitivity to the bitterness of aloin and saccharin. *Current Biology: CB*, *17*(16), 1403–1408.

Reyes, M. M., Gravina, S. A., & Hayes, J. E. (2019). Evaluation of sweetener synergy in humans by isobole analyses. *Chemical Senses*, *44*(8), 571–582.

Sainz, E., Cavenagh, M. M., LopezJimenez, N. D., Gutierrez, J. C., Battey, J. F., Northup, J. K., et al. (2007). The G-protein coupling properties of the human sweet and amino acid taste receptors. *Developmental Neurobiology*, *67*(7), 948–959.

Sainz, E., Korley, J. N., Battey, J. F., & Sullivan, S. L. (2001). Identification of a novel member of the T1R family of putative taste receptors. *Journal of Neurochemistry*, 77(3), 896–903.

Sanematsu, K., Kitagawa, M., Yoshida, R., Nirasawa, S., Shigemura, N., & Ninomiya, Y. (2016). Intracellular acidification is required for full activation of the sweet taste receptor by miraculin. *Scientific Reports*, *6*, 22807.

Schiffman, S. S., Booth, B. J., Carr, B. T., Losee, M. L., Sattely-Miller, E. A., & Graham, B. G. (1995). Investigation of synergism in binary mixtures of sweeteners. *Brain Research Bulletin*, *38*(2), 105–120.

Schiffman, S. S., Booth, B. J., Sattely-Miller, E. A., Graham, B. G., & Gibes, K. M. (1999). Selective inhibition of sweetness by the sodium salt of +/−2-(4-methoxyphenoxy) propanoic acid. *Chemical Senses*, *24*(4), 439–447.

Schiffman, S. S., Sattely-Miller, E. A., Graham, B. G., Booth, B. J., & Gibes, K. M. (2000). Synergism among ternary mixtures of fourteen sweeteners. *Chemical Senses*, *25*(2), 131–140.

Schou, K. B., Pedersen, L. B., & Christensen, S. T. (2015). Ins and outs of GPCR signaling in primary cilia. *EMBO Reports*, *16*(9), 1099–1113.

Servant, G., & Servant, N. (2019). 10,281,467. U. S. P. Office.

Servant, G., Tachdjian, C., Li, X., & Karanewsky, D. S. (2011). The sweet taste of true synergy: Positive allosteric modulation of the human sweet taste receptor. *Trends in Pharmacological Sciences*, *904*, 1–6.

Servant, G., Tachdjian, C., Tang, X. Q., Werner, S., Zhang, F., Li, X., et al. (2010). Positive allosteric modulators of the human sweet taste receptor enhance sweet taste. *Proceedings of the National Academy of Sciences of the United States of America*, *107*(10), 4746–4751.

Shim, J., Son, H. J., Kim, Y., Kim, K. H., Kim, J. T., Moon, H., et al. (2015). Modulation of sweet taste by umami compounds via sweet taste receptor subunit hT1R2. *PLoS One*, *10*(4), e0124030.

Sigoillot, M., Brockhoff, A., Meyerhof, W., & Briand, L. (2012). Sweet-taste-suppressing compounds: Current knowledge and perspectives of application. *Applied Microbiology and Biotechnology*, *96*(3), 619–630.

Slack, J. P. (2012). 8,124,360. U. S. P. Office.

Slack, J. P., Brockhoff, A., Batram, C., Menzel, S., Sonnabend, C., Born, S., et al. (2010). Modulation of bitter taste perception by a small molecule hTAS2R antagonist. *Current Biology: CB*, *20*(12), 1104–1109.

Tan, V. W. K., Wee, M. S. M., Tomic, O., & Forde, C. G. (2019). Temporal sweetness and side tastes profiles of 16 sweeteners using temporal check-all-that-apply (TCATA). *Food Research International*, *121*, 39–47.

Teng, B., Wilson, C. E., Tu, Y. H., Joshi, N. R., Kinnamon, S. C., & Liman, E. R. (2019). Cellular and neural responses to sour stimuli require the proton channel Otop1. *Current Biology*, *29*, 3647–3656.e5. https://doi.org/10.1016/j.cub.2019.08.077.

Tu, Y. H., Cooper, A. J., Teng, B., Chang, R. B., Artiga, D. J., Turner, H. N., et al. (2018). An evolutionarily conserved gene family encodes proton-selective ion channels. *Science*, *359*(6379), 1047–1050.

Vincent, H. C., Lynch, M. J., Pohley, F. M., Helgren, F. J., & Kirchmeyer, F. J. (1955). A taste panel study of cyclamate-saccharin mixture and of its components. *Journal of the American Pharmaceutical Association. American Pharmaceutical Association*, *44*(7), 442–446.

Walters, D. E., & Hellekant, G. (2006). Interactions of the sweet protein brazzein with the sweet taste receptor. *Journal of Agricultural and Food Chemistry*, *54*(26), 10129–10133.

Winnig, M., Bufe, B., Kratochwil, N. A., Slack, J. P., & Meyerhof, W. (2007). The binding site for neohesperidin dihydrochalcone at the human sweet taste receptor. *BMC Structural Biology*, *7*, 66.

Winnig, M., Bufe, B., & Meyerhof, W. (2005). Valine 738 and lysine 735 in the fifth transmembrane domain of rTas1r3 mediate insensitivity towards lactisole of the rat sweet taste receptor. *BMC Neuroscience*, *6*, 22.

Xu, H., Staszewski, L., Tang, H., Adler, E., Zoller, M., & Li, X. (2004). Different functional roles of T1R subunits in the heteromeric taste receptors. *Proceedings of the National Academy of Sciences of the United States of America*, *101*(39), 14258–14263.

Yasumatsu, K., Ogiwara, Y., Takai, S., Yoshida, R., Iwatsuki, K., Torii, K., et al. (2012). Umami taste in mice uses multiple receptors and transduction pathways. *The Journal of Physiology*, *590*(5), 1155–1170.

Yee, K. K., Sukumaran, S. K., Kotha, R., Gilbertson, T. A., & Margolskee, R. F. (2011). Glucose transporters and ATP-gated K+ (KATP) metabolic sensors are present in type 1 taste receptor 3 (T1r3)-expressing taste cells. *Proceedings of the National Academy of Sciences of the United States of America*, *108*(13), 5431–5436.

Zhang, J., Jin, H., Zhang, W., Ding, C., O'Keeffe, S., Ye, M., et al. (2019). Sour sensing from the tongue to the brain. *Cell*, *179*, 392–402.e15. https://doi.org/10.1016/j.cell.2019.08.031.

Zhang, F., Klebansky, B., Fine, R. M., Liu, H., Xu, H., Servant, G., et al. (2010). Molecular mechanism of the sweet taste enhancers. *Proceedings of the National Academy of Sciences of the United States of America*, *107*(10), 4752–4757.

Zhang, F., Klebansky, B., Fine, R. M., Xu, H., Pronin, A., Liu, H., et al. (2008). Molecular mechanism for the umami taste synergism. *Proceedings of the National Academy of Sciences of the United States of America*, *105*(52), 20930–20934.

Zhao, M., Xu, X. Q., Meng, X. Y., & Liu, B. (2018). The heptahelical domain of the sweet taste receptor T1R2 is a new allosteric binding site for the sweet taste modulator amiloride that modulates sweet taste in a species-dependent manner. *Journal of Molecular Neuroscience*, *66*(2), 207–213.

Zhao, G. Q., Zhang, Y., Hoon, M. A., Chandrashekar, J., Erlenbach, I., Ryba, N. J., et al. (2003). The receptors for mammalian sweet and umami taste. *Cell*, *115*(3), 255–266.

CHAPTER FOUR

The different aspects of the $GABA_B$ receptor allosteric modulation

Julie Kniazeff*

Institut de Génomique Fonctionnelle (IGF), Université de Montpellier, CNRS, INSERM, Montpellier, France

*Corresponding author: e-mail address: julie.kniazeff@igf.cnrs.fr

Contents

Abstract

The $GABA_B$ receptor is activated by the main inhibitory neurotransmitter of the central nervous system, the γ-aminobutyric acid (GABA). The receptor is expressed in almost all neuronal and glial cells and plays a central role in the modulation of many physiological and pathological processes. The $GABA_B$ receptor has been considered for years as an interesting target for the treatment of spasticity, pain, addiction, anxiety or depression. This has prompted many studies aiming at understanding the activation of the receptor and its modulation. While it belongs to the super-family of G protein-coupled receptors (GPCRs), it was rapidly evident that the $GABA_B$ receptor is peculiar in the variety of allosteric modulations governing its activation. Here, I wish to gather the different aspects of the $GABA_B$ receptor allosteric modulation. After presenting the main small molecule allosteric modulators known to date, the intramolecular transitions controlling

Advances in Pharmacology, Volume 88
ISSN 1054-3589
https://doi.org/10.1016/bs.apha.2020.02.003

the receptor activation will be summarized. In addition, recent findings obtained in the last decade on the existence of $GABA_B$ receptor complexes and their influence on the receptor function will be introduced, including the $GABA_B$ receptor oligomers and the auxiliary proteins associated with the receptor. These new concepts will certainly be of major interest in the future analysis of $GABA_B$ receptor allosteric modulation.

Abbreviations

7TM	heptahelical transmembrane domain
Ago-PAM	positive allosteric modulator with agonist property
APP	amyloid precursor protein
BRET	bioluminescence resonance energy transfer
Cav2.2	high voltage-activated calcium channel 2.2
CHO	Chinese hamster ovary cell line
ER	endoplasmic reticulum
FRET	Förster resonance energy transfer
GABA	γ-aminobutyric acid
$GABA_B$	γ-aminobutyric acid type B
GPCR	G protein-coupled receptor
HCN	hyperpolarization-activated cyclic nucleotide-gated cation channel
HEK293	human embryonic kidney 293 cell line
KCTD	potassium channel tetramerization domain-containing protein
Kir3	inward-rectifier potassium ion channels
NAM	negative allosteric modulator
NMDA receptor	ionotropic glutamate receptor activated by N-methyl-D-aspartate
PAM	positive allosteric modulator
sAPP	soluble amyloid precursor peptide
SNAP	self-labeling protein tag
VFT	venus flytrap domain

1. Introduction

The $GABA_B$ receptor is the G protein-coupled receptor (GPCR) activated by the main inhibitory neurotransmitter of the central nervous system, the γ-aminobutyric acid (GABA). It is broadly expressed in most brain structures and is involved in the modulation of many synapses and processes. At the presynaptic level, it acts as both an auto-receptor and a hetero-receptor by limiting neurotransmitter release through activation of Cav2.2 channels. At the postsynapse, it diminishes the neuronal excitability by a hyperpolarization of the membrane through the opening of the Kir3 channels.

The central role of the $GABA_B$ receptor is directly in line with its implication in many physiological and pathological processes (Bettler, Kaupmann, Mosbacher, & Gassmann, 2004; Bowery, 2010; Pinard, Seddik, & Bettler, 2010). To date, $GABA_B$ receptor agonists are used to treat muscle spasms, alcohol dependency and cataplexy. In addition, the $GABA_B$ receptor is considered a good target for anxiety, depression, chronic pain or addiction (Alexander, 2017; Jacobson, Vlachou, Slattery, Li, & Cryan, 2018; Malcangio, 2018).

Due to its physiological importance, the mechanism and the modulation of $GABA_B$ receptor activation has been the subject of several studies. A better comprehension of the molecular basis of its activation and regulation may help designing better strategies to target the receptor in a pathological condition.

The $GABA_B$ receptor belongs to the class C GPCRs together with the metabotropic glutamate (mGlu) receptors or the calcium sensing receptor (Bräuner-Osborne, Wellendorph, & Jensen, 2007; Kniazeff, Prezeau, Rondard, Pin, & Goudet, 2011). In addition to the heptahelical transmembrane domain (7TM) common to all GPCRs, most class C GPCRs have a large extracellular domain at the N-terminus of the 7TM. This domain, called the Venus flytrap domain (VFT), is constituted of two opposite lobes forming a cleft containing the agonist binding site (Frangaj & Fan, 2018; Galvez et al., 1999; Galvez, Prezeau, et al., 2000; Galvez, Urwyler, et al., 2000; Pin & Bettler, 2016). The VFT is in equilibrium between an open and a closed conformation. Upon agonist binding, the two lobes are stabilized in the closed conformation, trapping the ligand, while orthosteric antagonists stabilize the open VFT conformation. In addition, class C GPCRs are obligatory dimers. In the case of the $GABA_B$ receptor, it is a heterodimer composed of two topologically related subunits $GABA_{B1}$ and $GABA_{B2}$ (Jones et al., 1998; Kaupmann et al., 1997, 1998; White et al., 1998). Both subunits are constituted by a VFT, a 7TM and an intracellular C-terminus (Fig. 1A). $GABA_{B1}$ bears the agonist binding site while $GABA_{B2}$ is critical for G protein activation. The correct association between the two subunits is ensured by a quality control at the exit of the endoplasmic reticulum (ER). Indeed, the $GABA_{B1}$ subunit bears an ER retention/retrieval signal in its C-terminus that is masked only upon interaction with the $GABA_{B2}$ subunit through a coiled-coil interaction between the C-termini of both subunits (Doly et al., 2016; Margeta-Mitrovic, Jan, & Jan, 2000; Maurel et al., 2008; Pagano et al., 2001; Restituito et al., 2005).

A

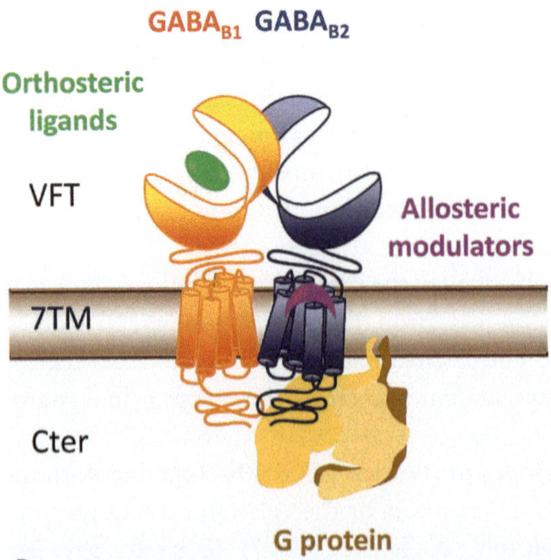

B

Compound name	Chemical structure	Pharmacol. class	Effect on GABA and $GABA_B$ receptor
GABA	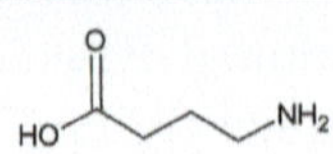	Agonist	
CGP7930	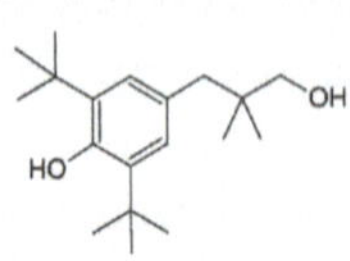	Ago-PAM	↗ GABA efficacy and potency ↗ GABA affinity
GS39783	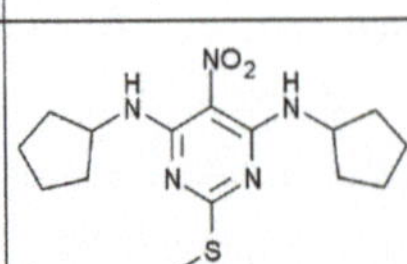	PAM	↗ GABA efficacy and potency ↗ GABA affinity
CLH304a	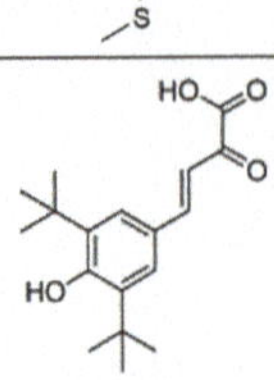	NAM	↘ GABA efficacy Inverse agonist properties

Fig. 1 The $GABA_B$ receptor and ligands. (A) Schematic representation of the heterodimeric $GABA_B$ receptor and the known orthosteric and allosteric binding sites (green and purple, respectively). (B) Chemical structure and properties of lead compounds of the $GABA_B$ receptor.

Structure resolution show that activation of class C receptors activation results from a general conformational change of the dimer. At the extracellular domain the agonist-bound VFT is stabilized in the closed conformation and a re-orientation occurs in the VFT dimer where the two VFTs get closer at the C-terminal ends. This conformation change is also associated with a re-orientation of the 7TM domains. This is well documented for mGlu receptors with a number of cryo-EM and crystal structures (Koehl et al., 2019; Kunishima et al., 2000). For the $GABA_B$ receptor, only structures of the isolated VFT dimer has been published to date. It confirms the re-orientation of the VFT dimer during activation where the N-termini of each VFT move apart while the C-termini get closer (Geng, Bush, Mosyak, Wang, & Fan, 2013).

Only two isoforms of the $GABA_B$ receptor exist. None of the subunits is submitted to alternative splicing but two variants of the $GABA_{B1}$ subunit, namely $GABA_{B1a}$ and $GABA_{B1b}$, are present in mammals and are generated by an alternate promoter usage resulting in two different first exons (Bischoff et al., 1999; Steiger, Bandyopadhyay, Farb, & Russek, 2004). As a result, the $GABA_{B1a}$ subunit bears two sushi domains that are absent in the $GABA_{B1b}$ subunit and that permit specific location of the heterodimer (Vigot et al., 2006). When associated with the $GABA_{B2}$ subunit, the resulting heterodimers did not show any detectable pharmacological differences in heterologous systems to date. However, pharmacologically different $GABA_B$ receptors have been proposed based on results obtained from native tissues (Bonanno & Raiteri, 1992, 1993; Raiteri, 2008). This illustrates that other parameters may play a role in modulating the pharmacology and the signaling of the $GABA_B$ receptor *in vivo*.

More recently, the ability of the $GABA_B$ receptor to form stable oligomers through the association of at least two heterodimers was reported (Calebiro et al., 2013; Maurel et al., 2008). The oligomers were initially detected in transfected cells using either a FRET-based approach or single molecule microscopy, their existence *in vivo* has since been suggested by various studies. First, the molecular size of the complex pulled-down using anti-$GABA_B$ receptor antibody directly from the mouse brain is fully compatible with the presence of at least two heterodimers together with accessory proteins (Schwenk et al., 2010). Second, spatial proximity between two $GABA_{B1a}$ was detected using FRET with anti-sushi domain antibodies on membrane preparations from the mouse brain (Comps-Agrar et al., 2011). Third, in transfected hippocampal neurons expressing the $GABA_B$ receptor at equivalent levels to endogenous expression, 2-photon fluctuation microscopy with scanning number and brightness analysis showed that the $GABA_B$ receptor is mainly oligomeric compared to the $mGlu_2$ receptor (Moller et al., 2018).

GPCRs are highly dynamic proteins which adopt a whole landscape of conformations, some being inactive and others active. The binding of a molecule or the interaction with a protein will differentially modify the equilibrium in the conformational landscape, thus favoring active or inactive conformations of the receptor. This relies on several micro-switches, or allosteric transitions, corresponding to a chain of small conformational changes within the receptor. All of these micro-switches play a role in the outcome of the receptor response. In addition, the binding of a molecule or a protein to a domain topologically different from the orthosteric binding site allosterically influences the conformational transitions, and are likely to result in an allosteric modulation of receptor signaling. Accordingly, pharmacologically positive and negative allosteric modulators (PAM and NAM, respectively), G proteins or oligomerization have all been reported to play a role in the allosteric transitions of GPCR signaling.

Considering the peculiar topology of the $GABA_B$ receptor—a heterodimer with each subunit composed of a VFT and a 7TM—and its ability to assemble in larger oligomers, the existence of a multifactorial allosteric modulation appears obvious. Over the last 20 years, we have gained an understanding of the molecular mechanisms involved in these transitions.

In this chapter, several aspects of the allosteric modulation of the $GABA_B$ receptor are considered starting with the modulation mediated by small molecule allosteric modulators. Then the allosteric transitions existing in the receptor dimer are explored. Finally, larger complexes, including oligomers and interacting partners, and their putative role in allosteric control of the receptor are introduced.

2. Pharmacologic allosteric modulation

Small molecule allosteric modulators have been reported for the $GABA_B$ receptor, mostly PAMs to date compared to NAMs (Brown, Roy, Hockerman, Doerksen, & Colby, 2015; Froestl, 2010; Mugnaini & Corelli, 2016).

The lead compounds of the two main $GABA_B$ PAM classes are the di-tert-butylbenzene CGP7930 and the pyrimidine GS39783 (Urwyler et al., 2001, 2003) (Fig. 1). Both have been identified and characterized by Novartis after the screening of a library of compounds on CHO cells using a [^{35}S]-GTPγS binding assay. CGP7930 and GS39783 increase the GTPγS binding induced by a sub-saturating concentration of GABA, confirming their PAM properties. GS39783 is better than CGP7930 to increase GABA potency. The PAM effect was also measured on native $GABA_B$ receptors using rat brain membrane (Urwyler et al., 2001, 2003). It was shown that both compounds increase not only the potency, but also the efficacy of GABA. In addition, partial agonists become more efficacious in the presence of PAMs and some neutral antagonists become partial agonists (Urwyler, Gjoni, Koljatić, & Dupuis, 2005). Hence, CGP7930 and GS39783 have a positive cooperativity both on agonist binding and agonist-induced activation of the G protein.

Surprisingly, in some functional assays, CGP7930 showed partial agonism in the absence of GABA. This was first reported by Binet et al. in a phosphoinositol turnover assay using a chimeric G protein to couple the $GABA_B$ receptor to the inositol pathway (Binet et al., 2004). In that assay, CGP7930 was able to promote inositol phosphate production in $GABA_B$ expressing HEK293 cells. The competitive antagonist CGP54626 failed to abolish the inositol phosphate production, indicating that CGP7930 is a PAM with partial agonist properties. Furthermore, in a cAMP assay, CGP7930 has shown a small activation independent of GABA. Indeed, on CHO cells expressing the $GABA_B$ receptor and stimulated by forskolin to promote cAMP production, CGP7930 significantly reduced the cAMP level in the absence of GABA (Urwyler et al., 2005). Of note, in that assay, a small agonist activity of GS39783 was also measured (Urwyler et al., 2005). Altogether, these observations indicate that CGP7930 has both positive allosteric modulator and partial agonist effects on the receptor and can be qualified as an 'ago-PAM'.

The effect of CGP7930 and GS39783 on the binding of orthosteric agonists and antagonists has been assessed. The total binding as well as the affinity of the agonist [^{3}H]-APPA are increased in the presence of either PAMs in both transfected cells and rat cortical membranes (Urwyler et al., 2001, 2003). Further analyses using GS39783 show that it decreases both the binding rate and the dissociation rate of the agonist—the latter to a larger extent—leading to a global increase in the agonist Kd (Urwyler et al., 2003). Displacement curves of tritiated antagonist ([^{3}H]-CGP62349) by GABA in the presence or absence of PAMs bring additional information (Urwyler et al., 2004, 2003). First, these studies highlight two populations of receptors in relation to GABA binding: a low-affinity state and a high affinity state, the latter being related to G protein binding to the receptor. PAMs increase GABA affinity in the two populations but they also increase the relative proportion of receptors coupled to G proteins. This indicates that, in addition to increasing agonist affinities, CGP7930 and GS39783 may promote G protein recruitment to the receptor.

Recently, the effect of CGP7930 and GS39783 was analyzed using a conformational FRET sensor that reveals the agonist-induced conformational rearrangement of $GABA_B$ receptor extracellular domains (Lecat-Guillet et al., 2017). As indicated above, during $GABA_B$ receptor activation the N-termini of each VFT move apart (Geng et al., 2013). The change in distance can be monitored by FRET and was used to develop FRET sensors. Using $GABA_B$ FRET sensors, both PAMs were shown to favor the conformational changes induced by GABA, albeit differently. CGP7930 mostly increases the efficacy of GABA and only has a small effect on GABA potency in this assay. GS39783 increases both efficacy and potency. This highlights that the two PAMs are likely stabilizing different conformations of the $GABA_B$ receptor. It has been already suggested that different PAMs for other class C receptors, mGlu and CaS receptors, stabilize distinct conformations and therefore are having different pharmacological effects (Leach et al., 2016; Rovira et al., 2014). Based on the results obtained with the FRET sensor, we may hypothesize that GS39783 has a cooperative effect on the stabilization of the GABA-induced closed conformation of the VFT while CGP7930 binding in $GABA_{B2}$ 7TM promotes a slightly different conformation of the closed VFT in the presence of GABA. Only structure resolution of the $GABA_B$ receptor in the presence of either PAM will help the determination of the differences of conformation.

When used alone, the PAMs did not promote any modulation of the FRET sensor. This suggests that neither CGP7930 nor GS39783 significantly alter the conformation of the extracellular domains of the $GABA_B$ receptor, in agreement with the proposed binding site of these compounds. Indeed, early observations led to the proposal that CGP7930 binds to the $GABA_{B2}$ subunit at the level of the 7TM domain. Indeed, in HEK293 cells transfected with only $GABA_{B2}$ subunit or even with the isolated $GABA_{B2}$ 7TM domain, CGP7930 could elicit G protein activation (Binet et al., 2004). Additionally, GS39783 was found to be active on rat $GABA_B$ receptor but without effect on the drosophila orthologue (Dupuis, Relkovic, Lhuillier, Mosbacher, & Kaupmann, 2006). Using chimera between the $GABA_{B2}$ subunits from both species, $GABA_{B2}$ 7TM domain and, more particularly, TM6 is likely to play an important role in the binding of GS39783.

Other FRET sensors to monitor $GABA_B$ receptor conformational change have been developed based on the conformational change of the 7TM dimer. These were obtained by fusion of fluorescent proteins, CFP and YFP, to the first or the second intracellular loops of $GABA_{B1}$ and $GABA_{B2}$ (Matsushita, Nakata, Kubo, & Tateyama, 2010). In these sensors, CGP7930 increased the modulation of FRET signal induced by sub-saturating concentration of GABA. Surprisingly, in the absence of GABA, CGP7930 did not change the FRET signal. This suggests that while the binding of either GABA or CGP7930 to the $GABA_B$ receptor promotes G protein activation, the conformation of the receptor is different depending on the compound. These conformations may correspond to the fully active and the partially active state of the receptor. GS39783 or other PAMs were not tested with these sensors.

Besides CGP7930 and GS39783, additional PAMs have been reported for the $GABA_B$ receptor. First, the two lead compounds have been derivatized. Rac-BHFF is a more potent derivative of CGP7930 while ADX71943 and ADX71441 are derivatives of GS39783 were considered as good candidate for clinical trials (Kalinichev, Donovan-Rodriguez, et al., 2014; Kalinichev, Palea, et al., 2014; Malherbe et al., 2008). In addition, other chemically unrelated compounds like quinoline, thiphenes and other heterocyclic compounds, are also $GABA_B$ receptor PAMs (Brown et al., 2015; Froestl, 2010; Mugnaini & Corelli, 2016). More recently, a sulfur-containing bicyclic compound ASP8062 was reported as a high potency $GABA_B$ PAM with high selectivity (Murai et al., 2019). Using this whole series of compounds, a recent modeling study aimed at determining the PAM binding site in the $GABA_{B2}$ 7TM (Freyd et al., 2017). Since no crystal structure of $GABA_B$ receptor 7TM domains is available, Freyd et al. used 6 templates of different GPCRs. After the initial modeling, docking of 5 PAMs from different chemical classes was performed. The bioinformatic analysis reveals the critical role of TM6 in PAM binding, with additional contributions from TM3, TM5, and the extracellular loop 2, depending on the individual molecule. The few mutations of the residues in the putative binding pharmacophore which have been published to date align with the predictions of the models. Nevertheless, additional extensive mutagenesis or high-resolution structure of PAM-bound $GABA_{B2}$ 7TM would be required to fully confirm these first models of PAM pharmacophores.

Only a few NAM compounds have been reported to date (Chen et al., 2014; Sun et al., 2016) (Fig. 1). These are based on CGP7930 that have been derivatized to obtain allosteric compounds which decrease GABA-induced activation of G proteins. Using phosphoinositol turnover in $GABA_B$ transfected HEK293 cells, CLH304a decreases GABA efficacy without modifying its potency. This compound is also effective on native receptors as measured by the decrease of baclofen-induced ERK1/2 phosphorylation in cultured mouse cerebellar granule cells. CLH304a does not compete with the binding of an orthosteric antagonist, confirming the allosteric nature of this compound. However, CHL304a abolishes the $GABA_B$ receptor activation mediated by CGP7930 both in transfected cells and in cultured neurons. The NAM also reduces GS39783-induced potentiation of GABA signaling in a Ca^{2+} release assay. In addition, CHL304a reduces the constitutive activity of the $GABA_B$ receptor. With regards to the binding site of CHL304a, it is not surprising that the molecule abolishes the CGP7930 mediated action of the isolated $GABA_{B2}$ 7TM domain. Accordingly, like CGP7930 and other PAMs, CHL304a likely binds to the $GABA_{B2}$ 7TM domain. The possibility to further derivatize this initial NAM has been explored, and the potential of obtaining additional NAMs with potentially different pharmacological properties has been confirmed.

To date, several chemically unrelated $GABA_B$ receptor PAMs, and a small family of NAMs, have been reported in the literature. However, it seems that the binding sites of all of these compounds are overlapping and are all located in $GABA_{B2}$ 7TM domain. Considering the other members of class C GPCR family and their allosteric modulators, one can imagine that PAMs or NAMs binding to other domains may be developed. First, PAMs acting at the VFT but outside the orthosteric binding sites exist for glutamate or taste receptors (Gee et al., 2014; Zhang et al., 2010, 2008). So far, in the $GABA_B$ receptor, Ca^{2+} has been reported to be critical for high affinity GABA binding to the $GABA_B$ receptor, as it directly interacts with a residue located in the orthosteric site (Galvez, Prezeau, et al., 2000; Galvez, Urwyler, et al., 2000). However, more distant VFT binders could be allosteric modulators, as reported for taste receptors with pyridine nucleotides and other molecules (Zhang et al., 2010, 2008). Another possibility would be to target the interface between $GABA_{B1}$ and $GABA_{B2}$ VFT to either favor or inhibit their re-orientation. Indeed, cations and nanobodies with PAM activity binding at the VFT interface have been described for the mGlu receptors (Scholler et al., 2017; Tsuchiya, Kunishima, Kamiya, Jingami, & Morikawa, 2002). Even though the conformational changes during $GABA_B$ receptor activation seem to be rather limited compared to mGlu receptors (Geng et al., 2013; Lecat-Guillet et al., 2017), it is still an interesting track to explore.

3. The $GABA_B$ receptor: An allosteric heterodimer

As indicated above, the $GABA_B$ receptor consists of two topologically related subunits, $GABA_{B1}$ and $GABA_{B2}$. Both are constituted by an extracellular VFT, a 7TM domain and a C-terminal intracellular tail. Interactions have been proposed to occur at all levels of the proteins. Indeed, isolated $GABA_{B1}$ and $GABA_{B2}$ VFTs have been co-crystalized, highlighting their large surface of interaction (Geng et al., 2013). The intracellular C-termini tightly interact through coiled-coil domains (Burmakina, Geng, Chen, & Fan, 2014). The 7TMs domains are likely to interact since only short segments separate them from the VFTs on one side, and from the coiled-coil domains on the other side. This has recently been confirmed in cross-linking experiment, where inserting cysteine residues in the 7TM of $GABA_{B1}$ and $GABA_{B2}$ led to the formation of disulfide bridges (Xue et al., 2019). Due to the tight interactions all along the subunits as well as the number of structural domains in the $GABA_B$ receptor, it becomes rather obvious that allosteric communications are likely occurring. A change of the conformation of one domain may propagate to the other domains and vice versa. Furthermore, GPCRs being highly dynamic proteins, conformational changes directly influence the thermodynamic equilibrium between active and resting states and, therefore, the function of the receptor.

3.1 Allosteric transitions modulating agonist affinity

If $GABA_{B1}$ VFT contains the orthosteric binding site, $GABA_{B2}$ VFT does not bind any ligand. Indeed, there is no pressure during evolution of the $GABA_{B2}$ putative binding site, and mutagenesis of the corresponding residues did not alter the $GABA_B$ receptor function (Kniazeff, Galvez, Labesse, & Pin, 2002). It is interesting to note that, in some species, the putative binding site is likely occluded by an N-glycosylation (Geng et al., 2012). More recently, the crystal structures of isolated $GABA_B$ VFT dimer confirmed the absence of any detectable ligand in $GABA_{B2}$ while $GABA_{B1}$ was bound to various agonists and antagonists (Geng et al., 2013). Despite the lack of endogenous ligand, $GABA_{B2}$ VFT was, however, proven to act allosterically on $GABA_{B1}$ VFT and ligand binding.

First, $GABA_{B2}$ was shown to exert positive cooperativity for agonist binding at $GABA_{B1}$ as initially reported after the cloning of the $GABA_{B2}$ subunit. Indeed, in binding experiments, the Ki measured for GABA is about 20 μM when $GABA_{B1}$ was expressed alone, and it decreases down to about 3 μM when $GABA_{B2}$ was co-expressed (Kaupmann et al., 1998).

This approximate 10-fold increase in agonist affinity in the presence of $GABA_{B2}$ was observed for all agonists. On the contrary, the affinity for antagonists remained unchanged. While the first set of experiments was performed on membrane preparations which may express immature receptors, a similar result was obtained from cell surface binding experiments (Galvez et al., 2001). Indeed, the $GABA_{B1}$ subunit does not traffic to the cell surface when expressed alone and shuffles between the ER and the Golgi, questioning its maturation level (Brock, Boudier, Maurel, Blahos, & Pin, 2005; Doly et al., 2016; Restituito et al., 2005). To promote $GABA_{B1}$ trafficking to the cell surface in the absence of $GABA_{B2}$, its ER retention/retrieval signal can be mutated and the resulting mutant $GABA_{B1}$-ASA is fully processed to the plasma membrane (Pagano et al., 2001). Using that mutant, the Ki measured for GABA on intact cells is 25 μM compared to 3 μM measured on cells co-expressing wild-type $GABA_{B1}$ and $GABA_{B2}$ subunits (for a schematic representation of the constructs and the combinations used in this chapter, see Table 1, here #1 and #2) (Galvez et al., 2001). Altogether, these observations show that $GABA_{B2}$ allosterically increases GABA affinity for $GABA_{B1}$. This was further confirmed using isolated VFTs. $GABA_{B2}$ VFT was shown to increase agonist binding affinity in $GABA_{B1}$ VFT with no effect on antagonist binding (Geng et al., 2012; Liu et al., 2004; Nomura, Suzuki, Kakizuka, & Jingami, 2008). This observation was obtained using either purified VFTs in solution (Table 1, #3 and #4), or plasma membrane-anchored VFT-TM1 constructs where a stop codon was inserted at the end of $GABA_{B1}$ and $GABA_{B2}$ TM1 (Table 1, #5 and #6). Of note, two additional pieces of information were obtained from these experiments. First, GABA affinity for the isolated $GABA_{B1}$ VFT was increased compared to that of the full length $GABA_{B1}$ subunit. Second, while $GABA_{B2}$ VFT increased GABA affinity measured in $GABA_{B1}$-VFT-TM1 + $GABA_{B2}$-VFT-TM1 combination, it remained smaller compared to $GABA_{B2}$-induced increase measured using the full length subunits. This information indicates that while $GABA_{B2}$ VFT plays a major role in governing agonist affinity in $GABA_{B1}$ VFT, the 7TM domains are likely to participate in the modulation of orthosteric ligand binding.

The specific contribution of $GABA_{B2}$ VFT to the modulation of agonist binding was also assessed in the context of a heterodimeric receptor. Two chimeras, GB1/2, consisting of the $GABA_{B1}$-VFT and $GABA_{B2}$-7TM, and GB2/1 consisting of the $GABA_{B2}$-VFT and $GABA_{B1}$-7TM, were generated. The chimeras were useful as they allowed the specific replacement of

Table 1 Schematic representation and main properties of the constructs described in part 3.

Agonist binding

	Expressed SU	Schem.	GABA Ki
#1	GABA$_{B1}$-ASA	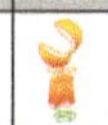	
#2	GABA$_{B1}$ GABA$_{B2}$	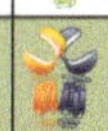	Ki ↘ 10-fold (vs #1)
#3	GABA$_{B1}$-VFT	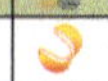	
#4	GABA$_{B1}$-VFT GABA$_{B2}$-VFT	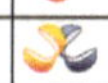	Ki ↘ (vs #3)
#5	GABA$_{B1}$-VFT-TM1	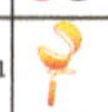	
#6	GABA$_{B1}$-VFT-TM1 GABA$_{B2}$-VFT-TM1	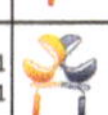	Ki ↘ (vs #5)
#7	GABA$_{B1}$ GB1/2	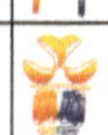	Similar to #1
#8	GABA$_{B1}$ GABA$_{B2}$-7TM	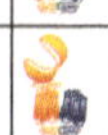	Similar to #1
#9	GABA$_{B1}$ GABA$_{B2}$ + PAM	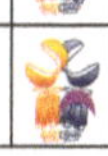	Ki ↘ (vs #2)

G protein coupling

	Expressed SU	Schem.	G prot activation
#2	GABA$_{B1}$ GABA$_{B2}$	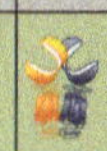	Reference
#10	GABA$_{B1}$ GABA$_{B2}$-Mut_i3	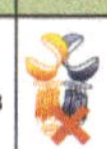	Not responsive
#11	GABA$_{B1}$-ASA GB2/1-ASA	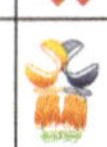	Not responsive
#12	GB1/2 GABA$_{B2}$	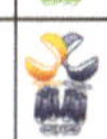	Decreased efficacy
#13	GABA$_{B1}$-CC-VFT GABA$_{B2}$	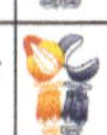	Constitutively active (100%)
#14	GABA$_{B1}$ GABA$_{B2}$-7TM	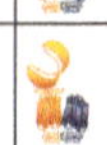	Decrease efficacy
#15	GABA$_{B1}$-NGly GABA$_{B2}$		Not responsive or decreased efficacy

Signal transduction

	Expressed SU	Schem.	G prot activation
#2	GABA$_{B1}$ GABA$_{B2}$	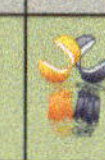	Reference
#16	GABA$_{B1}$-TM1 GABA$_{B2}$-7TM	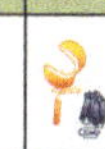	Not responsive
#17	GABA$_{B1}$-Mut_7TM GABA$_{B2}$-7TM	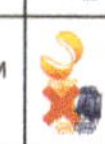	Not responsive
#18	GB1/2	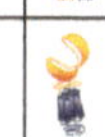	Not responsive
#8	GABA$_{B1}$ GABA$_{B2}$-7TM	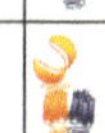	Decreased efficacy and potency
#19	GABA$_{B1}$-TM1 GABA$_{B2}$	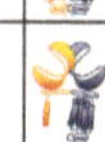	Decreased efficacy and potency
#20	GB1/2 GB2/1	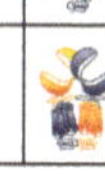	Similar to wt (#2)

one domain in the heterodimer when co-expressed with the wild-type subunits. Hence, a heterodimer where the VFT of GABA$_{B2}$ was substituted by GABA$_{B1}$ VFT could be obtained at the surface of HEK cells (co-expression of GABA$_{B1}$ + GB1/2, Table 1, #7) (Galvez et al., 2001; Margeta-Mitrovic, Jan, & Jan, 2001b). In this combination without GABA$_{B2}$ VFT, GABA Ki is intermediate (8 μM). In addition, the complete removal of GABA$_{B2}$ VFT, expressing GABA$_{B1}$ together with isolated 7TM domain of GABA$_{B2}$ (GABA$_{B1}$ + GABA$_{B2}$-7TM, Table 1, #8), abolished the increase in GABA affinity. Altogether these data confirm that GABA$_{B2}$ VFT plays an important role in controlling GABA affinity for GABA$_{B1}$ and that the 7TM domains are also involved (Fig. 2A).

Initial indications of the role of 7TM domains have been reported. First of all, in addition to increasing agonist potency for G protein activation, PAMs also increase agonist affinity in binding assays (Urwyler et al., 2001, 2003). PAMs likely stabilize an active-like conformation of GABA$_{B2}$ 7TM, indicating that the conformation of GABA$_{B2}$ 7TM has a direct influence on the stabilization of the active agonist-bond conformation of GABA$_{B1}$ VFT (Table 1, #9). Regarding the role of the GABA$_{B1}$ 7TM, as previously indicated, it appears that GABA$_{B1}$ VFT in the absence of GABA$_{B1}$ 7TM is more

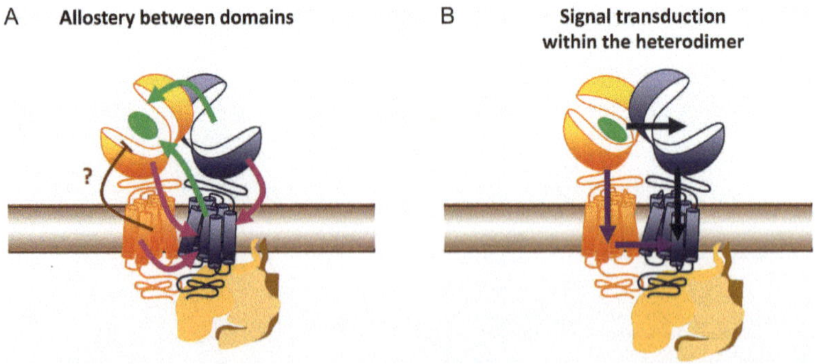

Fig. 2 Cooperativity between structural domains in the GABAB heterodimer. (A) Illustration of the positive (green arrows) and putative negative (brown) cooperativity for agonist binding and of positive cooperativity for G protein activation (pink arrows). (B) Transduction pathways from ligand binding in GABAB1 VFT to GABAB2 7TM in the heterodimer. Two concomitant pathways (illustrated by purple and black arrows) exist.

potent in binding GABA. This suggests that $GABA_{B1}$ 7TM may be directly involved in the stabilization of an inactive conformation of $GABA_{B1}$ VFT in the absence of $GABA_{B2}$ (Fig. 2A). However, the precise contribution of $GABA_{B1}$ 7TM to agonist binding remains to be fully characterized.

3.2 Allosteric transitions modulating G protein activation

With regards to G protein activation, the $GABA_B$ receptor heterodimer is peculiar in that agonists bind to one subunit while G protein activation requires the other subunit. This was proven by introducing point mutations in the intracellular loops of $GABA_{B2}$ 7TM (Table 1, #10) (Duthey et al., 2002; Margeta-Mitrovic, Jan, & Jan, 2001a; Robbins et al., 2001). It results in a heterodimer that does not activate G proteins, even though it binds GABA with high affinity. This indicates that $GABA_{B2}$ is critical for G protein activation. This has further been confirmed using the chimeras of $GABA_B$ subunits described above (Galvez et al., 2001; Margeta-Mitrovic et al., 2001b). Expressing a receptor in which $GABA_{B2}$ 7TM is replaced by that of $GABA_{B1}$ ($GABA_{B1}$-ASA + GB2/1-ASA; Table 1, #11) does not activate G proteins, while it does bind GABA with good affinity. On the contrary, the receptor in which both 7TM are those of $GABA_{B2}$ (GB1/2 + $GABA_{B2}$; Table 1, #12) stimulates G proteins in response to agonist binding. However, the efficacy and the potency of the agonists is significantly decreased. Therefore, while $GABA_{B2}$ 7TM is critical for G protein activation, the presence of $GABA_{B1}$ 7TM helps in activating G proteins.

In other words, $GABA_{B1}$ 7TM has a positive allosteric effect on $GABA_{B2}$-mediated G protein coupling. Of note, a cross-linking analysis of the relative organization of $GABA_{B1}$ and $GABA_{B2}$ 7TMs highlights that there is a re-orientation of the dimer during activation (Xue et al., 2019). When the receptor is not active, TM5s from each subunit are facing each other. In the presence of GABA, a re-orientation of the 7TMs occurs, bringing TM6s to face each other. Stabilizing the active interface increases the constitutive activity of the receptor. This further supports a coordinated function and the cooperativity of both $GABA_{B1}$ and $GABA_{B2}$ 7TMs (Fig. 2A).

Reciprocally to what is observed for ligand binding, it appears that $GABA_B$ receptor VFTs exert some allosteric control on G protein activation by 7TMs. First of all, unlike most GPCRs, the agonist binding site is not located in the 7TM. As such, it is obvious that $GABA_{B1}$ VFT is involved in G protein activation and, therefore, regulates the $GABA_{B2}$ 7TM conformation. First, it is the $GABA_{B1}$ VFT conformation that is important rather than the binding of agonists. In fact, when $GABA_{B1}$ is stabilized in its closed conformation by a disulfide bridge in the absence of agonist, G proteins are activated as efficiently as in the presence of GABA (Table 1, #13) (Kniazeff et al., 2004). Furthermore, the wild-type $GABA_B$ receptor shows a high constitutive activity that is reversed by an orthosteric antagonist known to stabilize the open conformation of $GABA_{B1}$ VFT (Kniazeff et al., 2004). In addition, the agonist effect of the PAM CGP7930 is not fully inhibited by an orthosteric antagonist, however, the efficacy of the compound is reduced (Binet et al., 2004). Altogether, this confirms that the conformation of $GABA_{B1}$ VFT modulates G protein activation at $GABA_{B2}$ 7TM. More surprisingly, even though $GABA_{B2}$ VFT does not bind a ligand and is not submitted to a large conformational change, it is also involved in the modulation of G protein activation. Indeed, when solely the $GABA_{B2}$ VFT is removed from a $GABA_B$ receptor dimer by co-expressing $GABA_{B1}$ with 7TM of $GABA_{B2}$ (Table 1, #14), GABA-induced G protein activation could be measured, but the maximal response was decreased and the EC_{50} was increased (Monnier et al., 2011). This highlights that the $GABA_{B2}$ VFT participates in the global shaping of GABA-induced G protein signaling. Additionally, the ability of $GABA_{B1}$ and $GABA_{B2}$ VFT to change conformation plays a part in the modulation of GABA-induced G protein activation. Indeed, the introduction of a glycosylation in the lobe 1 of $GABA_{B2}$ VFT near the interface with $GABA_{B1}$ decreases the efficacy and the affinity of the G protein response by GABA (Rondard et al., 2008). Furthermore, introduction of a glycosylation in lobe 2 of either $GABA_{B1}$ or $GABA_{B2}$ VFTs at positions facing the other protomer resulted in heterodimeric receptors with good cell surface expression and binding affinity, but unable to elicit a G protein response (Table 1, #15). Altogether, these data indicate that conformational changes in $GABA_B$ receptor VFTs allosterically modulate G protein signaling via $GABA_{B2}$ 7TM (Fig. 2A).

3.3 Signal transduction within $GABA_B$ receptor heterodimer

Considering that GABA binds to $GABA_{B1}$ VFT, that $GABA_{B2}$ 7TM is the main transducer for G protein activation, and that all domains have an allosteric effect on the others, one wonders how the signal is transduced from GABA binding to G protein activation. Three hypotheses may be drawn: 1—agonist binding to $GABA_{B1}$ VFT directly activates $GABA_{B2}$ 7TM; 2—agonist binding to $GABA_{B1}$ VFT is transduced to $GABA_{B2}$ 7TM through $GABA_{B1}$ 7TM; 3—agonist binding to $GABA_{B1}$ VFT is transduced to $GABA_{B2}$ 7TM through $GABA_{B2}$ VFT. A combination of 2 or 3 of the hypotheses may also be possible. These hypotheses were tested using truncated subunits or chimeras to express receptors where one or several domains were deleted or replaced.

The first hypothesis was dismissed since several combinations aiming at expressing only intact $GABA_{B1}$ VFT and $GABA_{B2}$ 7TM did not activate G protein despite efficiently binding GABA (Galvez et al., 2001; Monnier et al., 2011). The combinations included the co-expression of $GABA_{B2}$ 7TM with the $GABA_{B1}$ subunit truncated after TM1 ($GABA_{B1}$ VFT-TM1 + $GABA_{B2}$, Table 1, #16), or with a $GABA_{B1}$ in which the 7TM was invalidated by introducing a disulfide bridge between TM2 and TM3 locking $GABA_{B1}$ 7TM conformation (Table 1, #17). In addition, the chimera composed of $GABA_{B1}$ VFT and $GABA_{B2}$ 7TM, GB1/2 (Table 1, #18) was also unable to activate G protein, despite binding GABA (Galvez et al., 2001; Margeta-Mitrovic et al., 2001b).

The two other possibilities for the signal transduction are most probably concomitant in the wild-type heterodimer. This was demonstrated by deleting either the VFT of $GABA_{B2}$ (co-expression of $GABA_{B1}$ + $GABA_{B2}$ 7TM, Table 1, #8), or the 7TM of $GABA_{B1}$ (co-expression of $GABA_{B1}$ VFT-TM1 + $GABA_{B2}$, Table 1, #19). GABA application to cells expressing either combination promoted G protein signaling, albeit with lower efficacy and potency (Monnier et al., 2011). This result confirms that in the absence of either $GABA_{B1}$ 7TM or $GABA_{B2}$ VFT, the GABA-mediated activation of G protein still occurs through the remaining domains. Hence, in the wild-type receptor containing all four domains, the transduction may occur from $GABA_{B1}$ VFT to $GABA_{B2}$ 7TM either through $GABA_{B1}$ 7TM or through $GABA_{B2}$ VFT (Fig. 2B). Of note, the co-expression of the chimeras GB1/2 and GB2/1 (Table 1, #20), which contain all four domains, leads to a pattern of G protein activation upon agonist stimulation which is very similar to the wild-type receptor (Galvez et al., 2001; Margeta-Mitrovic et al., 2001b). Such similarity between wild-type receptors and the co-expression of GB1/2 and GB2/1 chimeras was also shown using the FRET sensors where CFP and YFP were inserted in the intracellular loops of the 7TM domains (Matsushita et al., 2010). It appears that the presence of the four domains is critical for optimal activation of the receptor and for all the allosteric transitions to occur. This further confirms that in the $GABA_B$ receptor heterodimer, both VFTs and both 7TMs are involved in the activation of the receptor either through the binding of ligands, interacting with G proteins or allosterically modulating the activation process of the receptor.

4. Oligomerization of the $GABA_B$ receptor: A putative manner for further allosteric control?

Over the years, many technical breakthroughs have led to the study of GPCR ability to form dimers or oligomers in living cells (Jonas, Huhtaniemi, & Hanyaloglu, 2016; Milligan, Ward, & Marsango, 2019; Nakamura, Ishii, & Kondo, 2016; Scarselli et al., 2016; Sleno & Hébert, 2018). This started with the use of BRET in transfected cells, shortly followed by FRET and, more recently, the use of single molecule microscopy. Even though the dimeric nature of the $GABA_B$ receptor and other class C GPCRs was never questioned, whether these receptors form oligomers remained to be determined. Several techniques have been employed to decipher the oligomeric status of the $GABA_B$ receptor. Initial data showing that FRET could be measured between two $GABA_B$ heterodimers as well as single molecule microscopy and biochemical experiments show that the $GABA_B$ receptors have the ability to form higher-ordered oligomers (Calebiro et al., 2013; Comps-Agrar et al., 2011; Maurel et al., 2008; Schwenk et al., 2010). Among the receptors tested, the $GABA_B$ receptor seems to form oligomers at very low concentrations both in transfected cell lines and primary neurons (Calebiro et al., 2013; Moller et al., 2018). Also, it seems that the complexes are likely to be larger than tetramers. While a definite proof that endogenous $GABA_B$ receptors exist as oligomers, this however questions the molecular organization and the putative role of the oligomeric entities. These questions were addressed in heterologous systems.

4.1 Molecular organization of $GABA_B$ higher ordered oligomers

Initial experiments leading to the discovery of the $GABA_B$ receptor oligomers using a FRET-based approach provide information regarding their organization (Maurel et al., 2008). When co-expressing $GABA_B$ heterodimers in which either a FRET donor or a FRET acceptor is inserted at the N-terminus of the $GABA_{B1}$ subunit, a strong FRET signal was measured. Indeed, the signal is comparable to that measured between $GABA_{B1}$ and $GABA_{B2}$ in the heterodimer. On the contrary, the insertion of the fluorophores at the N-terminus of $GABA_{B2}$ subunit produced only a small FRET signal. This initial data indicates that at least two $GABA_B$ receptor heterodimers can assemble at the surface of transfected cells. Additionally, it also supports an organization of the complex with $GABA_{B1}$ subunits directly interacting and the $GABA_{B2}$ counterparts being further apart (Fig. 3).

In these FRET experiments, the fluorophores are attached upstream of the VFT to a SNAP suicide enzyme fused at the N-terminus of the receptor. Accordingly, the data described above indicate that the VFT domains of $GABA_{B1}$ subunits are in proximity in the oligomers and are likely interacting. This hypothesis was tested in mutagenesis studies (Comps-Agrar et al., 2011; Stewart, Comps-Agrar, Norskov-Lauritsen, Pin, & Kniazeff, 2018). Based on the oligomeric organization of related VFT domains in

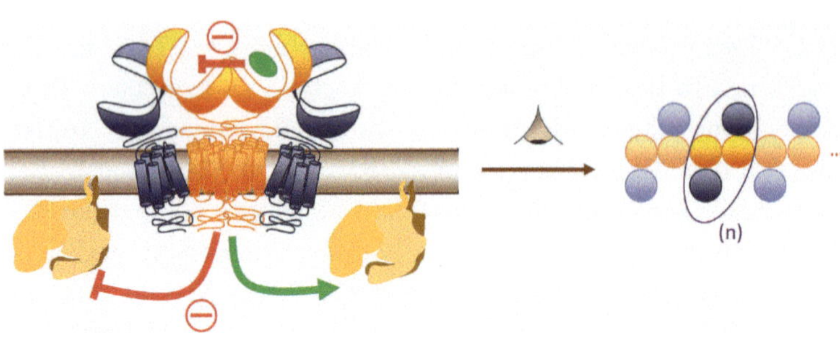

Fig. 3 Cooperativity between heterodimers in GABAB receptor oligomers. The GABAB receptor from high-ordered oligomers with the GABAB1 subunits interacting together (right panel). Pharmacological analysis and mutagenesis studies revealed a strong negative cooperativity for ligand binding leading to occupancy of only a fraction of the binding sites. In addition, G protein activation is limited in the oligomers.

the NMDA receptor, point mutations were introduced in $GABA_{B1}$ VFT at the putative interface between two $GABA_{B1}$ subunits. When expressed with $GABA_{B2}$, three mutants significantly reduced the FRET signal measured between $GABA_{B1}$ subunits. Accordingly, the mutations are destabilizing the $GABA_{B1}$—$GABA_{B1}$ interface at the VFT level even if they do not prevent the interaction. The proximity between $GABA_{B1}$ subunits at the 7TM level was also assessed (Xue et al., 2019). Using a cross-linking strategy, Xue et al. showed that in the absence of ligand, two $GABA_{B1}$ subunits are mainly cross-linked through their TM4 or TM6. In the presence of agonist, the conformational change in the heterodimers results in a concomitant re-organization of the oligomers which are mainly interacting through $GABA_{B1}$ TM1, TM5 or TM7. Of note, oligomers larger than tetramers were also detected in the cross-linking experiments involving trans-membrane helices on opposite region of the $GABA_{B1}$ subunits: TM4 and TM1, TM4 and TM6 or TM4 and TM7 in the absence of ligand or TM5 and TM1 in the presence of GABA. Altogether, these data strongly support that $GABA_{B1}$ are in close vicinity within $GABA_B$ oligomers.

4.2 Allosteric modulation of ligand binding in the oligomers

Since the $GABA_B$ receptor has a strong propensity for forming oligomers, the question of whether this brings additional allosteric control arises. This question was addressed in ligand binding assays using a fluorescent or a radioactive antagonist as a tracer (CGP54626A). A comparison of the binding properties of different oligomeric assemblies was performed (Stewart et al., 2018). The wild-type oligomer co-expressing $GABA_{B1}$ and $GABA_{B2}$ was compared to oligomers which were either destabilized by a mutation (see above), or where some of the $GABA_{B1}$ binding sites were invalidated by mutagenesis. Competition binding experiments showed that the Ki values for both the antagonist and GABA were similar in all three conditions. Surprisingly however, saturation binding experiments with the fluorescent antagonist revealed differences in the Bmax values. In cells expressing the mutant that destabilizes the oligomers, the Bmax is almost twice that measured in cells expressing the wild-type oligomers for a similar expression level. On the contrary, the K_D values were left unchanged in all conditions. Therefore, because the affinity of the tracer and the total number of binding sites are similar in both conditions, these observations indicate that only a fraction of the binding sites are actually occupied in the wild-type oligomers. When the interaction between $GABA_{B1}$ subunits is destabilized at the VFT level, the antagonist gets access to additional binding sites. In other words, this result indicates that there is a strong negative allostery between heterodimers in the oligomer when considering antagonist binding (Fig. 3). The mechanism is not yet well understood. We may hypothesize that steric hindrance or molecular switches allow the occupancy of only a fraction of the binding sites at a time. While a similar experiment could not be performed with a labeled agonist due to the low affinity of agonists, it is likely that the negative allostery also applies to agonist binding. However, further analyses are required to fully confirm this hypothesis.

4.3 Modulation of G protein activation in the oligomer

In addition to ligand binding, oligomerization also modulates G protein activation. Indeed, in cells expressing destabilized oligomers due to the mutation at the $GABA_{B1}$-$GABA_{B1}$ interface, the efficacy of G protein activation by GABA is increased by about twofold (Comps-Agrar et al., 2011; Stewart et al., 2018). On the contrary, the EC_{50} value remains unchanged. This was further supported when using a modified version of $GABA_{B1}$ to compete the $GABA_{B1}$-$GABA_{B1}$ interaction in the oligomer (Comps-Agrar et al., 2011). This competitor consists of the $GABA_{B1}$ subunit deleted of its C-terminus to allow cell surface targeting without $GABA_{B2}$, and in which the GABA binding site is invalidated to prevent agonist binding. The competitor was shown to efficiently reduce the interaction between $GABA_{B1}$ subunits, hence likely preventing oligomer formation. In these conditions, GABA efficacy in activating G proteins is significantly increased to about 250–300% of the wild-type oligomer E_{max}. These data could be directly related to the putative limitation of the number of binding sites occupied by agonists in the oligomer. However, because of the extent of E_{max} increase, we cannot exclude an additional negative cooperativity in the oligomer for G protein activation. The data, however, correlates with a limitation of heterodimers to become active in the oligomer. This hypothesis is further supported by an additional manipulation of the oligomers. Indeed, the co-expression of $GABA_{B1}$ with both wild-type and mutated $GABA_{B2}$ which cannot activate G protein results in random distribution of $GABA_{B2}$ subunits and, therefore, in oligomers where a part of the $GABA_{B2}$ is unable to activate G proteins. These oligomers had a similar efficacy in activating G protein compared to wild-type oligomers when normalized to the number of $GABA_{B1}$ subunits at the cell surface (Comps-Agrar et al., 2011). This confirms that not all heterodimers become active in the oligomers. Altogether, this indicates that G protein activation is limited in the oligomers through some kind of negative cooperativity. It may result either of a reciprocal influence on the conformation or of some steric hindrance for G protein accessibility where binding of a first G protein prevents the binding of additional ones to the surrounding dimers (Fig. 3). Further data is required to determine whether this phenomenon is only because of a negative cooperativity in agonist binding in the oligomer, or whether additional negative allostery for G protein binding and activation also exists.

5. Allosteric modulation of $GABA_B$ receptor by protein partners?

In addition to the allosteric transition which occurs within the receptor, protein partners may also influence the function of the $GABA_B$ receptor. Indeed, G proteins are well-known regulators of agonist affinity of GPCRs (Yao et al., 2009). In addition, other proteins have been identified to interact with the $GABA_B$ receptor and may, as such, have some allosteric effects on the receptor (Schwenk et al., 2010, 2016).

5.1 G proteins control of agonist affinity

G proteins are known to modulate the agonist affinity of GPCRs (Yao et al., 2009). Indeed, the recruitment of G proteins to the receptor is described to stabilize the active conformation of the receptor that has a high affinity for agonist. This explains why the potency of agonists measured in functional assays is usually greater than the affinity measured in binding assays. If the former type of experiments relies only on receptor bound to a G protein (i.e., high affinity state), in the latter all of the receptors contribute to binding whether or not they are coupled to a G protein. This phenomenon was also assessed for the $GABA_B$ receptor. Initial data mentioned by Kaupmann et al. when cloning the $GABA_{B1}$ subunit indicate that uncoupling the G protein through the addition of GTP or its stable analogue Gpp(NH)p reduces the affinity of the receptor for agonists (Kaupmann et al., 1997). More recently, the effect of G protein on agonist affinity was assessed using a FRET sensor developed to measure the conformational changes in the VFT domains (Lecat-Guillet et al., 2017). In this assay, the G protein—$GABA_B$ receptor complex was stabilized by overexpressing a G protein mutant. This mutant has a weak affinity for both GTP and GDP, and mainly remains in the empty state (Barren & Artemyev, 2007). When recruited to the receptor, it remains bound since it is inefficient in binding GTP. Overexpression of this G protein mutant has a dominant-negative effect of the recruitment of endogenous G proteins. In this context, GABA was more potent and slightly more efficacious in the FRET sensor. Altogether, these data confirm that, similar to other GPCRs, G protein allosterically potentiates the agonist binding to the $GABA_B$ receptor.

5.2 Do other auxiliary proteins modulate the $GABA_B$ receptor?

A question that remains unsolved in the context of the $GABA_B$ receptor is the discrepancy between heterologous systems and brain membrane. Indeed, pharmacologically distinct $GABA_B$ receptors are detected in the brain and the affinity measured on native tissues is largely better than that in heterologous expression systems (Bonanno & Raiteri, 1992, 1993; Cruz et al., 2004; Kaupmann et al., 1998; Raiteri, 2008). If the interaction with G proteins potentiates GABA affinity, it does not reach the range of values measured in brain membrane. This suggests that additional factors, likely auxiliary proteins, are involved in the control of GABA affinity.

Proteomic analyses of proteins associated with the $GABA_B$ receptor were performed by combining affinity purification of protein complexes and quantitative mass spectrometry (Schwenk et al., 2010, 2016). Using rodent brains and antibodies targeting various epitopes on the $GABA_B$ receptor, a panel of auxiliary proteins were identified. These belong to the complex immunoprecipitated with the receptor but may be directly or indirectly interacting with it. The analysis confirmed the interaction of the receptor with some $G\alpha$, $G\beta$ and $G\gamma$ subunits or subunits of the Cav2.2 channel. Other cytoplasmic proteins like some 14-3-3 isoforms or KCTDs (potassium channel tetramerization domain-containing) were also identified. In addition, a number of membrane proteins also belong to the complex such as the amyloid precursor protein (APP) or the hyperpolarization-activated cyclic nucleotide-gated cation channel (HCN). The precise organization, physiological role and consequence on the receptor function remains to be determined for most of these auxiliary proteins.

The most studied auxiliary proteins are probably KCTDs. KCTD8, 12, 12b and 16 which were reported to interact tightly to the $GABA_B$ receptor (Schwenk et al., 2010). They control the kinetics of the Kir3 currents induced by the $GABA_B$ receptor and, more particularly, increase the desensitization of the channel through interception of the $G\beta\gamma$ signaling

(Adelfinger et al., 2014; Fritzius et al., 2017; Turecek et al., 2014; Zheng, Abreu, Levitz, & Kruse, 2019; Zuo et al., 2019). The ability of these proteins to modulate the function of the $GABA_B$ receptor was studied. Initial data recording Kir3 currents in CHO cells suggest that KCTD12 and KCTD16 increase the baclofen potency (Rajalu et al., 2015; Schwenk et al., 2010). However, $[^3H]$-antagonist binding displacement by GABA on HEK293 cell membranes expressing the $GABA_B$ receptor showed a very small increase in agonist binding in the presence of KCTD8 or KCTD16 (Rajalu et al., 2015). In addition, the GABA Ki measured on brain membranes were similar between wild-type mice and mice invalidated for all three KCTDs. When considering G protein activation in a $[^{35}S]$-GTPγS binding assay, none of the KCTDs altered GABA efficacy or potency (Rajalu et al., 2015). Only the basal activity was slightly reduced when KCTD8 was expressed. Altogether, it appears that KCTDs have no or barely significant allosteric effect on the $GABA_B$ receptor itself. However, KCTD12 was shown to potentiate the PAM effect of CGP7930 on $GABA_B$-mediated activation of Kir3 currents in oocytes (Li et al., 2017). Further studies, and more precisely structural analyses are required to determine whether KCTDs have a direct influence on the $GABA_B$ receptor conformation.

With regards to the other proteins that were reported to interact with the $GABA_B$ receptor, no real analysis of their putative allosteric regulation of the receptor has been performed to date. An isoform of the 14-3-3 family, 14-3-3 ζ, was reported to dissociate $GABA_B$ receptor heterodimer in a specific neuropathic condition in the dorsal root ganglia (Laffray et al., 2012). This isoform was not identified in the proteomic analysis previously described and no other 14-3-3 protein has been reported to have such an effect on heterodimer association.

APP and its secreted version sAPPα bind to the first sushi domain of $GABA_{B1a}$ expressing $GABA_B$ receptor (Rice et al., 2019; Schwenk et al., 2016). It has recently been shown that sAPPα induces $GABA_B$-mediated signaling and that its effect is abolished by an orthosteric antagonist (Rice et al., 2019). The precise effect of sAPPα on GABA-mediated signaling has not been studied so far, but it may be possible that sAPPα allosterically potentiates the signaling of the receptor.

Other partners like HCN or ITM2B, for example, were found to be present in the $GABA_B$ receptor complex but do not interact directly with the receptor (Schwenk et al., 2016). HCN interacts with KCTD, while ITM2B interacts with APP. It is, therefore, more probable that these proteins play a role in modulating the signaling downstream of the $GABA_B$ receptor activation via their intracellular tail rather than on the receptor itself.

Additional studies are still required to fully elucidate the allosteric regulation of the $GABA_B$ receptor by auxiliary proteins, and to reconcile the affinity measured in heterologous expression systems and the ones measured on native receptors from brain membranes.

6. Conclusion

Over the last three decades, the panel of compounds targeting the $GABA_B$ receptor has evolved to include agonists, antagonists, inverse agonists and allosteric modulators. These molecules tightly and differently control the intracellular response of the receptor likely by stabilizing different conformation of the $GABA_B$ receptor dimer. Many studies were designed to decipher the molecular transitions underlying the receptor activation. They revealed that the $GABA_B$ receptor is a complex allosteric machine including many transitions between structural domains. Accordingly, binding of the molecule to one or another domain modifies the overall energetic landscape of the receptor and stabilizes a given conformation. Additionally, new concepts, like oligomerization and auxiliary proteins, were proposed that are likely to add more possibilities to control the activation of the $GABA_B$ receptor. To gain a better understanding of the molecular transition additional studies are still required. A first insight could be obtained with the resolution of the structure of the $GABA_B$ receptor heterodimer bound to various orthosteric and allosteric compound. In addition, further pharmacological and structural studies are required to characterize the role and the allosteric control within these large complexes with the final aim to reach an understanding of the discrepancy between the pharmacologically different $GABA_B$ receptors detected in the brain and the reconstitution of the complexes in heterologous systems. The comprehension of this phenomenon will open new avenues in developing better strategies to modulate the function of the $GABA_B$ receptor *in vivo*.

Acknowledgments

I wish to thank Drs Laurent Prézeau, Jean-Philippe Pin and Louise Lagerqvist for the critical reading of the manuscript. The work in Pin's laboratory is supported by CNRS, Inserm, the University of Montpellier, the Foundation pour la Recherche Médicale (DEQ20170336747) the Agence Nationale de la Recherche (ANR-12-BSV2-0015) and CisBio bioassays.

Conflict of interest

I declare no conflict of interest.

References

Adelfinger, L., Turecek, R., Ivankova, K., Jensen, A. A., Moss, S. J., Gassmann, M., et al. (2014). GABAB receptor phosphorylation regulates KCTD12-induced K^+ current desensitization. *Biochemical Pharmacology*, *91*(3), 369–379. https://doi.org/10.1016/j.bcp.2014.07.013.

Alexander, R. C. (2017). The potential efficacy of GABAB antagonists in depression. *Current Opinion in Pharmacology*, *35*, 101–104. https://doi.org/10.1016/j.coph.2017.07.009.

Barren, B., & Artemyev, N. O. (2007). Mechanisms of dominant negative G-protein α subunits. *Journal of Neuroscience Research*, *85*(16), 3505–3514. https://doi.org/10.1002/jnr.21414.

Bettler, B., Kaupmann, K., Mosbacher, J., & Gassmann, M. (2004). Molecular structure and physiological functions of GABA(B) receptors. *Physiological Reviews*, *84*(3), 835–867. https://doi.org/10.1152/physrev.00036.2003.

Binet, V., Brajon, C., Le Corre, L., Acher, F., Pin, J.-P., & Prézeau, L. (2004). The heptahelical domain of GABA(B2) is activated directly by CGP7930, a positive allosteric modulator of the GABA(B) receptor. *The Journal of Biological Chemistry*, *279*(28), 29085–29091. https://doi.org/10.1074/jbc.M400930200.

Bischoff, S., Leonhard, S., Reymann, N., Schuler, V., Shigemoto, R., Kaupmann, K., et al. (1999). Spatial distribution of GABABR1 receptor mRNA and binding sites in the rat brain. *Journal of Comparative Neurology*, *412*(1), 1–16.

Bonanno, G., & Raiteri, M. (1992). Functional evidence for multiple gamma-aminobutyric acidB receptor subtypes in the rat cerebral cortex. *Journal of Pharmacology and Experimental Therapeutics*, *262*(1), 114–118.

Bonanno, G., & Raiteri, M. (1993). Gamma-aminobutyric acid (GABA) autoreceptors in rat cerebral cortex and spinal cord represent pharmacologically distinct subtypes of the GABAB receptor. *Journal of Pharmacology and Experimental Therapeutics*, *265*(2), 765–770.

Bowery, N. G. (2010). Historical perspective and emergence of the GABAB receptor. *Advances in Pharmacology (San Diego, Calif.)*, *58*, 1–18. https://doi.org/10.1016/S1054-3589(10)58001-3.

Bräuner-Osborne, H., Wellendorph, P., & Jensen, A. A. (2007). Structure, pharmacology and therapeutic prospects of family C G-protein coupled receptors. *Current Drug Targets*, *8*(1), 169–184. https://doi.org/10.2174/138945007779315614.

Brock, C., Boudier, L., Maurel, D., Blahos, J., & Pin, J.-P. (2005). Assembly-dependent surface targeting of the heterodimeric GABAB receptor is controlled by COPI but not 14-3-3. *Molecular Biology of the Cell*, *16*(12), 5572–5578. https://doi.org/10.1091/mbc.e05-05-0400.

Brown, K. M., Roy, K. K., Hockerman, G. H., Doerksen, R. J., & Colby, D. A. (2015). Activation of the γ-aminobutyric acid type B (GABAB) receptor by agonists and positive allosteric modulators. *Journal of Medicinal Chemistry*, *58*(16), 6336–6347. https://doi.org/10.1021/jm5018913.

Burmakina, S., Geng, Y., Chen, Y., & Fan, Q. R. (2014). Heterodimeric coiled-coil interactions of human GABAB receptor. *Proceedings of the National Academy of Sciences of the United States of America*, *111*(19), 6958–6963. https://doi.org/10.1073/pnas.1400081111.

Calebiro, D., Rieken, F., Wagner, J., Sungkaworn, T., Zabel, U., Borzi, A., et al. (2013). Single-molecule analysis of fluorescently labeled G-protein-coupled receptors reveals complexes with distinct dynamics and organization. *Proceedings of the National Academy of Sciences of the United States of America*, *110*(2), 743–748. https://doi.org/10.1073/pnas.1205798110.

Chen, L.-H., Sun, B., Zhang, Y., Xu, T.-J., Xia, Z.-X., Liu, J.-F., et al. (2014). Discovery of a negative allosteric modulator of GABAB receptors. *ACS Medicinal Chemistry Letters*, *5*(7), 742–747. https://doi.org/10.1021/ml500162z.

Comps-Agrar, L., Kniazeff, J., Norskov-Lauritsen, L., Maurel, D., Gassmann, M., Gregor, N., et al. (2011). The oligomeric state sets GABA(B) receptor signalling efficacy. *The EMBO Journal*, *30*(12), 2336–2349. https://doi.org/10.1038/emboj.2011.143.

Cruz, H. G., Ivanova, T., Lunn, M.-L., Stoffel, M., Slesinger, P. A., & Lüscher, C. (2004). Bi-directional effects of GABA B receptor agonists on the mesolimbic dopamine system. *Nature Neuroscience*, 7(2), 153–159. https://doi.org/10.1038/nn1181.

Doly, S., Shirvani, H., Gäta, G., Meye, F. J., Emerit, M.-B., Enslen, H., et al. (2016). GABAB receptor cell-surface export is controlled by an endoplasmic reticulum gatekeeper. *Molecular Psychiatry*, *21*(4), 480–490. https://doi.org/10.1038/mp.2015.72.

Dupuis, D. S., Relkovic, D., Lhuillier, L., Mosbacher, J., & Kaupmann, K. (2006). Point mutations in the transmembrane region of GABAB2 facilitate activation by the positive modulator N,N'-dicyclopentyl-2-methylsulfanyl-5-nitro-pyrimidine-4,6-diamine (GS39783) in the absence of the GABAB1 subunit. *Molecular Pharmacology*, *70*(6), 2027–2036. https://doi.org/10.1124/mol.106.028183.

Duthey, B., Caudron, S., Perroy, J., Bettler, B., Fagni, L., Pin, J.-P., et al. (2002). A single subunit (GB2) is required for G-protein activation by the heterodimeric GABA(B) receptor. *The Journal of Biological Chemistry*, *277*(5), 3236–3241. https://doi.org/10.1074/jbc.M108900200.

Frangaj, A., & Fan, Q. R. (2018). Structural biology of GABAB receptor. *Neuropharmacology*, *136*(Pt. A), 68–79. https://doi.org/10.1016/j.neuropharm.2017.10.011.

Freyd, T., Warszycki, D., Mordalski, S., Bojarski, A. J., Sylte, I., & Gabrielsen, M. (2017). Ligand-guided homology modelling of the GABAB2 subunit of the GABAB receptor. *PLoS One*, *12*(3), e0173889. https://doi.org/10.1371/journal.pone.0173889.

Fritzius, T., Turecek, R., Seddik, R., Kobayashi, H., Tiao, J., Rem, P. D., et al. (2017). KCTD hetero-oligomers confer unique kinetic properties on hippocampal GABAB receptor-induced K^+ currents. *The Journal of Neuroscience: The Official Journal of the Society for Neuroscience*, *37*(5), 1162–1175. https://doi.org/10.1523/JNEUROSCI.2181-16.2016.

Froestl, W. (2010). Novel GABA(B) receptor positive modulators: A patent survey. *Expert Opinion on Therapeutic Patents*, *20*(8), 1007–1017. https://doi.org/10.1517/13543776.2010.506480.

Galvez, T., Duthey, B., Kniazeff, J., Blahos, J., Rovelli, G., Bettler, B., et al. (2001). Allosteric interactions between GB1 and GB2 subunits are required for optimal GABAB receptor function. *The EMBO Journal*, *20*(9), 2152–2159.

Galvez, T., Parmentier, M. L., Joly, C., Malitschek, B., Kaupmann, K., Kuhn, R., et al. (1999). Mutagenesis and modeling of the GABAB receptor extracellular domain support a venus flytrap mechanism for ligand binding. *The Journal of Biological Chemistry*, 274(19), 13362–13369. https://doi.org/10.1074/jbc.274.19.13362.

Galvez, T., Prezeau, L., Milioti, G., Franek, M., Joly, C., Froestl, W., et al. (2000). Mapping the agonist-binding site of GABAB type 1 subunit sheds light on the activation process of GABAB receptors. *The Journal of Biological Chemistry*, *275*(52), 41166–41174. https://doi.org/10.1074/jbc.M007848200.

Galvez, T., Urwyler, S., Prézeau, L., Mosbacher, J., Joly, C., Malitschek, B., et al. (2000). Ca(2+) requirement for high-affinity gamma-aminobutyric acid (GABA) binding at GABA(B) receptors: Involvement of serine 269 of the GABA(B)R1 subunit. *Molecular Pharmacology*, *57*(3), 419–426. https://doi.org/10.1124/mol.57.3.419.

Gee, C. E., Peterlik, D., Neuhäuser, C., Bouhelal, R., Kaupmann, K., Laue, G., et al. (2014). Blocking metabotropic glutamate receptor subtype 7 (mGlu7) via the Venus flytrap domain (VFTD) inhibits amygdala plasticity, stress, and anxiety-related behavior. *Journal of Biological Chemistry*, *289*(16), 10975–10987. https://doi.org/10.1074/jbc.M113.542654.

Geng, Y., Bush, M., Mosyak, L., Wang, F., & Fan, Q. R. (2013). Structural mechanism of ligand activation in human GABA(B) receptor. *Nature*, *504*(7479), 254–259. https://doi.org/10.1038/nature12725.

Geng, Y., Xiong, D., Mosyak, L., Malito, D. L., Kniazeff, J., Chen, Y., et al. (2012). Structure and functional interaction of the extracellular domain of human GABA(B) receptor GBR2. *Nature Neuroscience*, *15*(7), 970–978. https://doi.org/10.1038/nn.3133.

Jacobson, L. H., Vlachou, S., Slattery, D. A., Li, X., & Cryan, J. F. (2018). The gamma-aminobutyric acid B receptor in depression and reward. *Biological Psychiatry*, *83*(11), 963–976. https://doi.org/10.1016/j.biopsych.2018.02.006.

Jonas, K. C., Huhtaniemi, I., & Hanyaloglu, A. C. (2016). Chapter 4—Single-molecule resolution of G protein-coupled receptor (GPCR) complexes. In A. K. Shukla (Ed.), *Vol. 132. Methods in cell biology* (pp. 55–72): Academic Press. http://www.sciencedirect.com/science/article/pii/S0091679X1500206X.

Jones, K. A., Borowsky, B., Tamm, J. A., Craig, D. A., Durkin, M. M., Dai, M., et al. (1998). GABA(B) receptors function as a heteromeric assembly of the subunits GABA(B)R1 and GABA(B)R2. *Nature*, *396*(6712), 674–679. https://doi.org/10.1038/25348.

Kalinichev, M., Donovan-Rodriguez, T., Girard, F., Riguet, E., Rouillier, M., Bournique, B., et al. (2014). Evaluation of peripheral versus central effects of GABAB receptor activation using a novel, positive allosteric modulator of the GABAB receptor ADX71943, a pharmacological tool compound with a fully peripheral activity profile. *British Journal of Pharmacology*, *171*(21), 4941–4954. https://doi.org/10.1111/bph.12812.

Kalinichev, M., Palea, S., Haddouk, H., Royer-Urios, I., Guilloteau, V., Lluel, P., et al. (2014). ADX71441, a novel, potent and selective positive allosteric modulator of the GABAB receptor, shows efficacy in rodent models of overactive bladder. *British Journal of Pharmacology*, *171*(4), 995–1006. https://doi.org/10.1111/bph.12517.

Kaupmann, K., Huggel, K., Heid, J., Flor, P. J., Bischoff, S., Mickel, S. J., et al. (1997). Expression cloning of GABA(B) receptors uncovers similarity to metabotropic glutamate receptors. *Nature*, *386*(6622), 239–246. https://doi.org/10.1038/386239a0.

Kaupmann, K., Malitschek, B., Schuler, V., Heid, J., Froestl, W., Beck, P., et al. (1998). GABA(B)-receptor subtypes assemble into functional heteromeric complexes. *Nature*, *396*(6712), 683–687. https://doi.org/10.1038/25360.

Kniazeff, J., Galvez, T., Labesse, G., & Pin, J.-P. (2002). No ligand binding in the GB2 subunit of the GABA(B) receptor is required for activation and allosteric interaction between the subunits. *The Journal of Neuroscience: The Official Journal of the Society for Neuroscience*, *22*(17), 7352–7361.

Kniazeff, J., Prezeau, L., Rondard, P., Pin, J.-P., & Goudet, C. (2011). Dimers and beyond: The functional puzzles of class C GPCRs. *Pharmacology & Therapeutics*, *130*(1), 9–25. https://doi.org/10.1016/j.pharmthera.2011.01.006.

Kniazeff, J., Saintot, P.-P., Goudet, C., Liu, J., Charnet, A., Guillon, G., et al. (2004). Locking the dimeric GABA(B) G-protein-coupled receptor in its active state. *The Journal of Neuroscience: The Official Journal of the Society for Neuroscience*, *24*(2), 370–377. https://doi.org/10.1523/JNEUROSCI.3141-03.2004.

Koehl, A., Hu, H., Feng, D., Sun, B., Zhang, Y., Robertson, M. J., et al. (2019). Structural insights into the activation of metabotropic glutamate receptors. *Nature*, *566*(7742), 79–84. https://doi.org/10.1038/s41586-019-0881-4.

Kunishima, N., Shimada, Y., Tsuji, Y., Sato, T., Yamamoto, M., Kumasaka, T., et al. (2000). Structural basis of glutamate recognition by a dimeric metabotropic glutamate receptor. *Nature*, *407*(6807), 971–977. https://doi.org/10.1038/35039564.

Laffray, S., Bouali-Benazzouz, R., Papon, M.-A., Favereaux, A., Jiang, Y., Holm, T., et al. (2012). Impairment of GABAB receptor dimer by endogenous 14-3-3ζ in chronic pain conditions. *The EMBO Journal*, *31*(15), 3239–3251. https://doi.org/10.1038/emboj.2012.161.

Leach, K., Gregory, K. J., Kufareva, I., Khajehali, E., Cook, A. E., Abagyan, R., et al. (2016). Towards a structural understanding of allosteric drugs at the human calcium-sensing receptor. *Cell Research*, *26*(5), 574–592. https://doi.org/10.1038/cr.2016.36.

Lecat-Guillet, N., Monnier, C., Rovira, X., Kniazeff, J., Lamarque, L., Zwier, J. M., et al. (2017). FRET-based sensors unravel activation and allosteric modulation of the GABAB receptor. *Cell Chemical Biology*, 24(3), 360–370. https://doi.org/10.1016/j.chembiol.2017.02.011.

Li, M., Milligan, C. J., Wang, H., Walker, A., Churilov, L., Lawrence, A. J., et al. (2017). KCTD12 modulation of GABA(B) receptor function. *Pharmacology Research & Perspectives*, *5*(4), e00319. https://doi.org/10.1002/prp2.319.

Liu, J., Maurel, D., Etzol, S., Brabet, I., Ansanay, H., Pin, J.-P., et al. (2004). Molecular determinants involved in the allosteric control of agonist affinity in the GABAB receptor by the GABAB2 subunit. *The Journal of Biological Chemistry*, *279*(16), 15824–15830. https://doi.org/10.1074/jbc.M313639200.

Malcangio, M. (2018). GABAB receptors and pain. *Neuropharmacology*, *136*(Pt. A), 102–105. https://doi.org/10.1016/j.neuropharm.2017.05.012.

Malherbe, P., Masciadri, R., Norcross, R. D., Knoflach, F., Kratzeisen, C., Zenner, M.-T., et al. (2008). Characterization of (R,S)-5,7-di-tert-butyl-3-hydroxy-3-trifluoromethyl-3H-benzofuran-2-one as a positive allosteric modulator of GABAB receptors. *British Journal of Pharmacology*, *154*(4), 797–811. https://doi.org/10.1038/bjp.2008.135.

Margeta-Mitrovic, M., Jan, Y. N., & Jan, L. Y. (2000). A trafficking checkpoint controls GABA(B) receptor heterodimerization. *Neuron*, *27*(1), 97–106. https://doi.org/10.1016/s0896-6273(00)00012-x.

Margeta-Mitrovic, M., Jan, Y. N., & Jan, L. Y. (2001a). Function of GB1 and GB2 subunits in G protein coupling of GABA(B) receptors. *Proceedings of the National Academy of Sciences of the United States of America*, *98*(25), 14649–14654. https://doi.org/10.1073/pnas.251554498.

Margeta-Mitrovic, M., Jan, Y. N., & Jan, L. Y. (2001b). Ligand-induced signal transduction within heterodimeric GABA(B) receptor. *Proceedings of the National Academy of Sciences of the United States of America*, *98*(25), 14643–14648. https://doi.org/10.1073/pnas.251554798.

Matsushita, S., Nakata, H., Kubo, Y., & Tateyama, M. (2010). Ligand-induced rearrangements of the GABAB receptor revealed by fluorescence resonance energy transfer. *Journal of Biological Chemistry*, *285*(14), 10291–10299. https://doi.org/10.1074/jbc.M109.077990.

Maurel, D., Comps-Agrar, L., Brock, C., Rives, M.-L., Bourrier, E., Ayoub, M. A., et al. (2008). Cell-surface protein-protein interaction analysis with time-resolved FRET and snap-tag technologies: Application to GPCR oligomerization. *Nature Methods*, *5*(6), 561–567. https://doi.org/10.1038/nmeth.1213.

Milligan, G., Ward, R. J., & Marsango, S. (2019). GPCR homo-oligomerization. *Current Opinion in Cell Biology*, *57*, 40–47. https://doi.org/10.1016/j.ceb.2018.10.007.

Moller, T. C., Hottin, J., Clerte, C., Zwier, J. M., Durroux, T., Rondard, P., et al. (2018). Oligomerization of a G protein-coupled receptor in neurons controlled by its structural dynamics. *Scientific Reports*, *8*(1), 10414. https://doi.org/10.1038/s41598-018-28682-6.

Monnier, C., Tu, H., Bourrier, E., Vol, C., Lamarque, L., Trinquet, E., et al. (2011). Trans-activation between 7TM domains: Implication in heterodimeric GABAB receptor activation. *The EMBO Journal*, *30*(1), 32–42. https://doi.org/10.1038/emboj.2010.270.

Mugnaini, C., & Corelli, F. (2016). The allosteric modulation of the GABAB receptor: A medicinal chemistry perspective. In G. Colombo (Ed.), *GABAB receptor* (pp. 33–52): Springer International Publishing. https://doi.org/10.1007/978-3-319-46044-4_3.

Murai, N., Kondo, Y., Akuzawa, S., Mihara, T., Shiraishi, N., Kakimoto, S., et al. (2019). A novel GABAB receptor positive allosteric modulator, ASP8062, exerts analgesic effects in a rat model of fibromyalgia. *European Journal of Pharmacology, 865*, 172750. https://doi.org/10.1016/j.ejphar.2019.172750.

Nakamura, Y., Ishii, J., & Kondo, A. (2016). Current techniques for studying oligomer formations of G-protein-coupled receptors using mammalian and yeast cells. *Current Medicinal Chemistry, 23*(16), 1638–1656. https://doi.org/10.2174/0929867323666160407113353.

Nomura, R., Suzuki, Y., Kakizuka, A., & Jingami, H. (2008). Direct detection of the interaction between recombinant soluble extracellular regions in the heterodimeric metabotropic γ-aminobutyric acid receptor. *Journal of Biological Chemistry, 283*(8), 4665–4673. https://doi.org/10.1074/jbc.M705202200.

Pagano, A., Rovelli, G., Mosbacher, J., Lohmann, T., Duthey, B., Stauffer, D., et al. (2001). C-terminal interaction is essential for surface trafficking but not for heteromeric assembly of GABA(b) receptors. *The Journal of Neuroscience: The Official Journal of the Society for Neuroscience, 21*(4), 1189–1202.

Pin, J.-P., & Bettler, B. (2016). Organization and functions of mGlu and GABAB receptor complexes. *Nature, 540*(7631), 60–68. https://doi.org/10.1038/nature20566.

Pinard, A., Seddik, R., & Bettler, B. (2010). GABAB receptors: Physiological functions and mechanisms of diversity. In T. P. Blackburn (Ed.), *Vol. 58. Advances in pharmacology* (pp. 231–255): Academic Press. http://www.sciencedirect.com/science/article/pii/S1054358910580104.

Raiteri, M. (2008). Presynaptic metabotropic glutamate and GABAB receptors. *Handbook of Experimental Pharmacology, 184*, 373–407. https://doi.org/10.1007/978-3-540-74805-2_12.

Rajalu, M., Fritzius, T., Adelfinger, L., Jacquier, V., Besseyrias, V., Gassmann, M., et al. (2015). Pharmacological characterization of GABAB receptor subtypes assembled with auxiliary KCTD subunits. *Neuropharmacology, 88*, 145–154. https://doi.org/10.1016/j.neuropharm.2014.08.020.

Restituito, S., Couve, A., Bawagan, H., Jourdain, S., Pangalos, M. N., Calver, A. R., et al. (2005). Multiple motifs regulate the trafficking of GABA(B) receptors at distinct checkpoints within the secretory pathway. *Molecular and Cellular Neurosciences, 28*(4), 747–756. https://doi.org/10.1016/j.mcn.2004.12.006.

Rice, H. C., de Malmazet, D., Schreurs, A., Frere, S., Van Molle, I., Volkov, A. N., et al. (2019). Secreted amyloid-β precursor protein functions as a GABABR1a ligand to modulate synaptic transmission. *Science (New York, N.Y.), 363*(6423), eaao4827. https://doi.org/10.1126/science.aao4827.

Robbins, M. J., Calver, A. R., Filippov, A. K., Hirst, W. D., Russell, R. B., Wood, M. D., et al. (2001). GABAB2 is essential for G-protein coupling of the GABAB receptor heterodimer. *Journal of Neuroscience, 21*(20), 8043–8052. https://doi.org/10.1523/JNEUROSCI.21-20-08043.2001.

Rondard, P., Huang, S., Monnier, C., Tu, H., Blanchard, B., Oueslati, N., et al. (2008). Functioning of the dimeric GABA(B) receptor extracellular domain revealed by glycan wedge scanning. *The EMBO Journal, 27*(9), 1321–1332. https://doi.org/10.1038/emboj.2008.64.

Rovira, X., Malhaire, F., Scholler, P., Rodrigo, J., Gonzalez-Bulnes, P., Llebaria, A., et al. (2014). Overlapping binding sites drive allosteric agonism and positive cooperativity in type 4 metabotropic glutamate receptors. *The FASEB Journal, 29*(1), 116–130. https://doi.org/10.1096/fj.14-257287.

Scarselli, M., Annibale, P., McCormick, P. J., Kolachalam, S., Aringhieri, S., Radenovic, A., et al. (2016). Revealing G-protein-coupled receptor oligomerization at the single-molecule level through a nanoscopic lens: Methods, dynamics and biological function. *The FEBS Journal, 283*(7), 1197–1217. https://doi.org/10.1111/febs.13577.

Scholler, P., Nevoltris, D., de Bundel, D., Bossi, S., Moreno-Delgado, D., Rovira, X., et al. (2017). Allosteric nanobodies uncover a role of hippocampal mGlu2 receptor homodimers in contextual fear consolidation. *Nature Communications*, *8*(1), 1967. https://doi.org/10.1038/s41467-017-01489-1.

Schwenk, J., Metz, M., Zolles, G., Turecek, R., Fritzius, T., Bildl, W., et al. (2010). Native GABA(B) receptors are heteromultimers with a family of auxiliary subunits. *Nature*, *465*(7295), 231–235. https://doi.org/10.1038/nature08964.

Schwenk, J., Pérez-Garci, E., Schneider, A., Kollewe, A., Gauthier-Kemper, A., Fritzius, T., et al. (2016). Modular composition and dynamics of native GABAB receptors identified by high-resolution proteomics. *Nature Neuroscience*, *19*(2), 233–242. https://doi.org/10.1038/nn.4198.

Sleno, R., & Hébert, T. E. (2018). The dynamics of GPCR oligomerization and their functional consequences. *International Review of Cell and Molecular Biology*, *338*, 141–171. https://doi.org/10.1016/bs.ircmb.2018.02.005.

Steiger, J. L., Bandyopadhyay, S., Farb, D. H., & Russek, S. J. (2004). cAMP response element-binding protein, activating transcription factor-4, and upstream stimulatory factor differentially control hippocampal GABABR1a and GABABR1b subunit gene expression through alternative promoters. *The Journal of Neuroscience: The Official Journal of the Society for Neuroscience*, *24*(27), 6115–6126. https://doi.org/10.1523/JNEUROSCI.1200-04.2004.

Stewart, G. D., Comps-Agrar, L., Norskov-Lauritsen, L. B., Pin, J.-P., & Kniazeff, J. (2018). Allosteric interactions between GABAB1 subunits control orthosteric binding sites occupancy within GABAB oligomers. *Neuropharmacology*, *136*(Pt. A), 92–101. https://doi.org/10.1016/j.neuropharm.2017.12.042.

Sun, B., Chen, L., Liu, L., Xia, Z., Pin, J.-P., Nan, F., et al. (2016). A negative allosteric modulator modulates GABAB-receptor signalling through GB2 subunits. *Biochemical Journal*, *473*(6), 779–787. https://doi.org/10.1042/BJ20150979.

Tsuchiya, D., Kunishima, N., Kamiya, N., Jingami, H., & Morikawa, K. (2002). Structural views of the ligand-binding cores of a metabotropic glutamate receptor complexed with an antagonist and both glutamate and Gd^{3+}. *Proceedings of the National Academy of Sciences of the United States of America*, *99*(5), 2660–2665. https://doi.org/10.1073/pnas.052708599.

Turecek, R., Schwenk, J., Fritzius, T., Ivankova, K., Zolles, G., Adelfinger, L., et al. (2014). Auxiliary GABAB receptor subunits uncouple G protein βγ subunits from effector channels to induce desensitization. *Neuron*, *82*(5), 1032–1044. https://doi.org/10.1016/j.neuron.2014.04.015.

Urwyler, S., Gjoni, T., Kaupmann, K., Pozza, M. F., & Mosbacher, J. (2004). Selected amino acids, dipeptides and arylalkylamine derivatives do not act as allosteric modulators at GABAB receptors. *European Journal of Pharmacology*, *483*(2–3), 147–153. https://doi.org/10.1016/j.ejphar.2003.10.024.

Urwyler, S., Gjoni, T., Koljatić, J., & Dupuis, D. S. (2005). Mechanisms of allosteric modulation at GABAB receptors by CGP7930 and GS39783: Effects on affinities and efficacies of orthosteric ligands with distinct intrinsic properties. *Neuropharmacology*, *48*(3), 343–353. https://doi.org/10.1016/j.neuropharm.2004.10.013.

Urwyler, S., Mosbacher, J., Lingenhoehl, K., Heid, J., Hofstetter, K., Froestl, W., et al. (2001). Positive allosteric modulation of native and recombinant gamma-aminobutyric acid(B) receptors by 2,6-Di-tert-butyl-4-(3-hydroxy-2,2-dimethyl-propyl)-phenol (CGP7930) and its aldehyde analog CGP13501. *Molecular Pharmacology*, *60*(5), 963–971.

Urwyler, S., Pozza, M. F., Lingenhoehl, K., Mosbacher, J., Lampert, C., Froestl, W., et al. (2003). N,N'-Dicyclopentyl-2-methylsulfanyl-5-nitro-pyrimidine-4,6-diamine (GS39783) and structurally related compounds: Novel allosteric enhancers of gamma-aminobutyric acidB receptor function. *The Journal of Pharmacology and Experimental Therapeutics*, *307*(1), 322–330. https://doi.org/10.1124/jpet.103.053074.

Vigot, R., Barbieri, S., Bräuner-Osborne, H., Turecek, R., Shigemoto, R., Zhang, Y.-P., et al. (2006). Differential compartmentalization and distinct functions of GABAB receptor variants. *Neuron, 50*(4), 589–601. https://doi.org/10.1016/j.neuron.2006.04.014.

White, J. H., Wise, A., Main, M. J., Green, A., Fraser, N. J., Disney, G. H., et al. (1998). Heterodimerization is required for the formation of a functional GABA(B) receptor. *Nature, 396*(6712), 679–682. https://doi.org/10.1038/25354.

Xue, L., Sun, Q., Zhao, H., Rovira, X., Gai, S., He, Q., et al. (2019). Rearrangement of the transmembrane domain interfaces associated with the activation of a GPCR hetero-oligomer. *Nature Communications, 10*(1), 2765. https://doi.org/10.1038/s41467-019-10834-5.

Yao, X. J., Ruiz, G. V., Whorton, M. R., Rasmussen, S. G. F., DeVree, B. T., Deupi, X., et al. (2009). The effect of ligand efficacy on the formation and stability of a GPCR-G protein complex. *Proceedings of the National Academy of Sciences, 106*(23), 9501–9506. https://doi.org/10.1073/pnas.0811437106.

Zhang, F., Klebansky, B., Fine, R. M., Liu, H., Xu, H., Servant, G., et al. (2010). Molecular mechanism of the sweet taste enhancers. *Proceedings of the National Academy of Sciences of the United States of America, 107*(10), 4752–4757. https://doi.org/10.1073/pnas.0911660107.

Zhang, F., Klebansky, B., Fine, R. M., Xu, H., Pronin, A., Liu, H., et al. (2008). Molecular mechanism for the umami taste synergism. *Proceedings of the National Academy of Sciences, 105*(52), 20930–20934. https://doi.org/10.1073/pnas.0810174106.

Zheng, S., Abreu, N., Levitz, J., & Kruse, A. C. (2019). Structural basis for KCTD-mediated rapid desensitization of GABAB signalling. *Nature, 567*(7746), 127–131. https://doi.org/10.1038/s41586-019-0990-0.

Zuo, H., Glaaser, I., Zhao, Y., Kurinov, I., Mosyak, L., Wang, H., et al. (2019). Structural basis for auxiliary subunit KCTD16 regulation of the GABAB receptor. *Proceedings of the National Academy of Sciences of the United States of America, 116*(17), 8370–8379. https://doi.org/10.1073/pnas.1903024116.

CHAPTER FIVE

RAMPs as allosteric modulators of the calcitonin and calcitonin-like class B G protein-coupled receptors

Augen A. Pioszak[a,*], **Debbie L. Hay**[b,c]
[a]Department of Biochemistry and Molecular Biology, The University of Oklahoma Health Sciences Center, Oklahoma City, OK, United States
[b]School of Biological Sciences, University of Auckland, Auckland, New Zealand
[c]Maurice Wilkins Centre for Molecular Biodiscovery, University of Auckland, Auckland, New Zealand
*Corresponding author: e-mail address: augen-pioszak@ouhsc.edu

Contents

Abstract

Receptor activity-modifying proteins (RAMPs) are a family of three single span transmembrane proteins in humans that interact with many GPCRs and can modulate their function. RAMPs were discovered as key components of the calcitonin gene-related peptide and adrenomedullin receptors. They are required for transport of this class B GPCR, calcitonin receptor-like receptor (CLR), to the cell surface and determine its peptide ligand binding preferences. Soon thereafter RAMPs were shown to modulate the binding of calcitonin and amylin peptides to the related calcitonin receptor (CTR) and in the years since an ever-growing number of RAMP-interacting receptors have been identified including most if not all of the 15 class B GPCRs and several GPCRs from other families. Studies of CLR, CTR, and a handful of other GPCRs revealed that RAMPs are

Advances in Pharmacology, Volume 88
ISSN 1054-3589
https://doi.org/10.1016/bs.apha.2020.01.001

able to modulate various aspects of receptor function including trafficking, ligand binding, and signaling. Here, we review RAMP interactions and functions with an emphasis on class B receptors for which our understanding is most advanced. A key focus is to discuss recent evidence that RAMPs serve as endogenous allosteric modulators of CLR and CTR. We discuss structural studies of RAMP-CLR complexes and CTR and biochemical and pharmacological studies that collectively have significantly expanded our understanding of the mechanistic basis for RAMP modulation of these class B GPCRs. Last, we consider the implications of these findings for drug development targeting RAMP-CLR/CTR complexes.

Abbreviations

AM adrenomedullin
AM2/IMD adrenomedullin 2/intermedin
CGRP calcitonin gene-related peptide
CLR calcitonin receptor-like receptor
CT calcitonin
CTR calcitonin receptor
ECD extracellular domain
RAMP receptor activity-modifying protein
TMD transmembrane domain

1. Introduction

The class B/Secretin family of G protein-coupled receptors (GPCRs) comprises 15 receptors in humans that mediate responses to a diverse collection of peptides that signal in an endocrine, paracrine, or autocrine manner (Hoare, 2005). This family includes two receptors for the calcitonin family peptides (CTR and CLR), two receptors for parathyroid hormone and related peptides (PTH1R and PTH2R), two receptors for the corticotropin releasing factor/urocortin peptide family (CRFR1 and CRFR2), four receptors for glucagon family peptides (GCGR, GLP1R, GLP2R, and GIPR), three receptors for pituitary adenylate cyclase-activating peptide and related peptides (PAC1R, VPAC1R, VPAC2R), and the receptors for secretin (SECR) and growth hormone-releasing hormone (GHRHR). Receptors in this family have clinical relevance for many diseases including migraine, diabetes, cardiovascular disorders, osteoporosis, depression, and cancer. Several peptide therapeutics targeting class B receptors are on the market; with the most successful example being the GLP1R agonists used for type II diabetes (Drucker, 2018). Enormous potential remains for developing novel therapeutics targeting this receptor family and it is expected that recent breakthroughs in the structural biology of class B receptors will facilitate progress in this area (Wootten & Miller, 2020). Most of these receptors, if not all (see Section 3), can be modulated by receptor activity-modifying proteins (RAMPs) that are the focus of this chapter. These accessory membrane proteins can affect various aspects of receptor function, which adds considerable complexity to their pharmacology, but also significantly expands opportunities for drug discovery.

Class B receptors have a two-domain structure with an N-terminal extracellular domain (ECD) followed by a transmembrane domain (TMD). The ECD is ~120 amino acids and forms a conserved α/β fold with an N-terminal α-helix connected to a series of β-strands and loops, all stabilized by three conserved disulfide bonds (Pal, Melcher, & Xu, 2012). The TMD forms a 7-transmembrane helical bundle with a single conserved disulfide bond connecting ECL2 and the top of TM3 (Hollenstein et al., 2014). The bundle is similar to that of the class A GPCRs except that the top half is more open to accommodate the binding of large peptides (Hollenstein et al., 2013; Siu et al., 2013). The peptide ligands, which are generally ~30–40 amino acids in length, engage both receptor domains in what is known as the "two-domain" binding model and is thought to occur in two steps (Hoare, 2005). The C-terminal half of the peptide first binds the ECD in a somewhat high-affinity interaction and this then promotes binding of the N-terminal half of the peptide to the TMD, which is otherwise a low-affinity interaction. The latter interaction is responsible for receptor activation. Class B receptors predominantly couple to G_s, but they also couple to G_i and G_q and many signal through β-arrestins.

Structural studies of class B receptors have advanced our understanding of peptide binding and receptor activation, particularly with the recent determinations of full-length CTR, CLR, GCGR, GLP1R, and PTH1R structures by X-ray crystallography or cryo-EM methods (Ehrenmann et al., 2018; Jazayeri et al., 2017; Liang, Khoshouei, Deganutti, et al., 2018; Liang, Khoshouei, Glukhova, et al., 2018; Liang et al., 2017; Zhang, Quia, et al., 2018, 2017; Zhang, Sun, et al., 2017; Zhao et al., 2019). Most of the peptide ligands adopt continuous α-helical conformations spanning both receptor domains, except for the calcitonin family peptides for which the TMD-binding portions are α-helical and the ECD-binding portions are relatively unstructured (Sections 5 and 6). Receptor activation involves TM helix movements similar to those observed in class A GPCRs

(Weis & Kobilka, 2018), except that the changes in TM6 are more dramatic with a nearly 90° bend in the middle resulting in the outward movement of TM6 needed to accommodate G_s binding (Liang, Khoshouei, Deganutti, et al., 2018; Liang, Khoshouei, Glukhova, et al., 2018; Liang et al., 2017; Zhang, Sun, et al., 2017; Zhao et al., 2019). A consistent theme emerging from these structures is that there is inter-domain flexibility in the class B receptors and this can be considerable even in the agonist-bound active state as observed for CTR (Liang et al., 2017; Wootten & Miller, 2020).

The calcitonin and calcitonin-like receptors, CTR and CLR, are the best-studied class B receptors in terms of their modulation by RAMPs so much of this chapter focuses on them. The most notable effect of the RAMPs on CTR and CLR is modulation of their binding preferences for the six calcitonin family peptides: calcitonin (CT), amylin, calcitonin gene-related peptides α and β (αCGRP and βCGRP), adrenomedullin (AM) and adrenomedullin 2/intermedin (AM2/IMD). Here, we introduce the functions and clinical applications of these peptides and refer the reader to excellent reviews for more information. The endocrine hormone CT inhibits osteoclast activity and high affinity forms such as salmon CT (sCT) are used to treat hypercalcemia, Paget's disease, and osteoporosis (Naot, Musson, & Cornish, 2019). Amylin is a glucoregulatory endocrine hormone co-secreted with insulin that decreases food intake, gastric emptying, and glucagon secretion (Hay, Chen, Lutz, Parkes, & Roth, 2015). The amylin analog pramlintide is used as an insulin adjunct therapy for types I and II diabetes. α/βCGRP (hereafter CGRP) are neuropeptides with vasodilator and cardioprotective activities and roles in pain transmission and neurogenic inflammation (Kee, Kodji, & Brain, 2018; Russell, King, Smillie, Kodji, & Brain, 2014). CGRP contributes to migraine headache pathogenesis and monoclonal antibodies that either bind to CGRP or a CGRP receptor have recently obtained regulatory approval for this condition (Edvinsson, Haanes, Warfvinge, & Krause, 2018). AM is critical for lymphatic vasculature and heart development and its functions in the adult include vasodilation, cardioprotection, and promotion of embryo implantation (Kato & Kitamura, 2015; Klein & Caron, 2015; Lenhart & Caron, 2012; Tsuruda, Kato, Kuwasako, & Kitamura, 2019). AM holds promise for treating heart attack, heart failure, lymphedema, infertility, sepsis, and inflammatory bowel disease. AM2/IMD is a vasodilator and it has cardioprotective activity, promotes endothelial barrier integrity, and has roles in angiogenesis and metabolism (Holmes, Campbell, Harbinson, & Bell, 2013; Zhang, Xu, & Wang, 2018). AM2/IMD may be of value for cardiovascular disorders, sepsis, and metabolic syndrome.

In the sections below, we begin with a brief history of the discovery of the RAMPs followed by discussion of their interacting GPCR partners identified to date. After this we discuss mechanisms by which the RAMPs modulate class B GPCRs with an emphasis on how they determine CTR/CLR ligand selectivity. We discuss recent studies that provide evidence that an important component of the mechanism involves allosteric modulation by the RAMPs. Last, we discuss the implications of these findings for drug development targeting RAMP-CLR/CTR complexes.

2. Discovery of RAMPs as accessory proteins for CLR and CTR

The RAMPs were discovered through an expression-cloning strategy seeking to identify the CGRP receptor (McLatchie et al., 1998). Using a cDNA library from a human neuroblastoma cell line a clone encoding RAMP1 was found that conferred enhanced CGRP responses in *Xenopus* oocytes. Rather than encoding a GPCR, RAMP1 encoded a single span transmembrane protein with a small ECD and a short cytoplasmic tail. It was realized that RAMP1 must potentiate the CGRP receptor and co-expression of RAMP1 and CLR in HEK293T cells was shown to yield a functional CGRP receptor at the cell surface. This explained earlier findings that CLR could act as a CGRP receptor in some cell lines, but not others, likely due to differential expression of RAMP1. RAMP2 and -3 were identified based on sequence similarity and co-expression of RAMP2 with CLR conferred preferential response to AM over CGRP. This original landmark report thus identified a novel family of accessory single span transmembrane proteins and showed that they can aid the transport of a class B GPCR to the cell surface and alter its ligand binding preferences.

Soon after the discovery of the RAMPs several groups reported that RAMP1 and -3 confer high-affinity amylin binding and signaling responses when co-expressed with CTR (Armour, Foord, Kenakin, & Chen, 1999; Christopoulos et al., 1999; Muff, Buhlmann, Fischer, & Born, 1999). RAMP1 also confers high affinity CGRP binding on CTR (Hay, Christopoulos, Christopoulos, Poyner, & Sexton, 2005; Tilakaratne, Christopoulos, Zumpe, Foord, & Sexton, 2000). RAMP2 could also elicit an amylin receptor when co-expressed with CTR, but this phenotype is harder to observe and was cell-type dependent indicating that cellular context can affect RAMP-GPCR interactions (Tilakaratne et al., 2000). In contrast to CLR, which is dependent on RAMPs for cell surface expression,

CTR transports to the cell surface on its own and functions independently of RAMPs as the receptor for CT (Purdue, Tilakaratne, & Sexton, 2002).

The pharmacology of the CT family peptides at the receptors arising from CLR/CTR and their complexes with RAMPs has been thoroughly reviewed (Hay, Garelja, Poyner, & Walker, 2018; Hong, Hay, Quirion, & Poyner, 2012; Poyner et al., 2002). Here, we briefly summarize the receptors and their ligand selectivity profiles. Rank orders are for cAMP production, which tends to mirror affinity for radioligand binding experiments, where available. CLR-RAMP1 is the CGRP receptor that is activated with a potency rank order of CGRP > AM ≈ AM2/IMD. CLR-RAMP2 is the AM_1 receptor that is activated with the rank order AM > AM2/IMD > CGRP. CLR-RAMP3 is the AM_2 receptor that is activated with the rank order AM ≥ AM2/IMD > CGRP. CGRP has a clear preference for the CGRP receptor, whereas AM and AM2/IMD discriminate the three receptors to lesser extents. CTR alone is the CT receptor that is activated with the rank order CT > Amy. CTR-RAMP1 is the AMY_1 receptor that is activated roughly equivalently by amylin and CGRP. CTR-RAMP2 and CTR-RAMP3 are the AMY_2 and AMY_3 receptors that are both activated by amylin.

3. RAMP modulation of additional class B GPCRs

Early efforts to identify additional RAMP interactions took advantage of the poor cell surface expression of the RAMPs when expressed on their own. Thus, cell surface expression of the RAMP when co-expressed with a receptor is indicative of an interaction between the two. Using this assay, RAMPs were reported to interact with the GCGR, the PTH1R and PTH2R, and the VPAC1R (Christopoulos et al., 2003). Subsequent studies demonstrated further RAMP interactions with the CRFR1, SCTR, and VPAC2R (Bailey et al., 2019; Harikumar, Simms, Christopoulos, Sexton, & Miller, 2009; Wootten et al., 2013). Notably, in contrast to CLR and CTR, some of the other class B receptors seemed to selectively interact with a subset of the RAMPs (Table 1). The effects of these interactions on the receptors' functions, where known, are discussed in Section 7.

Newer approaches to catalog putative RAMP-GPCR interactions appear to significantly expand the number of RAMP partners. A bioinformatics study analyzed phylogenetic trees in various organisms and expression correlations of RAMPs and GPCRs and found that RAMPs and GPCRs co-evolved, suggesting that RAMP-GPCR interactions are widespread

Table 1 RAMP interactions with human class B GPCRs.

Receptor	Interacting RAMP	Modulation of	Reference(s)
CLR	RAMP1, -2, -3	Trafficking, ligand selectivity, signaling	Hay et al. (2018), McLatchie et al. (1998), Roehrkasse, Booe, Lee, Warner, and Pioszak (2018), and Weston et al. (2016)
CTR	RAMP1, -2, -3	Ligand selectivity, signaling	Armour et al. (1999), Christopoulos et al. (1999), Lee, Hay, and Pioszak (2016), Morfis et al. (2008), and Muff et al. (1999)
PTH1R	RAMP1[a], -2, -3[a]	Unknown	Christopoulos et al. (2003) and Lorenzen et al. (2019)
PTH2R	RAMP1[a], -2[a], -3	Unknown	Christopoulos et al. (2003) and Lorenzen et al. (2019)
CRFR1	RAMP2, -3[a]	Trafficking, signaling	Bailey et al. (2019), Lorenzen et al. (2019), and Wootten et al. (2013)
CRFR2	RAMP3[a]	Unknown	Lorenzen et al. (2019)
GCGR	RAMP1[a], -2, -3[a]	Trafficking, ligand selectivity, signaling	Cegla et al. (2017), Christopoulos et al. (2003), Lorenzen et al. (2019), and Weston et al. (2015)
GLP1R	RAMP1[a], -2[a], -3[a]	Unknown	Lorenzen et al. (2019)
GLP2R	RAMP1[a], -2[a], -3[a]	Unknown	Lorenzen et al. (2019)
GIPR	RAMP1[a], -2[a], -3[a]	Unknown	Lorenzen et al. (2019)
SCTR	RAMP1[a], -2[a], -3	Rescue trafficking of mutant receptor	Harikumar et al. (2009) and Lorenzen et al. (2019)
GHRHR	RAMP2[a], -3[a]	Unknown	Lorenzen et al. (2019)
PAC1R	RAMP1[a], -2[a], -3[a]	Unknown	Lorenzen et al. (2019)
VPAC1R	RAMP1, -2, -3	Signaling	Christopoulos et al. (2003)
VPAC2R	RAMP1, -2, -3	Signaling	Wootten et al. (2013)

[a]These interactions have only been observed in a high-throughput multiplexed suspension bead immunoassay using dodecylmaltoside-solubilized cells transfected with epitope tagged receptor components.

(Barbash, Lorenzen, Persson, Huber, & Sakmar, 2017). A follow-up study used an experimental high-throughput approach to examine the interactions of the human RAMPs with 23 different GPCRs and identified RAMP interactions with all 15 class B receptors (Lorenzen et al., 2019) (Table 1). This study used a high throughput bead-based immunoassay with detergent-solubilized lysates from cells transfected with epitope-tagged receptors. As intriguing as these findings are, only a few interactions were further validated by an independent assay and the functional consequences of these interactions remains to be tested.

4. RAMP modulation beyond class B receptors

It is worth noting that RAMP effects are not limited to class B GPCRs (Hay & Pioszak, 2016). The first demonstration involved the class C calcium sensing receptor where RAMP1 and -3 facilitated its trafficking to the cell surface in model cell lines (Bouschet, Martin, & Henley, 2005). This finding was confirmed in human thyroid carcinoma cells (Desai, Roberts, Richards, & Skerry, 2014). The class A GPR30 estrogen receptor interacts with RAMP3 and this association may also be important for receptor trafficking. RAMP3 was required for GPR30-mediated sex-dependent cardioprotection in a mouse model demonstrating the relevance of this interaction (Lenhart, Broselid, Barrick, Leeb-Lundberg, & Caron, 2013). The bioinformatics study mentioned above suggested that RAMPs may interact with GPCRs on a widespread scale involving members from each of the GPCR families, but most of these putative interactions have not been validated (Barbash et al., 2017). Last, application of the high-throughput bead-based immunoassay mentioned above found RAMP interactions with several class A chemokine receptors, class A receptors GPR4 and GPR182, and the adhesion receptor ADGRF5 (Lorenzen et al., 2019). These findings await further confirmation.

5. Mechanisms of RAMP modulation of CLR ligand binding

How the RAMPs determine the peptide ligand binding preferences of CLR has been a fundamental question since their discovery. A priori one can imagine that they might perform this function by three possible mechanisms: (1) the RAMPs directly contribute some portion of the peptide binding site and thereby make direct contacts with the ligand, (2) the RAMPs allosterically modulate the conformation and/or dynamics of the receptor without directly contacting the ligand, or (3) the RAMPs provide both direct contacts to the ligand and allosteric modulation of the receptor. There is now good evidence that RAMP modulation of CLR peptide binding involves mechanism 3.

An obvious first question is what are the roles of the ECD and TMD. Chimeric RAMP experiments indicated that the RAMP ECD largely drives peptide preference at CLR (Fitzsimmons, Zhao, & Wank, 2003; Fraser et al., 1999). Bacterial expression and purification of the isolated RAMP1-CLR and RAMP2-CLR ECD complexes showed that the ECDs associate in the absence of the TMDs and the CGRP and AM binding preferences of these complexes generally reflected those of the intact receptors (Hill & Pioszak, 2013; Koth et al., 2010; Moad & Pioszak, 2013; Watkins et al., 2013). We characterized the binding of CGRP, AM, and AM2/IMD to purified, N-glycosylated RAMP1-, RAMP2-, and RAMP3-CLR ECD complexes produced in mammalian cells and found that the peptide selectivity profiles of these complexes were similar, although not identical to those of the intact CGRP, AM_1, and AM_2 receptors (Roehrkasse et al., 2018). Thus, the RAMP ECD is a primary determinant of peptide selectivity, but other regions also contribute.

Structural studies considerably advanced our understanding of RAMP modulation of CLR peptide binding (Table 2). The RAMP1 and -2 ECDs form 3-helix bundles held together by conserved disulfide bonds and their α2-α3 face binds the α1 helix of the CLR ECD (Kusano et al., 2008, 2012; ter Haar et al., 2010). We determined ECD complex structures with bound C-terminal antagonist peptide fragments including a high-affinity CGRP analog bound to RAMP1-CLR ECD, AM bound to RAMP2-CLR ECD, and AM2/IMD bound to RAMP1-CLR ECD (Booe et al., 2015; Roehrkasse et al., 2018) (Fig. 1A–C). The three peptides occupy a common peptide-binding site that is primarily on CLR and they adopt distinct, relatively unstructured conformations influenced by Pro residues. They share a type I β-turn prior to the C-terminal residue. CT family peptides are C-terminally amidated and this modification is important for activity. The C-terminal F37-amide of CGRP, Y52-amide of AM, and Y47-amide of AM2/IMD anchor the interactions by occupying a pocket in the CLR ECD over the W72 "trp shelf" (Fig. 1A). The amide group hydrogen bonds with the main chain of CLR T122 at the base of the "turret loop" and the side chain rests on the trp shelf. Small molecule CGRP receptor antagonists developed for migraine occupy this same pocket (ter Haar et al., 2010).

Table 2 Experimentally determined structures of RAMPs, CLR, and CTR.

Modulator/receptor/ transducer protein(s)	Ligand	Resolution Å (method)	PDB ID	References
RAMP1 ECD	None	2.4 (X-ray)	2YX8	Kusano et al. (2008)
RAMP2 ECD	None	2.1, 2.0 (X-ray)	2XVT, 3AQE	Unpublished, Kusano et al. (2012)
RAMP1 ECD:CLR ECD complex	None	2.8 (X-ray)	3N7P	ter Haar et al. (2010)
RAMP1 ECD:CLR ECD complex	Telcagepant (small molecule antagonist)	2.9 (X-ray)	3N7R	ter Haar et al. (2010)
RAMP1 ECD:CLR ECD complex	Olcegepant (small molecule antagonist)	2.1 (X-ray)	3N7S	ter Haar et al. (2010)
RAMP2 ECD:CLR ECD complex	None	2.6 (X-ray)	3AQF	Kusano et al. (2012)
[a]MBP-RAMP1 ECD-CLR ECD fusion	CGRP(27–37) N31D/S34P/K35F (high-affinity antagonist)	2.4 (X-ray)	4RWG	Booe et al. (2015)
[a]MBP-RAMP2 ECD-CLR ECD fusion	AM(25–52) (peptide antagonist)	1.8 (X-ray)	4RWF	Booe et al. (2015)
[a]MBP-RAMP1 ECD-CLR ECD fusion	AM2/IMD(29–47) (peptide antagonist)	2.1 (X-ray)	6D1U	Roehrkasse et al. (2018)
[a]MBP-RAMP1 ECD-CLR ECD fusion	AM(37–52) S45W/ K46L/Q50W/Y52F (high-affinity, altered selectivity peptide antagonist)	2.8 (X-ray)	5V6Y	Booe, Warner, Roehrkasse, Hay, and Pioszak (2018)
CTR ECD	Salmon CT(8–32) BrPhe22 (peptide antagonist)	2.1 (X-ray)	5II0	Johansson et al. (2016)
CTR:Gs heterotrimer:[b]Nb35 complex	Salmon CT(1 − 32) (high-affinity peptide agonist)	4.1, 3.3 (Cryo-EM)	5UZ7, 6NIY	Dal Maso et al. (2019), Liang et al. (2017)
CLR: RAMP1:[c]DNGs heterotrimer:[b]Nb35 complex	CGRP(1–37) (peptide agonist)	3.3 (Cryo-EM)	6E3Y	Liang, Khoshouei, Deganutti, et al. (2018)

[a]Maltose binding protein (MBP) in the fusion was used to promote crystallization.
[b]Nanobody 35 was used to stabilize the Gs heterotrimer for structural studies.
[c]DN = dominant negative mutant of G alpha used to increase complex stability.

The RAMP subunits augment the pocket with residues from their α2-α3 loop and α2 helix, with some of these shared and some unique among the RAMPs (Fig. 1E). A conserved *cis*-proline in the α2-α3 loop (P85 or P112) makes contact with the peptide C-terminal residue (Fig. 1A–C). Prior to the *cis*-proline RAMP1 and -3 share W84 and in RAMP1 this can contact CGRP F37 and AM2/IMD Y47 (Fig. 1A and C), whereas RAMP2 has F111 that does not reach the C-terminal residue (Fig. 1B). Three residues from RAMP2 α2, R97, E101, and E105, augment the pocket and are within hydrogen bonding distance of AM Y52 and/or K46 (Fig. 1B). Of these, only E101 significantly contributes to peptide binding because its mutation to Ala diminishes AM cAMP signaling whereas the R97A and E105A mutants had no effect (Booe et al., 2015). At the position equivalent to RAMP2 E101, RAMP1 has W74, which does not contact CGRP or AM2/IMD, and RAMP3 has E74, which presumably would hydrogen bond with AM Y52 and AM2/IMD Y47 (Fig. 1E). So RAMP1 W84 and RAMP2 E101 each provide unique contacts to the peptide that the other RAMP cannot and RAMP3 appears to be a hybrid with E74 and W84 able to provide either contact. This at least partially explains why peptides with a C-terminal Phe show reduced binding at RAMP2-CLR (Booe et al., 2018; Roehrkasse et al., 2018).

Consistent with the structures, mutagenesis experiments indicated that the C-terminal residue of each of the peptides and RAMP1 W84, RAMP2 E101, and RAMP3 E74 are important for peptide-receptor interactions and that RAMP2 E101 and RAMP3 E74 promote AM binding (Moad & Pioszak, 2013; Moore, Gingell, Kane, Hay, & Salvatore, 2010; Qi et al., 2008, 2011; Roehrkasse et al., 2018; Watkins et al., 2013, 2014). AM K46 mutagenesis also indicated its importance for receptor binding (Moad & Pioszak, 2013; Watkins et al., 2013), but its unclear if this is due to its packing against AM Y52 and CLR W72 or contact with RAMP2. Notably, the ECD-complex binding properties of peptides having reciprocal C-terminal residue exchange and the signaling activity of wild-type agonist peptides at receptors bearing reciprocal exchange of RAMP1/2 residues near the CLR ECD pocket confirmed the importance of AM Y52-RAMP2 E101 contact for binding the AM_1 receptor, but the reciprocal peptide and RAMP exchanges were insufficient to swap selectivity (Booe et al., 2015). These data suggested that there must be an allosteric component to RAMP modulation of CLR.

Comparisons of the peptide-bound ECD complexes revealed conformational differences in CLR between the RAMP1- and RAMP2-bound states.

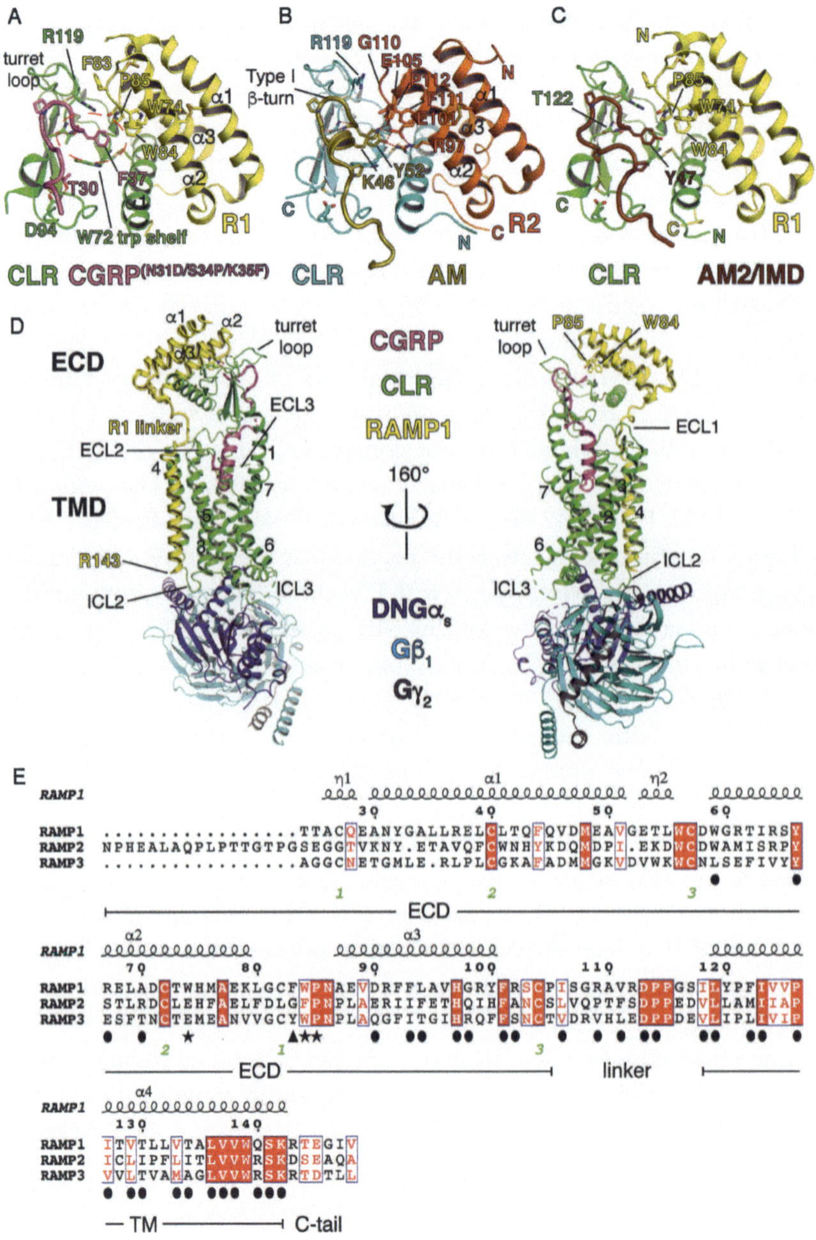

Fig. 1 Structures of peptide-bound RAMP-CLR complexes. (A) RAMP1-CLR ECD in complex with a high-affinity variant CGRP C-terminal fragment (PDB 4RWG). The dotted ellipse highlights the pocket that is occupied by the peptide C-terminal residue. (B) RAMP2-CLR ECD in complex with an AM C-terminal fragment (PDB 4RWF). (C) RAMP1-CLR ECD in complex with an AM2/IMD C-terminal fragment (PDB 6D1U).

The RAMP1/2 helical bundles are shifted in their position against CLR α1 and this shifts α1 (Fig. 2A). These changes likely result from differences in RAMP1/2 residues at the α2-α3 interface (Figs. 2B and 1E), and appear to propagate to the CLR pocket resulting in subtle shape changes that may affect the position of the peptide C-terminal residue (Fig. 2C). There is also a dramatic movement of CLR R119 that seems to be controlled by the RAMPs with RAMP1 F83 pushing it down toward the pocket and RAMP2 G110 allowing it to point up (Fig. 2C). Notably, the CLR R119A mutant is more deleterious in the RAMP1 complex than in the RAMP2 complex (Booe et al., 2015). The contour of the CLR pocket is different in the RAMP1- and RAMP-2 bound states (Fig. 2D and E) and this may impact selectivity because we were able to engineer an AM antagonist variant with altered preference for RAMP1-CLR over RAMP2-CLR via the K46L mutation designed to exploit the pocket shape changes and Y52F to remove RAMP2 E101 contact (Booe et al., 2018). A crystal structure of this variant bound to RAMP1-CLR ECD suggested that it filled out the pocket better than AM would and it may have been able to overcome the R119 down position because of additional affinity-enhancing mutations (Fig. 2F). We cannot rule out the possibility that the K46L effect on selectivity stemmed from loss of K46 contact with RAMP2; however, there is also evidence for an allosteric component to RAMP function from an engineered high-affinity CGRP antagonist variant with the F37Y substitution designed to enable contact with RAMP2 E101. This variant retained better binding to RAMP1-CLR than RAMP2-CLR, which was likely due to CLR ECD conformational differences because only the C-terminal residue of CGRP contacts the RAMP (Booe et al., 2018). The structural, biochemical, and pharmacological data thus support a mechanism in which direct RAMP-peptide contacts and allosteric modulation of CLR cooperate at the level of the ECDs to determine peptide-binding preferences.

(D) Full-length RAMP1-CLR complex (CGRP receptor) with full-length CGRP and Gs heterotrimer (PDB 6E3Y). (E) Amino acid sequence alignment of the three human RAMPs. The signal peptides are omitted for clarity. Residue numbering above the sequences corresponds to RAMP1 and numbers below indicate disulfide bond connectivity. Filled ovals mark residues at the interface with CLR, stars indicate key residues that augment the ECD binding pocket and in some cases directly contact the peptide ligands, and the filled triangle indicates the residue that appears to determine the position of R119 in the CLR turret loop. The alignment was performed with Clustal Omega (Madeira et al., 2019) and the depiction was made with ESpript 3 (Robert & Gouet, 2014).

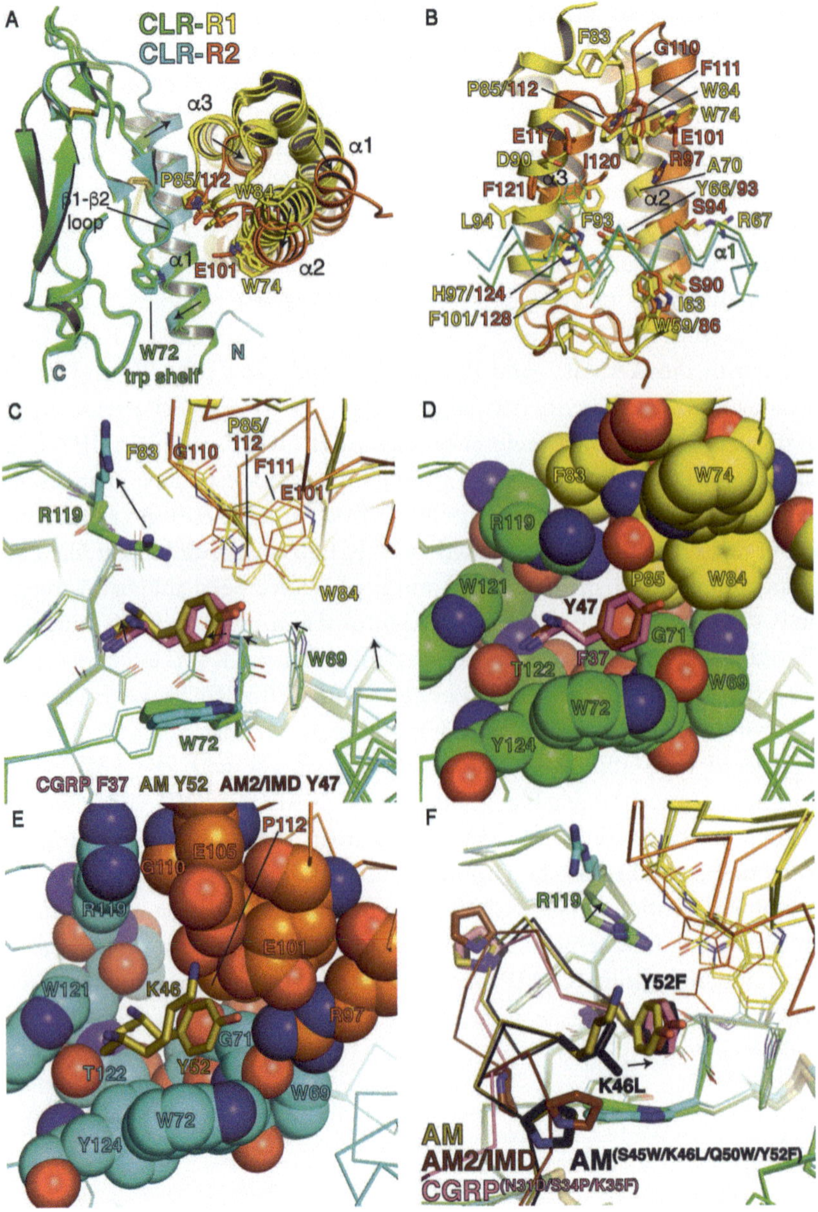

Fig. 2 Allosteric modulation of CLR ECD conformation by RAMP1 and RAMP2. (A) Superimpositions of the high-affinity CGRP variant-bound RAMP1-CLR ECD (PDB 4RWG), AM-bound RAMP2-CLR ECD (PDB 4RWF), and AM2/IMD-bound RAMP1-CLR ECD (PDB 6D1U) complexes. For clarity the CLR turret loop is omitted. Arrows indicate shifts occurring from the RAMP1 complexes to the RAMP2 complex. (B) View of the RAMP1/2 α2-α3 interface with the CLR α1 helix (shown as α-carbon trace).

The cryo-EM structure of the full-length CGRP receptor with bound CGRP and G_s heterotrimer showed that other than CGRP F37 being near RAMP1 W84 and P85 in the ECD, there were no direct contacts between RAMP1 and the CGRP agonist (Liang, Khoshouei, Deganutti, et al., 2018) (Fig. 1D). Additional modulation of peptide binding arising beyond the level of the ECD complex must therefore be allosteric. The RAMP1 TMD packs against CLR TM3, 4, and 5 and the RAMP linker connecting the ECD and TMD contacts CLR ECL2, which in turn contacts CGRP. RAMP2 and -3 likely occupy the same TM3/4/5 interface given the sequence similarity in the RAMP TMD (Fig. 1E). Differences among the RAMPs in the linker might differentially affect ECL2 to alter peptide binding. Pharmacological studies indicated that some mutations in the CLR TMD, including several in ECL2, have RAMP-dependent effects consistent with allosteric modulation of the CLR TMD and ECL2 by the RAMPs (Watkins et al., 2016; Woolley et al., 2017). Mutagenesis and modeling studies also support RAMP-dependent effects on ECL3, which is distant from the RAMP TMD (Watkins et al., 2016). Notably, allosteric modulation of a GPCR via the extra-helical bundle TM3/4/5 site is not without precedent. A small molecule agoPAM of the class A free fatty acid receptor GPR40 binds in this region (Lu et al., 2017). Last, given the inter-domain flexibility of the class B GPCRs it seems reasonable to speculate that the RAMPs might differentially modulate CLR inter-domain dynamics and this could also affect peptide selectivity. MD simulations indicated that RAMP1 restricts the flexibility of the CLR ECD relative to the TMD (Liang, Khoshouei, Deganutti, et al., 2018), so the other RAMPs probably have similar, although not identical effects. Additional cryo-EM structures of the AM_1 and AM_2 receptors expected in the near future should provide further insights into how the RAMPs allosterically modulate the CLR TMD and ECD-TMD dynamics.

(C) Close-up view of the pocket occupied by the peptides' C-terminal residues, which are shown as sticks. Arrows indicate shifts occurring from the RAMP1 complexes to the RAMP2 complex. (D) View of the pocket in the RAMP1-CLR ECD complexes with residues in space-filling representation. The CGRP F37 and AM2/IMD Y47 C-terminal residues are shown as sticks. (E) View of the pocket in the RAMP2-CLR ECD complex with pocket residues in space-filling representation and the AM K46 and Y52 residues as sticks. (F) Superimpositions of the three structures in panels (A) and (C) with RAMP1-CLR ECD bound to a rationally-designed high-affinity, altered selectivity AM variant (PDB 5V6Y). Arrows indicate shifts in the positions of the AM variant C-terminal residue and CLR R119. In all panels the structures were aligned based on the CLR ECD.

6. Mechanisms of RAMP modulation of CTR ligand binding

Our understanding of the mechanisms of RAMP modulation of CTR peptide binding is less advanced than for CLR. Structures of CTR alone are available, but we lack structures of CTR-RAMP complexes (Table 2). Biochemical and pharmacological studies revealed similarities with CLR including evidence for an allosteric role of the RAMPs, but there are also differences and unresolved puzzles particularly regarding the role of the peptide C-terminus and its possible contact with RAMPs. The high-affinity ligands for CTR and the CTR-RAMP complexes, CT, amylin, and CGRP, are more similar to each other than the adrenomedullins, but those that require RAMPs (amylin, CGRP) and those that do not (CT) differ at their C-terminus. CT ends with a Pro-amide that is critical for activity, whereas amylin ends with a Tyr-amide as in the adrenomedullins and similar to the Phe-amide of CGRP.

Chimeric RAMP1/2 studies indicated that the RAMP ECD dictated CTR peptide selectivity (Udawela, Christopoulos, Tilakaratne, et al., 2006; Zumpe et al., 2000) and binding studies with purified CTR ECD and RAMP1-CTR and RAMP2-CTR ECD complexes showed that the RAMPs enhanced affinity for amylin and CGRP (Hay & Pioszak, 2016; Lee et al., 2017). A crystal structure of the CTR ECD with a C-terminal antagonist fragment of sCT revealed that it occupied a binding site very similar to that in CLR and adopted a CGRP-like conformation except with a type II turn (Fig. 3A) (Johansson et al., 2016). The C-terminal Pro-amide occupied the pocket over the W79 trp shelf with the side chain packing against the shelf and the amide hydrogen bonding with the S129 backbone. Modeling suggested that the RAMPs augment the pocket with the conserved *cis*-proline and the α2-α3 loop/α2 helix residues described in Section 5 (Fig. 1E), and peptide mutagenesis supported a CGRP-like ECD-bound conformation for amylin (Lee et al., 2016).

One might predict that the RAMPs enhance amylin affinity in part through contact of RAMP1 W84, RAMP2 E101, or RAMP3 W84/E74 with the amylin C-terminal Y37; however, mutation of RAMP1 W84 or RAMP2 E101 in the purified ECD complexes had no effect on amylin analog binding and the amylin Y37A mutation only modestly diminished binding and signaling at intact $AMY_{1/3}$ receptors (Bower et al., 2018; Lee et al., 2016). In contrast, loss of the amylin C-terminal amide dramatically

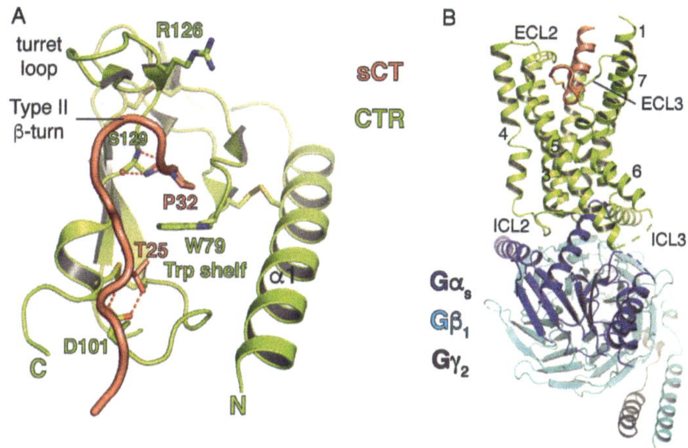

Fig. 3 Structures of sCT-bound CTR. (A) CTR ECD in complex with a sCT C-terminal fragment (PDB 5II0). (B) Full-length CTR with full-length sCT and Gs heterotrimer (PDB 6NIY). The ECD and C-terminal half of sCT were not modeled because of weak cryo-EM density for this region, apparently due to significant inter-domain flexibility.

diminished binding and signaling at $AMY_{1/3}$ (Bower et al., 2018). A C-terminal Tyr may contribute to AMY receptor selectivity as in the traditional antagonists AC187 and AC413 (Hay et al., 2005; Young et al., 1994), but substitution of the C-terminal Tyr with Pro in amylin or amylin analogs enhanced RAMP-CTR ECD complex binding and signaling at $AMY_{1/3}$ (Bower et al., 2018; Lee et al., 2016). Overall, the amylin C-terminal residue side chain appears to be less important to receptor binding than those of CT or CGRP, AM, and AM2/IMD at the CLR complexes and its role in selectivity and RAMP contact remains unresolved. A crystal structure of an amylin-bound RAMP-CTR ECD complex would clarify these issues.

The diminished role of the amylin C-terminal Tyr may reflect more importance of allostery as a mechanism for RAMP modulation of CTR peptide binding. In the CTR ECD structure R126 in the turret loop was in the up position (Fig. 3A) similar to CLR R119 in the RAMP2 complex structure, so RAMP1 would be expected to alter R126 position to reshape the pocket. Consistent with this, mutation of R126 had little effect on signaling at CTR while significantly diminishing signaling at AMY_1 (Gingell et al., 2016). In this study, RAMP-dependent effects on ligand pharmacology were also observed with mutation of predicted CTR-RAMP interface residues, which may reflect disruption of an allosteric pathway. Moreover, modeling and MD simulations provided support for RAMP1 altering the dynamics of the CTR ECD such that two loops and the C-terminus of the CTR ECD near the peptide-binding site became more flexible in the presence of the RAMP. These results were interpreted in light of the concept of "dynamic" allostery whereby entropically driven changes in flexibility alter global domain dynamics to regulate function (Gingell et al., 2016).

The cryo-EM structure of full-length CTR with bound sCT agonist and G_s heterotrimer showed how the agonist binds the TMD and revealed substantial inter-domain flexibility such that the ECD was not modeled in this structure (Fig. 3B) (Dal Maso et al., 2019; Liang et al., 2017). Sequence similarity of CTR and CLR supports the RAMP TMD occupying the same TM3/4/5 site observed in the CGRP receptor so the RAMPs likely contact ECL2 and have no direct contact with the N-terminal half of the peptide. The RAMPs probably restrict the flexibility of the CTR ECD relative to the TMD and this modulation of inter-domain dynamics along with direct modulation of the CTR TMD may contribute to peptide selectivity. Support for the latter comes from extensive pharmacological studies assessing the impacts of mutagenesis of CTR ECL2 and ECL3 in the context of the CTR and the AMY_3 receptors (Dal Maso et al., 2019, 2018; Pham et al., 2019). These provided evidence for RAMP3-mediated changes in ECL2 and ECL3, the latter of which is likely distant from the RAMP. Cryo-EM structures of full-length CTR-RAMP complexes are needed to further advance our understanding of RAMP allosteric modulation of the CTR TMD and ECD-TMD dynamics.

7. RAMP modulation of class B GPCR signaling

RAMPs modulate the signaling of several class B GPCRs, but the mechanistic bases for these effects are poorly understood. Early studies on CTR indicated that RAMP1 and -3 alter G protein coupling efficiency in the AMY receptors and at least part of this is likely due to direct interaction of the RAMP C-tail with the transducer proteins (Morfis et al., 2008; Udawela, Christopoulos, Morfis, et al., 2006; Udawela, Christopoulos, Tilakaratne, et al., 2006). A more recent study provided support for an allosteric role of RAMP3 in altering the CTR signaling profile in the AMY_3 receptor (Pham et al., 2019). RAMPs were also reported to bias coupling of CLR to G_s, G_i, and G_q (Weston et al., 2016). RAMP2 alters the G protein coupling efficiency of both VPAC receptors and CRFR1 while having no effect on ligand binding (Christopoulos et al., 2003; Wootten et al., 2013). Mixed results have been reported for RAMP2 modulation of GCGR signaling and ligand binding. In one study RAMP2 increased potency and efficacy of cAMP signaling, decreased G_i coupling, and decreased binding of a subset of peptide ligands (Weston et al., 2015). In another study, RAMP2 decreased potency while enhancing efficacy of cAMP signaling, decreased efficacy of Ca^{2+} signaling, abolished β-arrestin recruitment, and had no effect on the binding of several peptide ligands (Cegla et al., 2017). Differences in these studies may be attributable in part to the different cell lines used and/or the use of stable vs. transient expression.

In most cases other than CLR/CTR it is unclear how the RAMPs interact with GPCRs. However, the interaction interface was mapped for the RAMP3-SECR pair (Harikumar et al., 2009). RAMP3 had no effect on the ligand binding and signaling of the SECR, but it did alter trafficking of a mutant receptor. Chimeric and truncated receptor and peptide TMD competition experiments were consistent with the interaction being mediated solely by the TMDs with the RAMP3 TMD contacting SECR TM6/7. This study raises the interesting possibility that the RAMPs may utilize various faces of the GPCR helical bundle for interaction depending on the receptor. It is unclear if any other class B GPCR-RAMP associations involve ECD-ECD interactions.

8. RAMPs in lower organisms

The CT family peptides and their receptors have been mostly studied in vertebrates, but recent work identified their existence in invertebrates (Sekiguchi, 2018). This has implications for understanding the mechanistic basis for RAMP modulation of GPCRs throughout evolution. The amphioxus *Branchiostoma floridae* (Bf) has a family of three CT-like peptides, a CTR/CLR-like receptor, and three RAMP-like proteins (Sekiguchi et al., 2016). Heterologous expression of the Bf receptor in mammalian cells enabled pharmacological characterization of this system. The three CT-like peptides stimulated cAMP accumulation when the Bf receptor was co-expressed with any one of the three Bf RAMPs, but not in their absence, and the RAMPs differentially modulated the responses to the peptides. Notably, the three Bf peptides all end with a Pro-amide like CT, rather than the Phe- or Tyr-amide residues in CGRP, the adrenomedullins, and amylin. As noted in a recent review by Poyner and colleagues (Simms, Routledge, Uddin, & Poyner, 2019), if the Bf receptors and their peptides are structurally similar to those in humans, then it would appear that the

Bf RAMPs do not directly contact the peptides and instead probably function through an allosteric mechanism. The RAMPs may have started as trafficking chaperones and allosteric modulators and the utilization of direct RAMP-ligand contacts in the modulation mechanism may have emerged only as the peptide family expanded in complexity in higher organisms.

9. Drug development outlook for RAMP-CLR/CTR complexes

Novel opportunities for drug development provided by RAMP association with GPCRs has been reviewed (Sexton, Poyner, Simms, Christopoulos, & Hay, 2012; Wootten & Miller, 2020), but it is worth emphasizing a couple of aspects in light of our increasing understanding of the mechanisms of RAMP modulation of CLR and CTR. First, the RAMP-GPCR interface provides expanded opportunities for targeting with small molecules, peptides, and antibodies. This was first demonstrated with the development of small molecule CGRP receptor antagonists for migraine that occupy the pocket in the CLR ECD and make contacts with RAMP1 that enable selectivity (ter Haar et al., 2010). More recently this concept was confirmed and expanded with the development and FDA approval of a monoclonal antibody that binds the CGRP receptor ECD complex to antagonize CGRP signaling for migraine (Edvinsson et al., 2018; Shi et al., 2016). Going forward it should be possible to develop allosteric modulators that bind to various areas at the RAMP-CLR/CTR interface to modulate peptide binding and signaling. The additional protein, RAMP, in RAMP-GPCR complexes presumably creates many more allosteric ligand pockets that could be exploited with different types of molecules.

Second, the structural advances are enabling structure-guided drug design approaches to be applied to these receptors. Our work on this front has yielded short ECD complex binding CGRP, AM, and AM2/IMD antagonist variants with enhanced affinity for the CGRP and AM receptors (Booe et al., 2018; Roehrkasse et al., 2018). In a few cases, we have been able to engineer receptor selectivity into these variants, but in general this is very challenging because the endogenous peptides make so few contacts with the RAMP subunits that determine receptor phenotype. Nonetheless, future developments have the potential to lead to agonist peptide variants with enhanced potencies or perhaps long-duration signaling capabilities. It might even become possible to engineer kinetic selectivity into these variants as we obtain a better understanding of the kinetics of their receptor binding. We anticipate significant advances in the coming years for the development of novel therapeutics targeting RAMP-CLR/CTR complexes.

10. Conclusion

Recent advances in our understanding of the biochemistry, pharmacology, and structural biology of RAMP-CLR/CTR complexes has revealed that RAMPs act as endogenous allosteric modulators of these class B GPCRs. Allosteric modulation by the RAMPs involves conformational effects on both the ECD and TMD of the receptors and alteration of receptor dynamics is likely also important. RAMP modulation of CLR and CTR determines their peptide binding phenotype and also has the capacity to alter their signaling. With the expanding list of GPCRs that appear to interact with RAMPs it is possible that allosteric modulation of GPCRs by RAMPs is widespread, but more studies are needed in this area. Although RAMP interactions complicate GPCR pharmacology, they provide new opportunities for drug development.

Acknowledgments

Research in the Pioszak laboratory is supported by National Institutes of Health grant R01GM104251.

Conflict of interest

A.A.P. is inventor on a patent describing enhanced affinity and altered selectivity AM and CGRP variant peptides.

References

Armour, S. L., Foord, S., Kenakin, T., & Chen, W. J. (1999). Pharmacological characterization of receptor-activity-modifying proteins (RAMPs) and the human calcitonin receptor. *Journal of Pharmacological and Toxicological Methods*, *42*(4), 217–224. Retrieved from https://www.ncbi.nlm.nih.gov/pubmed/11033437.

Bailey, S., Harris, M., Barkan, K., Winfield, I., Harper, M. T., Simms, J., et al. (2019). Interactions between RAMP2 and CRF receptors: The effect of receptor subtypes, splice variants and cell context. *Biochimica et Biophysica Acta—Biomembranes*, *1861*(5), 997–1003. https://doi.org/10.1016/j.bbamem.2019.02.008.

Barbash, S., Lorenzen, E., Persson, T., Huber, T., & Sakmar, T. P. (2017). GPCRs globally coevolved with receptor activity-modifying proteins, RAMPs. *Proceedings of the National Academy of Sciences of the United States of America*, *114*(45), 12015–12020. https://doi.org/10.1073/pnas.1713074114.

Booe, J. M., Walker, C. S., Barwell, J., Kuteyi, G., Simms, J., Jamaluddin, M. A., et al. (2015). Structural basis for receptor activity-modifying protein-dependent selective peptide recognition by a G protein-coupled receptor. *Molecular Cell*, *58*(6), 1040–1052. https://doi.org/10.1016/j.molcel.2015.04.018.

Booe, J. M., Warner, M. L., Roehrkasse, A. M., Hay, D. L., & Pioszak, A. A. (2018). Probing the mechanism of receptor activity-modifying protein modulation of GPCR ligand selectivity through rational design of potent adrenomedullin and calcitonin gene-related peptide antagonists. *Molecular Pharmacology*, *93*(4), 355–367. https://doi.org/10.1124/mol.117.110916.
Bouschet, T., Martin, S., & Henley, J. M. (2005). Receptor-activity-modifying proteins are required for forward trafficking of the calcium-sensing receptor to the plasma membrane. *Journal of Cell Science*, *118*(Pt. 20), 4709–4720. https://doi.org/10.1242/jcs.02598.
Bower, R. L., Yule, L., Rees, T. A., Deganutti, G., Hendrikse, E. R., Harris, P. W. R., et al. (2018). Molecular signature for receptor engagement in the metabolic peptide hormone amylin. *ACS Pharmacology & Translational Science*, *1*(1), 32–49. https://doi.org/10.1021/acsptsci.8b00002.
Cegla, J., Jones, B. J., Gardiner, J. V., Hodson, D. J., Marjot, T., McGlone, E. R., et al. (2017). RAMP2 influences glucagon receptor pharmacology via trafficking and signaling. *Endocrinology*, *158*(8), 2680–2693. https://doi.org/10.1210/en.2016-1755.
Christopoulos, A., Christopoulos, G., Morfis, M., Udawela, M., Laburthe, M., Couvineau, A., et al. (2003). Novel receptor partners and function of receptor activity-modifying proteins. *The Journal of Biological Chemistry*, *278*(5), 3293–3297. https://doi.org/10.1074/jbc.C200629200.
Christopoulos, G., Perry, K. J., Morfis, M., Tilakaratne, N., Gao, Y., Fraser, N. J., et al. (1999). Multiple amylin receptors arise from receptor activity-modifying protein interaction with the calcitonin receptor gene product. *Molecular Pharmacology*, *56*(1), 235–242. https://doi.org/10.1124/mol.56.1.235.
Dal Maso, E., Glukhova, A., Zhu, Y., Garcia-Nafria, J., Tate, C. G., Atanasio, S., et al. (2019). The molecular control of calcitonin receptor signaling. *ACS Pharmacology & Translational Science*, *2*(1), 31–51. https://doi.org/10.1021/acsptsci.8b00056.
Dal Maso, E., Zhu, Y., Pham, V., Reynolds, C. A., Deganutti, G., Hick, C. A., et al. (2018). Extracellular loops 2 and 3 of the calcitonin receptor selectively modify agonist binding and efficacy. *Biochemical Pharmacology*, *150*, 214–244. https://doi.org/10.1016/j.bcp.2018.02.005.
Desai, A. J., Roberts, D. J., Richards, G. O., & Skerry, T. M. (2014). Role of receptor activity modifying protein 1 in function of the calcium sensing receptor in the human TT thyroid carcinoma cell line. *PLoS One*, *9*(1), e85237. https://doi.org/10.1371/journal.pone.0085237.
Drucker, D. J. (2018). Mechanisms of action and therapeutic application of glucagon-like peptide-1. *Cell Metabolism*, *27*(4), 740–756. https://doi.org/10.1016/j.cmet.2018.03.001.
Edvinsson, L., Haanes, K. A., Warfvinge, K., & Krause, D. N. (2018). CGRP as the target of new migraine therapies—Successful translation from bench to clinic. *Nature Reviews Neurology*, *14*(6), 338–350. https://doi.org/10.1038/s41582-018-0003-1.
Ehrenmann, J., Schoppe, J., Klenk, C., Rappas, M., Kummer, L., Dore, A. S., et al. (2018). High-resolution crystal structure of parathyroid hormone 1 receptor in complex with a peptide agonist. *Nature Structural & Molecular Biology*, *25*(12), 1086–1092. https://doi.org/10.1038/s41594-018-0151-4.
Fitzsimmons, T. J., Zhao, X., & Wank, S. A. (2003). The extracellular domain of receptor activity-modifying protein 1 is sufficient for calcitonin receptor-like receptor function. *The Journal of Biological Chemistry*, *278*(16), 14313–14320. https://doi.org/10.1074/jbc.M211946200.
Fraser, N. J., Wise, A., Brown, J., McLatchie, L. M., Main, M. J., & Foord, S. M. (1999). The amino terminus of receptor activity modifying proteins is a critical determinant of glycosylation state and ligand binding of calcitonin receptor-like receptor. *Molecular Pharmacology*, *55*(6), 1054–1059. https://doi.org/10.1124/mol.55.6.1054.

Gingell, J. J., Simms, J., Barwell, J., Poyner, D. R., Watkins, H. A., Pioszak, A. A., et al. (2016). An allosteric role for receptor activity-modifying proteins in defining GPCR pharmacology. *Cell Discovery*, *2*, 16012. https://doi.org/10.1038/celldisc.2016.12.

Harikumar, K. G., Simms, J., Christopoulos, G., Sexton, P. M., & Miller, L. J. (2009). Molecular basis of association of receptor activity-modifying protein 3 with the family B G protein-coupled secretin receptor. *Biochemistry*, *48*(49), 11773–11785. https://doi.org/10.1021/bi901326k.

Hay, D. L., Chen, S., Lutz, T. A., Parkes, D. G., & Roth, J. D. (2015). Amylin: Pharmacology, physiology, and clinical potential. *Pharmacological Reviews*, *67*(3), 564–600. https://doi.org/10.1124/pr.115.010629.

Hay, D. L., Christopoulos, G., Christopoulos, A., Poyner, D. R., & Sexton, P. M. (2005). Pharmacological discrimination of calcitonin receptor: Receptor activity-modifying protein complexes. *Molecular Pharmacology*, *67*(5), 1655–1665. https://doi.org/10.1124/mol.104.008615.

Hay, D. L., Garelja, M. L., Poyner, D. R., & Walker, C. S. (2018). Update on the pharmacology of calcitonin/CGRP family of peptides: IUPHAR review 25. *British Journal of Pharmacology*, *175*(1), 3–17. https://doi.org/10.1111/bph.14075.

Hay, D. L., & Pioszak, A. A. (2016). Receptor activity-modifying proteins (RAMPs): New insights and roles. *Annual Review of Pharmacology and Toxicology*, *56*, 469–487. https://doi.org/10.1146/annurev-pharmtox-010715-103120.

Hill, H. E., & Pioszak, A. A. (2013). Bacterial expression and purification of a heterodimeric adrenomedullin receptor extracellular domain complex using DsbC-assisted disulfide shuffling. *Protein Expression and Purification*, *88*(1), 107–113. https://doi.org/10.1016/j.pep.2012.11.019.

Hoare, S. R. (2005). Mechanisms of peptide and nonpeptide ligand binding to Class B G-protein-coupled receptors. *Drug Discovery Today*, *10*(6), 417–427. https://doi.org/10.1016/S1359-6446(05)03370-2.

Hollenstein, K., de Graaf, C., Bortolato, A., Wang, M. W., Marshall, F. H., & Stevens, R. C. (2014). Insights into the structure of class B GPCRs. *Trends in Pharmacological Sciences*, *35*(1), 12–22. https://doi.org/10.1016/j.tips.2013.11.001.

Hollenstein, K., Kean, J., Bortolato, A., Cheng, R. K., Dore, A. S., Jazayeri, A., et al. (2013). Structure of class B GPCR corticotropin-releasing factor receptor 1. *Nature*, *499*(7459), 438–443. https://doi.org/10.1038/nature12357.

Holmes, D., Campbell, M., Harbinson, M., & Bell, D. (2013). Protective effects of intermedin on cardiovascular, pulmonary and renal diseases: Comparison with adrenomedullin and CGRP. *Current Protein & Peptide Science*, *14*(4), 294–329. Retrieved from https://www.ncbi.nlm.nih.gov/pubmed/23745696.

Hong, Y., Hay, D. L., Quirion, R., & Poyner, D. R. (2012). The pharmacology of adrenomedullin 2/intermedin. *British Journal of Pharmacology*, *166*(1), 110–120. https://doi.org/10.1111/j.1476-5381.2011.01530.x.

Jazayeri, A., Rappas, M., Brown, A. J. H., Kean, J., Errey, J. C., Robertson, N. J., et al. (2017). Crystal structure of the GLP-1 receptor bound to a peptide agonist. *Nature*, *546*(7657), 254–258. https://doi.org/10.1038/nature22800.

Johansson, E., Hansen, J. L., Hansen, A. M., Shaw, A. C., Becker, P., Schaffer, L., et al. (2016). Type II turn of receptor-bound salmon calcitonin revealed by X-ray crystallography. *The Journal of Biological Chemistry*, *291*(26), 13689–13698. https://doi.org/10.1074/jbc.M116.726034.

Kato, J., & Kitamura, K. (2015). Bench-to-bedside pharmacology of adrenomedullin. *European Journal of Pharmacology*, *764*, 140–148. https://doi.org/10.1016/j.ejphar.2015.06.061.

Kee, Z., Kodji, X., & Brain, S. D. (2018). The role of calcitonin gene related peptide (CGRP) in neurogenic vasodilation and its cardioprotective effects. *Frontiers in Physiology*, *9*, 1249. https://doi.org/10.3389/fphys.2018.01249.

Klein, K. R., & Caron, K. M. (2015). Adrenomedullin in lymphangiogenesis: From development to disease. *Cellular and Molecular Life Sciences*, *72*(16), 3115–3126. https://doi.org/10.1007/s00018-015-1921-3.

Koth, C. M., Abdul-Manan, N., Lepre, C. A., Connolly, P. J., Yoo, S., Mohanty, A. K., et al. (2010). Refolding and characterization of a soluble ectodomain complex of the calcitonin gene-related peptide receptor. *Biochemistry*, *49*(9), 1862–1872. https://doi.org/10.1021/bi901848m.

Kusano, S., Kukimoto-Niino, M., Akasaka, R., Toyama, M., Terada, T., Shirouzu, M., et al. (2008). Crystal structure of the human receptor activity-modifying protein 1 extracellular domain. *Protein Science*, *17*(11), 1907–1914. https://doi.org/10.1110/ps.036012.108.

Kusano, S., Kukimoto-Niino, M., Hino, N., Ohsawa, N., Okuda, K., Sakamoto, K., et al. (2012). Structural basis for extracellular interactions between calcitonin receptor-like receptor and receptor activity-modifying protein 2 for adrenomedullin-specific binding. *Protein Science*, *21*(2), 199–210. https://doi.org/10.1002/pro.2003.

Lee, S. M., Booe, J. M., Gingell, J. J., Sjoelund, V., Hay, D. L., & Pioszak, A. A. (2017). N-Glycosylation of asparagine 130 in the extracellular domain of the human calcitonin receptor significantly increases peptide hormone affinity. *Biochemistry*, *56*(26), 3380–3393. https://doi.org/10.1021/acs.biochem.7b00256.

Lee, S. M., Hay, D. L., & Pioszak, A. A. (2016). Calcitonin and amylin receptor peptide interaction mechanisms: Insights into peptide-binding modes and allosteric modulation of the calcitonin receptor by receptor activity-modifying proteins. *The Journal of Biological Chemistry*, *291*(16), 8686–8700. https://doi.org/10.1074/jbc.M115.713628.

Lenhart, P. M., Broselid, S., Barrick, C. J., Leeb-Lundberg, L. M., & Caron, K. M. (2013). G-protein-coupled receptor 30 interacts with receptor activity-modifying protein 3 and confers sex-dependent cardioprotection. *Journal of Molecular Endocrinology*, *51*(1), 191–202. https://doi.org/10.1530/JME-13-0021.

Lenhart, P. M., & Caron, K. M. (2012). Adrenomedullin and pregnancy: Perspectives from animal models to humans. *Trends in Endocrinology and Metabolism*, *23*(10), 524–532. https://doi.org/10.1016/j.tem.2012.02.007.

Liang, Y. L., Khoshouei, M., Deganutti, G., Glukhova, A., Koole, C., Peat, T. S., et al. (2018). Cryo-EM structure of the active, Gs-protein complexed, human CGRP receptor. *Nature*, *561*(7724), 492–497. https://doi.org/10.1038/s41586-018-0535-y.

Liang, Y. L., Khoshouei, M., Glukhova, A., Furness, S. G. B., Zhao, P., Clydesdale, L., et al. (2018). Phase-plate cryo-EM structure of a biased agonist-bound human GLP-1 receptor-Gs complex. *Nature*, *555*(7694), 121–125. https://doi.org/10.1038/nature25773.

Liang, Y. L., Khoshouei, M., Radjainia, M., Zhang, Y., Glukhova, A., Tarrasch, J., et al. (2017). Phase-plate cryo-EM structure of a class B GPCR-G-protein complex. *Nature*, *546*(7656), 118–123. https://doi.org/10.1038/nature22327.

Lorenzen, E., Dodig-Crnkovic, T., Kotliar, I. B., Pin, E., Ceraudo, E., Vaughan, R. D., et al. (2019). Multiplexed analysis of the secretin-like GPCR-RAMP interactome. *Science Advances*, *5*(9). eaaw2778https://doi.org/10.1126/sciadv.aaw2778.

Lu, J., Byrne, N., Wang, J., Bricogne, G., Brown, F. K., Chobanian, H. R., et al. (2017). Structural basis for the cooperative allosteric activation of the free fatty acid receptor GPR40. *Nature Structural & Molecular Biology*, *24*(7), 570–577. https://doi.org/10.1038/nsmb.3417.

Madeira, F., Park, Y. M., Lee, J., Buso, N., Gur, T., Madhusoodanan, N., et al. (2019). The EMBL-EBI search and sequence analysis tools APIs in 2019. *Nucleic Acids Research*, *47*(W1), W636–W641. https://doi.org/10.1093/nar/gkz268.

McLatchie, L. M., Fraser, N. J., Main, M. J., Wise, A., Brown, J., Thompson, N., et al. (1998). RAMPs regulate the transport and ligand specificity of the calcitonin-receptor-like receptor. *Nature*, *393*(6683), 333–339. https://doi.org/10.1038/30666.

Moad, H. E., & Pioszak, A. A. (2013). Selective CGRP and adrenomedullin peptide binding by tethered RAMP-calcitonin receptor-like receptor extracellular domain fusion proteins. *Protein Science, 22*(12), 1775–1785. https://doi.org/10.1002/pro.2377.

Moore, E. L., Gingell, J. J., Kane, S. A., Hay, D. L., & Salvatore, C. A. (2010). Mapping the CGRP receptor ligand binding domain: Tryptophan-84 of RAMP1 is critical for agonist and antagonist binding. *Biochemical and Biophysical Research Communications, 394*(1), 141–145. https://doi.org/10.1016/j.bbrc.2010.02.131.

Morfis, M., Tilakaratne, N., Furness, S. G., Christopoulos, G., Werry, T. D., Christopoulos, A., et al. (2008). Receptor activity-modifying proteins differentially modulate the G protein-coupling efficiency of amylin receptors. *Endocrinology, 149*(11), 5423–5431. https://doi.org/10.1210/en.2007-1735.

Muff, R., Buhlmann, N., Fischer, J. A., & Born, W. (1999). An amylin receptor is revealed following co-transfection of a calcitonin receptor with receptor activity modifying proteins-1 or -3. *Endocrinology, 140*(6), 2924–2927. https://doi.org/10.1210/endo.140.6.6930.

Naot, D., Musson, D. S., & Cornish, J. (2019). The activity of peptides of the calcitonin family in bone. *Physiological Reviews, 99*(1), 781–805. https://doi.org/10.1152/physrev.00066.2017.

Pal, K., Melcher, K., & Xu, H. E. (2012). Structure and mechanism for recognition of peptide hormones by Class B G-protein-coupled receptors. *Acta Pharmacologica Sinica, 33*(3), 300–311. https://doi.org/10.1038/aps.2011.170.

Pham, V., Zhu, Y., Dal Maso, E., Reynolds, C. A., Deganutti, G., Atanasio, S., et al. (2019). Deconvoluting the molecular control of binding and signaling at the amylin 3 receptor: RAMP3 alters signal propagation through extracellular loops of the calcitonin receptor. *ACS Pharmacology & Translational Science, 2*(3), 183–197. https://doi.org/10.1021/acsptsci.9b00010.

Poyner, D. R., Sexton, P. M., Marshall, I., Smith, D. M., Quirion, R., Born, W., et al. (2002). International Union of Pharmacology. XXXII. The mammalian calcitonin gene-related peptides, adrenomedullin, amylin, and calcitonin receptors. *Pharmacological Reviews, 54*(2), 233–246. Retrieved from https://www.ncbi.nlm.nih.gov/pubmed/12037140.

Purdue, B. W., Tilakaratne, N., & Sexton, P. M. (2002). Molecular pharmacology of the calcitonin receptor. *Receptors & Channels, 8*(3–4), 243–255. Retrieved from https://www.ncbi.nlm.nih.gov/pubmed/12529940.

Qi, T., Christopoulos, G., Bailey, R. J., Christopoulos, A., Sexton, P. M., & Hay, D. L. (2008). Identification of N-terminal receptor activity-modifying protein residues important for calcitonin gene-related peptide, adrenomedullin, and amylin receptor function. *Molecular Pharmacology, 74*(4), 1059–1071. https://doi.org/10.1124/mol.108.047142.

Qi, T., Ly, K., Poyner, D. R., Christopoulos, G., Sexton, P. M., & Hay, D. L. (2011). Structure-function analysis of amino acid 74 of human RAMP1 and RAMP3 and its role in peptide interactions with adrenomedullin and calcitonin gene-related peptide receptors. *Peptides, 32*(5), 1060–1067. https://doi.org/10.1016/j.peptides.2011.03.004.

Robert, X., & Gouet, P. (2014). Deciphering key features in protein structures with the new ENDscript server. *Nucleic Acids Research, 42*(Web Server issue), W320–W324. https://doi.org/10.1093/nar/gku316.

Roehrkasse, A. M., Booe, J. M., Lee, S. M., Warner, M. L., & Pioszak, A. A. (2018). Structure-function analyses reveal a triple beta-turn receptor-bound conformation of adrenomedullin 2/intermedin and enable peptide antagonist design. *The Journal of Biological Chemistry, 293*(41), 15840–15854. https://doi.org/10.1074/jbc.RA118.005062.

Russell, F. A., King, R., Smillie, S. J., Kodji, X., & Brain, S. D. (2014). Calcitonin gene-related peptide: Physiology and pathophysiology. *Physiological Reviews, 94*(4), 1099–1142. https://doi.org/10.1152/physrev.00034.2013.

Sekiguchi, T. (2018). The calcitonin/calcitonin gene-related peptide family in invertebrate deuterostomes. *Frontiers in Endocrinology*, *9*, 695. https://doi.org/10.3389/fendo.2018.00695.

Sekiguchi, T., Kuwasako, K., Ogasawara, M., Takahashi, H., Matsubara, S., Osugi, T., et al. (2016). Evidence for conservation of the calcitonin superfamily and activity-regulating mechanisms in the basal chordate *Branchiostoma floridae*: Insights into the molecular and functional evolution in chordates. *The Journal of Biological Chemistry*, *291*(5), 2345–2356. https://doi.org/10.1074/jbc.M115.664003.

Sexton, P. M., Poyner, D. R., Simms, J., Christopoulos, A., & Hay, D. L. (2012). RAMPs as drug targets. *Advances in Experimental Medicine and Biology*, *744*, 61–74. https://doi.org/10.1007/978-1-4614-2364-5_6.

Shi, L., Lehto, S. G., Zhu, D. X., Sun, H., Zhang, J., Smith, B. P., et al. (2016). Pharmacologic characterization of AMG 334, a potent and selective human monoclonal antibody against the calcitonin gene-related peptide receptor. *The Journal of Pharmacology and Experimental Therapeutics*, *356*(1), 223–231. https://doi.org/10.1124/jpet.115.227793.

Simms, J., Routledge, S., Uddin, R., & Poyner, D. (2019). The structure of the CGRP and related receptors. *Handbook of Experimental Pharmacology*, *255*, 23–36. https://doi.org/10.1007/164_2018_132.

Siu, F. Y., He, M., de Graaf, C., Han, G. W., Yang, D., Zhang, Z., et al. (2013). Structure of the human glucagon class B G-protein-coupled receptor. *Nature*, *499*(7459), 444–449. https://doi.org/10.1038/nature12393.

ter Haar, E., Koth, C. M., Abdul-Manan, N., Swenson, L., Coll, J. T., Lippke, J. A., et al. (2010). Crystal structure of the ectodomain complex of the CGRP receptor, a class-B GPCR, reveals the site of drug antagonism. *Structure*, *18*(9), 1083–1093. https://doi.org/10.1016/j.str.2010.05.014.

Tilakaratne, N., Christopoulos, G., Zumpe, E. T., Foord, S. M., & Sexton, P. M. (2000). Amylin receptor phenotypes derived from human calcitonin receptor/RAMP coexpression exhibit pharmacological differences dependent on receptor isoform and host cell environment. *The Journal of Pharmacology and Experimental Therapeutics*, *294*(1), 61–72. Retrieved from https://www.ncbi.nlm.nih.gov/pubmed/10871296.

Tsuruda, T., Kato, J., Kuwasako, K., & Kitamura, K. (2019). Adrenomedullin: Continuing to explore cardioprotection. *Peptides*, *111*, 47–54. https://doi.org/10.1016/j.peptides.2018.03.012.

Udawela, M., Christopoulos, G., Morfis, M., Christopoulos, A., Ye, S., Tilakaratne, N., et al. (2006). A critical role for the short intracellular C terminus in receptor activity-modifying protein function. *Molecular Pharmacology*, *70*(5), 1750–1760. https://doi.org/10.1124/mol.106.024257.

Udawela, M., Christopoulos, G., Tilakaratne, N., Christopoulos, A., Albiston, A., & Sexton, P. M. (2006). Distinct receptor activity-modifying protein domains differentially modulate interaction with calcitonin receptors. *Molecular Pharmacology*, *69*(6), 1984–1989. https://doi.org/10.1124/mol.105.021915.

Watkins, H. A., Au, M., Bobby, R., Archbold, J. K., Abdul-Manan, N., Moore, J. M., et al. (2013). Identification of key residues involved in adrenomedullin binding to the AM1 receptor. *British Journal of Pharmacology*, *169*(1), 143–155. https://doi.org/10.1111/bph.12118.

Watkins, H. A., Chakravarthy, M., Abhayawardana, R. S., Gingell, J. J., Garelja, M., Pardamwar, M., et al. (2016). Receptor activity-modifying proteins 2 and 3 generate adrenomedullin receptor subtypes with distinct molecular properties. *The Journal of Biological Chemistry*, *291*(22), 11657–11675. https://doi.org/10.1074/jbc.M115.688218.

Watkins, H. A., Walker, C. S., Ly, K. N., Bailey, R. J., Barwell, J., Poyner, D. R., et al. (2014). Receptor activity-modifying protein-dependent effects of mutations in the calcitonin receptor-like receptor: Implications for adrenomedullin and calcitonin gene-related peptide pharmacology. *British Journal of Pharmacology, 171*(3), 772–788. https://doi.org/10.1111/bph.12508.

Weis, W. I., & Kobilka, B. K. (2018). The molecular basis of G protein-coupled receptor activation. *Annual Review of Biochemistry, 87*, 897–919. https://doi.org/10.1146/annurev-biochem-060614-033910.

Weston, C., Lu, J., Li, N., Barkan, K., Richards, G. O., Roberts, D. J., et al. (2015). Modulation of glucagon receptor pharmacology by receptor activity-modifying protein-2 (RAMP2). *The Journal of Biological Chemistry, 290*(38), 23009–23022. https://doi.org/10.1074/jbc.M114.624601.

Weston, C., Winfield, I., Harris, M., Hodgson, R., Shah, A., Dowell, S. J., et al. (2016). Receptor activity-modifying protein-directed G protein signaling specificity for the calcitonin gene-related peptide family of receptors. *The Journal of Biological Chemistry, 291*(42), 21925–21944. https://doi.org/10.1074/jbc.M116.751362.

Woolley, M. J., Reynolds, C. A., Simms, J., Walker, C. S., Mobarec, J. C., Garelja, M. L., et al. (2017). Receptor activity-modifying protein dependent and independent activation mechanisms in the coupling of calcitonin gene-related peptide and adrenomedullin receptors to Gs. *Biochemical Pharmacology, 142*, 96–110. https://doi.org/10.1016/j.bcp.2017.07.005.

Wootten, D., Lindmark, H., Kadmiel, M., Willcockson, H., Caron, K. M., Barwell, J., et al. (2013). Receptor activity modifying proteins (RAMPs) interact with the VPAC2 receptor and CRF1 receptors and modulate their function. *British Journal of Pharmacology, 168*(4), 822–834. https://doi.org/10.1111/j.1476-5381.2012.02202.x.

Wootten, D., & Miller, L. J. (2020). Structural basis for allosteric modulation of Class B G protein-coupled receptors. *Annual Review of Pharmacology and Toxicology, 60*, 89–107. https://doi.org/10.1146/annurev-pharmtox-010919-023301. Epub 2019 Aug 27.

Young, A. A., Gedulin, B., Gaeta, L. S., Prickett, K. S., Beaumont, K., Larson, E., et al. (1994). Selective amylin antagonist suppresses rise in plasma lactate after intravenous glucose in the rat. Evidence for a metabolic role of endogenous amylin. *FEBS Letters, 343*(3), 237–241. https://doi.org/10.1016/0014-5793(94)80563-6.

Zhang, H., Qiao, A., Yang, L., Van Eps, N., Frederiksen, K. S., Yang, D., et al. (2018). Structure of the glucagon receptor in complex with a glucagon analogue. *Nature, 553*(7686), 106–110. https://doi.org/10.1038/nature25153.

Zhang, H., Qiao, A., Yang, D., Yang, L., Dai, A., de Graaf, C., et al. (2017). Structure of the full-length glucagon class B G-protein-coupled receptor. *Nature, 546*(7657), 259–264. https://doi.org/10.1038/nature22363.

Zhang, Y., Sun, B., Feng, D., Hu, H., Chu, M., Qu, Q., et al. (2017). Cryo-EM structure of the activated GLP-1 receptor in complex with a G protein. *Nature, 546*(7657), 248–253. https://doi.org/10.1038/nature22394.

Zhang, S. Y., Xu, M. J., & Wang, X. (2018). Adrenomedullin 2/intermedin: A putative drug candidate for treatment of cardiometabolic diseases. *British Journal of Pharmacology, 175*(8), 1230–1240. https://doi.org/10.1111/bph.13814.

Zhao, L. H., Ma, S., Sutkeviciute, I., Shen, D. D., Zhou, X. E., de Waal, P. W., et al. (2019). Structure and dynamics of the active human parathyroid hormone receptor-1. *Science, 364*(6436), 148–153. https://doi.org/10.1126/science.aav7942.

Zumpe, E. T., Tilakaratne, N., Fraser, N. J., Christopoulos, G., Foord, S. M., & Sexton, P. M. (2000). Multiple ramp domains are required for generation of amylin receptor phenotype from the calcitonin receptor gene product. *Biochemical and Biophysical Research Communications, 267*(1), 368–372. https://doi.org/10.1006/bbrc.1999.1943.

CHAPTER SIX

Strategies and considerations of G-protein-coupled receptor photopharmacology

Alice E. Berizzi*, Cyril Goudet*
IGF, CNRS, INSERM, Univ. de Montpellier, Montpellier, France
*Corresponding authors: e-mail address: alice.berizzi@igf.cnrs.fr; cyril.goudet@igf.cnrs.fr

Contents

Abstract

G-protein-coupled receptor (GPCR) pharmacology tends to be complex and at times poorly understood. This has led to the development of GPCR-targeting agents that often demonstrate poor pharmacokinetic properties and poor selectivity for their target receptors. One approach that is emerging as a means of addressing these limitations is the use of molecules whose activity can be controlled by light. Photopharmacology involves the incorporation of a photoswitch into the structure of a given compound, cage or linker and following irradiation with light, undergoes a structural rearrangement, which changes its biological activity. The use of light-regulated ligands offers the opportunity to modulate and understand GPCR signaling in a more spatiotemporal manner than classical pharmacological approaches. In this chapter we will discuss some of the advancements that have been made in photopharmacology, particularly in developing photoswitchable ligands that target class A GPCRs, e.g., muscarinic acetylcholine receptors, class B GPCRs, e.g., glucagon-like peptide-1 receptor, and class C GPCRs, e.g., metabotrobic glutamate

Advances in Pharmacology, Volume 88
ISSN 1054-3589
https://doi.org/10.1016/bs.apha.2019.12.001

receptors. Given the intricacy of GPCR pharmacology, this chapter will also discuss some of the challenges the field faces when designing photopharmacological tools. Furthermore, it will propose that it is with a full appreciation of the spectrum of pharmacological and pharmacokinetic properties of photoswitchable ligands that research will be better placed to develop ligands with a reduced risk of failure during preclinical progression. This will likely enable photopharmacological approaches to continue to find novel applications and offer new perspectives in understanding (patho)physiology to ultimately inform future GPCR drug discovery efforts.

Nonstandard abbreviations

ADME	absorption, distribution, metabolism, and excretion
cAMP	cyclic adenosine monophosphate
EC_{80}	80% effective concentration
GLP-1R	glucagon-like peptide-1 receptor
GPCR	guanine nucleotide-binding protein-coupled receptor
GTPγS	guanosine 5′-*O*-[γ-thio]triphosphate
^{1}H NMR	proton nuclear magnetic resonance
mAChR	muscarinic acetylcholine receptor
maPORTL	membrane anchored photoswitchable orthogonal remotely tethered ligands
mGlu	metabotropic glutamate receptor
NAL	neutral allosteric ligand
NAM	negative allosteric modulator
NMS	*N*-methylscopolamine
PAM	positive allosteric modulator
PCL	photochromic ligands
pIC_{50}	the concentration require to cause 50% inhibition
PIS	photoisomerization score
PORTL	photoswitchable orthogonal remotely tethered ligands
pPPS	negative logarithm of the photoinduced potency shift
PTL	photoswitchable tethered ligands
QNB	quinuclidinyl benzilate
S1P	sphingosine-1-phosphate
SAR	structure-activity relationship
UV	ultraviolet

1. Introduction

G-protein-coupled receptors (GPCRs) represent the largest family of cell-surface receptors encoded by the human genome, and are necessary for the proper functioning of physiological responses (Lagerstrom & Schioth, 2008). Unsurprisingly, GPCRs have emerged as a major target class of drug discovery programs with drugs targeting GPCRs making-up a third of the total market share of therapeutics (Hauser, Attwood, Rask-Andersen, Schioth, & Gloriam, 2017; Overington, Al-Lazikani, & Hopkins, 2006). Despite their attractiveness as drug targets, one of the major challenges in GPCR drug discovery endeavors is the high attrition rate. Indeed, less than one-third of GPCR-targeting agents entering phase III clinical trials receive FDA approval (Hauser et al., 2017). Poor selectivity, sub-optimal pharmacokinetic properties and a lack of efficacy remain the greatest obstacles for clinical candidates to overcome. For GPCRs, many of these issues are due to receptor pharmacology, (patho)physiology and candidate compound properties tending to be poorly understood prior to clinical advancement. Moreover, candidate molecules have historically been developed to exploit GPCR pharmacology via unidimensional approaches, which may be insufficient when attempting to treat complex diseases where multiple systems are affected.

To address these limitations there has been increased interest in the development of small molecules that use novel mechanisms to dynamically control their activity, and that are also well characterized in different pharmacological systems—considering (patho)physiological contexts and the effects of ligands on multiple signaling partners downstream from their target receptor. It is anticipated that research will be better equipped to recognize predictors of preclinical efficacy in the absence of adverse effects.

To this end, one approach gaining popularity is the development of molecules and technologies whose activity can be controlled by light. The use of light in this way, particularly in biological applications, can be advantageous as it is non-invasive, non-contaminating and photons are associated with low or negligible toxicity as compared to chemicals. Critically, light can be delivered in a highly controlled manner in space and time, and the extent of its effect can be controlled through the adjustment of wavelength and intensity.

Historically, using light to control and manipulate biological processes has been important to the advancement of a number of fields of science, including neuroscience and pharmacology. For example, optogenetics is a method that utilizes light to modulate the activity of specific cell types or organisms in a genetically targeted manner. Since its inception, it has helped address many fundamental research questions. However, this technique requires genetic manipulation of a system and so it may not be suitable for clinical advancement in all situations. Furthermore, since classical optogenetics often replaces a protein with a different, non-mammalian protein in order to allow for light modulation, its behavior may differ from the endogenous protein, so direct conclusions about the endogenous system cannot be drawn with complete confidence. Irrespective of some of the limitations associated with optogenetics, other techniques have emerged that utilize light, which have become more commonplace in the clinic. Indeed, photodynamic therapy is approved for use in humans and is a minimally invasive therapeutic approach toward selectively killing malignant cells (Chilakamarthi & Giribabu, 2017). This technique relies on the use of photosensitizers to form reactive oxygen species in living tissue, which leads to non-specific cell death. Due to its non-selective nature though, its application is limited.

More recently, the use of small, light-regulated ligands has emerged as an interesting alternative for the modulation of physiological systems and signaling pathways. Unlike optogenetics, the application of photopharmacology allows for the modulation of native proteins with minimal to no genetic manipulation, allowing easier translation into the clinic. Furthermore, many classical pharmacological approaches are unable to target proteins in a temporal and tissue-dependent manner. For this reason, photopharmacological strategies may be advantageous; since precise drug delivery and activity can be achieved.

In principal, photopharmacology involves the manipulation of a given biological process with a synthetic photoswitch; a moiety that undergoes a change in its structure upon irradiation with light, which can either irreversibly release an active compound or reversibly control a ligand's activity at its target. To date, photopharmacology approaches have been implemented in the design of candidate drug-like compounds for a number of biological targets, including GPCRs, ion channels, transporters, lipids, enzymes and elements of cytoskeleton (Cheng, Shchepakin, Kavanaugh, & Trauner, 2017; Damijonaitis et al., 2015; Gomez-Santacana et al., 2017; Hull, Morstein, & Trauner, 2018; Liu, Xie, Shao, & Jiang, 2009; Pittolo et al., 2014; Rastogi et al., 2018; Tsai, Essig, James, Lang, & Chin, 2015; Velema, Szymanski, & Feringa, 2014). In this chapter, discussion will be restricted to light-regulated ligands that target GPCRs.

2. Modality of photoactivable ligands

At present, photopharmacology strategies targeting GPCRs can be designed to be either irreversible or reversible. Irreversible photopharmacological approaches including the development of photocaged compounds have grown in popularity, since they allow for greater control over the delivery and activity of a given drug at its site of action. For example, a photoactivable ligand can be administered systemically, but activated locally with the use of light and in this way can reduce the risk of adverse consequences in unwanted tissues. Photoactive caged-compounds possess a photoreactive component that is covalently bound to an active molecule, rendering it inactive to its target receptor. However, when exposed to irradiation of a select wavelength the active molecule is irreversibly released in a rapid and localized manner (Fig. 1), thereby controlling the location and extent of its therapeutic effects and reducing the risk of adverse side-effects at other locations in the body.

Since the first demonstration of the suitability of photocaged compounds to modulate biological systems in the late 1970s, a multitude of molecules employing this mechanism of action have emerged and shown promise in preclinical studies (Font et al., 2017; Kaplan, Forbush, & Hoffman, 1978; Taura et al., 2018). For example, techniques incorporating photocaged compounds have found utility in describing the functional connectivity of circuits within the central nervous system. The use of photocaged-glutamate has indeed allowed for the mapping of circuits that connect with the hippocampus and cortex, while also bypassing some of the limitations associated with conventional stimulatory approaches, such as desensitization effects and artifacts of current (Callaway & Katz, 1993). Many photoactive caged-compounds have also been designed to be sensitive to two-photon excitation and uncaging, which allows for high spatial resolution and minimal toxicity as compared to standard ultraviolet (UV) light excitation (Warther et al., 2010). Moreover, the photoactive caged compound, JF-NP-026 (caged-raseglurant; Fig. 1B), which was based on the selective

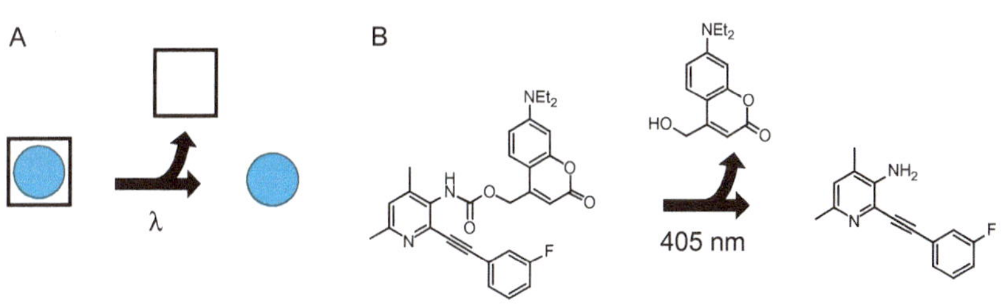

Fig. 1 (A) Schematic representation of the photo-uncaging approach. The photoactive caged compound is inactive under dark light conditions, but when exposed to a select wavelength of light the active molecule is irreversibly released and allowed to interact with its target receptor. (B) Structure and photochemistry of the photo-caged compound, JF-NP-026 (caged-raseglurant). Upon irradiation with 405 nm of light the mGlu5 NAM, raseglurant, is irreversibly released.

negative allosteric modulator (NAM) for the metabotropic glutamate receptor 5 (mGlu5), raseglurant, exhibits preclinical efficacy in mouse models of acute and neuropathic inflammatory pain (Font et al., 2017; Lopez-Cano, Font, Llebaria, Fernandez-Duenas, & Ciruela, 2019). In this study, the authors demonstrated that caged-raseglurant had no effect on pain prior to illumination, but following photolysis with violet light either peripherally on the hind paw, or centrally in the thalamus, it demonstrated analgesic effects (Font et al., 2017). In this way, the authors of the study were able to examine targeted and localized effects of the ligand at the mGlu5 in a light-directed manner that otherwise could not be achieved with conventional pharmacological approaches. They were also able to demonstrate the potential therapeutic efficacy of targeting this receptor with a selective photocaged NAM in different aspects of neuropathic pain. Another study has recently shown that the photocaged A_{2A} antagonist, MRS7145, shows efficacy in a number of animal models that represent aspects of the symptomology of Parkinson's disease (Taura et al., 2018). Thereby demonstrating the potential efficacy of photocaged A_{2A} antagonists to manage the symptomology of movement disorders including, Parkinson's disease. More recently, a series of photocaged lipid metabolites enabling the optical control of GPCRs (FFAR1, PTGER1, LPA2, LPA3, PTFAR) have also been designed (Wagner, Schuhmacher, Lohmann, & Nadler, 2019). For a more comprehensive list of GPCR-targeting photocaged compounds the reader is referred to another review (Ricart-Ortega, Font, & Llebaria, 2019).

Irrespective of these and other proof-of-concept studies, the use of photocaged compounds are limited by their irreversibility and care must be taken in their design to ensure efficient uncaging upon irradiation. For example, scenarios may arise where prior to irradiation the photocaged molecule is unreactive, but following illumination the biological activity of the parent ligand cannot be restored, or falls below the necessary threshold for biological activity due to incomplete uncaging (Deiters, 2010). The opposite may also occur, with a photocaged compound demonstrating activity prior to illumination leading to potential off-target or on-target effects in undesired tissues (Deiters, 2010).

3. Modality of photoswitchable ligands

In general, the design of reversible photoswitchable ligands involves the incorporation of an active moiety that can be selectively recognized by the target receptor and a photoswitchable core that reversibly isomerises under different light conditions. Following irradiation with distinct wavelengths of light the resulting photoisomers can interact differently with the target GPCR as a result of differences in pharmacological, chemical and/or physical properties. This results in the reversible control of a receptor from a state of activity to inactivity in a precisely timed manner. Often there is one photoisomer that is more thermodynamically stable. One wavelength of light will typically be used to switch the ligand to the less-stable isomer, and it may return to the more thermodynamically stable isomer in darkness via thermal relaxation or by irradiation with a second wavelength.

3.1 Tethered photoswitchable ligands

Reversible photoswitchable ligands are classified depending on their interaction with their target protein. To date, photoswitchable molecules have been designed that can covalently attach to receptors via a bioconjugation, which can be synthetic or native to the receptor (Broichhagen & Trauner, 2014; Donthamsetti et al., 2017; Hermanson, 2013). Tethered photoswitchable ligand approaches include hybrid methods that exploit genetic and chemical technologies to control protein function, including the incorporation of unnatural amino acids into a receptor (Noren, Anthony-Cahill, Griffith, & Schultz, 1989). The promise of this strategy is that it allows for greater selectivity for a target receptor and can rapidly oscillate between activating and inactivating a receptor, since its tether enables close proximity to its binding site (Fig. 2) (Leippe, Koehler Leman, & Trauner, 2017). This approach also allows any point on a receptor to be selectively targeted, but it does require genetic manipulation and the incorporation of unnatural amino acids can lead to decreased protein expression (Klippenstein, Ghisi, Wietstruk, & Plested, 2014).

Tethered ligands are classified based on the proximity of the covalent attachment site to the ligand binding site. Photoswitchable tethered ligands (PTLs) possess a photoswitch and a covalent attachment, via a single cysteine amino acid in very close proximity to the ligand binding site, so when switching occurs the local concentration at the active site of the molecule is affected (Fig. 2A). Alternatively, the bioconjugation to the receptor may occur with the use of larger protein tags, as is the case with photoswitchable orthogonal remotely tethered ligands (PORTLs; Fig. 2B). For both PTLs and PORTLs, the active component binds to and elicits a pharmacological response at the receptor in one conformation, but does not bind in the second conformation following photoisomerization (Fig. 2A and B).

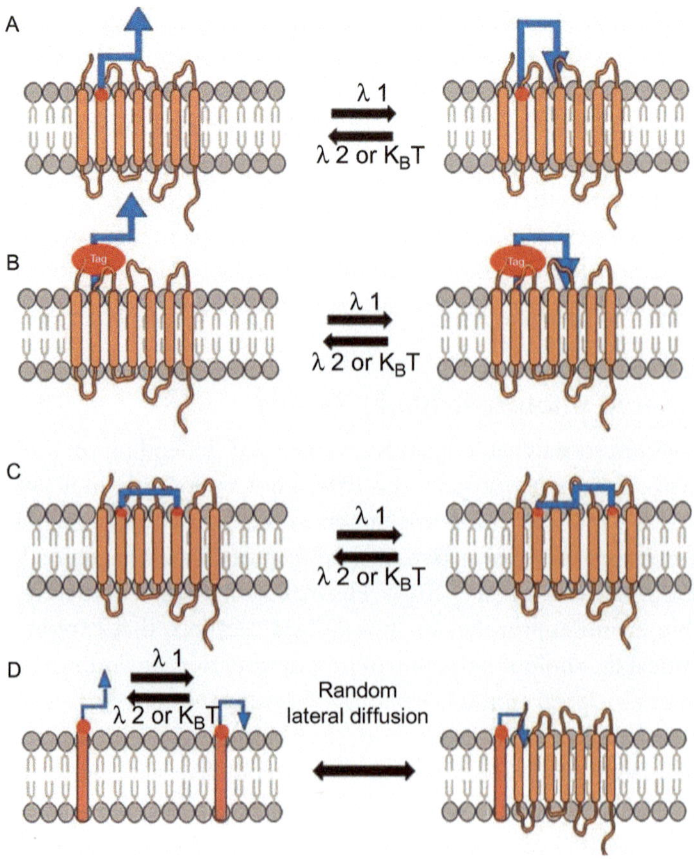

Fig. 2 Schematic representations of the different classes of tethered photoswitchable ligands available for targeting GPCRs. (A) Photoswitchable tethered ligands (PTLs), (B) photoswitchable orthogonal remotely tethered ligands (PORTLs), (C) nanotweezer, (D) membrane anchored photoswitchable orthogonal remotely tethered ligands (maPORTL).

Both strategies have been successfully applied to metabotropic glutamate receptors (Acosta-Ruiz, Broichhagen, & Levitz, 2019; Broichhagen, Damijonaitis et al., 2015; Carroll et al., 2015; Levitz et al., 2013). To date, the PORTL approach utilizes a number of different noncovalent binders, including antibodies and nanobodies, as a means of attaching a photoswitchable ligand to a receptor with very high selectivity (Farrants et al., 2018).

Nanotweezers are another class of tethered photoswitchable ligand that employ light-responsive cross-linkers, where each attachment point of the ligand to the receptor possesses a photoswitchable unit (Habermacher et al., 2016). Following isomerization, the binding and functional activity of the ligand is affected at the receptor (Fig. 2B). More recently, tethered ligands have been designed to genetically-target the plasma membrane of a cell instead of a target receptor and are named membrane anchored photoswitchable orthogonal remotely tethered ligands (maPORTL) (Donthamsetti et al., 2019). These ligands anchor to the plasma membrane and via lateral diffusion become close in proximity to their target receptor to enable interaction (Fig. 2C).

The action of tethered photoswitchable ligands tend to be rapid since the local concentration and/or activity at the receptor can be switched from being very high to very low depending on the light condition. Unfortunately, the tethered ligand approach is also limited. They are often restricted to targeting points on a receptor that can only be accessed by the solvent; limiting interactions to the extracellular environment, photoswitching between each isomer is often inefficient, which can lead to reduced activity if photoisomerization is required for ligand binding, and the nature of the ligand's attachment to the receptor can increase the potential for non-specific reactions to occur, e.g., non-specific cysteine conjugations. To date though, no adverse effects have been reported and this approach has been successfully implemented to control some GPCRs in a light-dependent manner, including mGlu receptors and dopamine receptors (Broichhagen, Damijonaitis et al., 2015; Donthamsetti et al., 2017). Research groups are beginning to address some of the limitations associated with this approach. For instance, a recent report describes the design of branched PORTLs as a means to improve the photoisomerization efficiency and affinity of tethered ligands (Acosta-Ruiz, Gutzeit, et al., 2019; Acosta-Ruiz, Broichhagen, & Levitz, 2019). Continued improvements of this type may lead to a set of tool compounds suitable for addressing a number of different mechanistic questions of receptor function in the future.

3.2 Freely-diffusible photoswitchable ligands

Of particular interest to this review, are photochromic ligands (PCLs). These are photoswitchable ligands that have been developed to interact with a receptor via noncovalent bonds. Like with covalently tethered compounds, photoswitchable molecules of this type can be designed so that following irradiation, photoisomers have opposing pharmacological interactions with the target receptor, which is a product of differences in isomer binding,

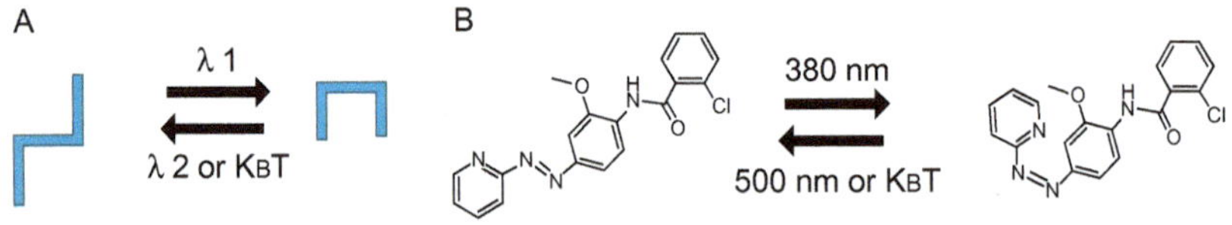

Fig. 3 (A) Schematic representation of the photoisomerization of a photochromic ligand (PCL). Following irradiation with a select wavelength of light, photoisomerization of a PCL is promoted, and the PCL can then return back to the more stable isomer via thermal relaxation or irradiation with a second wavelength. (B) Structure and photochemistry of the photoswitchable, mGlu5 NAM, alloswitch-1, which interconverts from *trans* to *cis* isomeric forms following irradiation with UV light, and from *cis* to *trans* upon exposure to green light or via thermal relaxation.

activity and/or pharmacokinetic properties (Fig. 3). In contrast, PCLs are freely diffusible and can be slower in switching between pharmacological responses. At present, PCLs have been synthesized to target all major GPCR classes and do so by many different mechanisms of action, including via orthosteric interactions (e.g., VUF15000 is a photoswitchable Histamine H_3 receptor agonist and photoiperoxo is a photoswitchable muscarinic acetylcholine receptor [mAChR] partial agonist), allosteric interactions (e.g., alloswitch-1 is a photoswitchable mGlu5 NAM and PhotoETP is a photoswitchable positive allosteric modulator (PAM) of the glucagon-like peptide-1 receptor (GLP-1R)), and by connections that engage aspects of both the orthosteric and allosteric sites of a receptor; that is by bitopic interactions (e.g., BQCAAI is a bitopic ligand for the M_1 mAChR) (Agnetta et al., 2017; Broichhagen, Johnston, von Ohlen, & Meyer-Berg, et al., 2016; Broichhagen, Podewin, et al., 2015; Gomez-Santacana et al., 2017; Hauwert et al., 2019; Jones et al., 2017; Schonberger & Trauner, 2014). For a comprehensive list of currently available, GPCR-targeting PCLs the reader is referred to other reviews (Hull et al., 2018; Ricart-Ortega et al., 2019).

3.3 Types of photoswitchable cores

Photoreactive ligands incorporate photoswitchable cores, which are classified into two distinct groups—based on their mechanism of isomerization. Following irradiation, molecules that incorporate azobenzene-, hemithioindigos- or stilbenes-based photoswitches into their structure will be interconverted between *trans* and *cis* isomers; leading to a substantial change in the overall shape and polarity of the molecule (Ricart-Ortega et al., 2019) (Fig. 4A–C). Spiropyrans-, diarylethenes- or fulgides-based

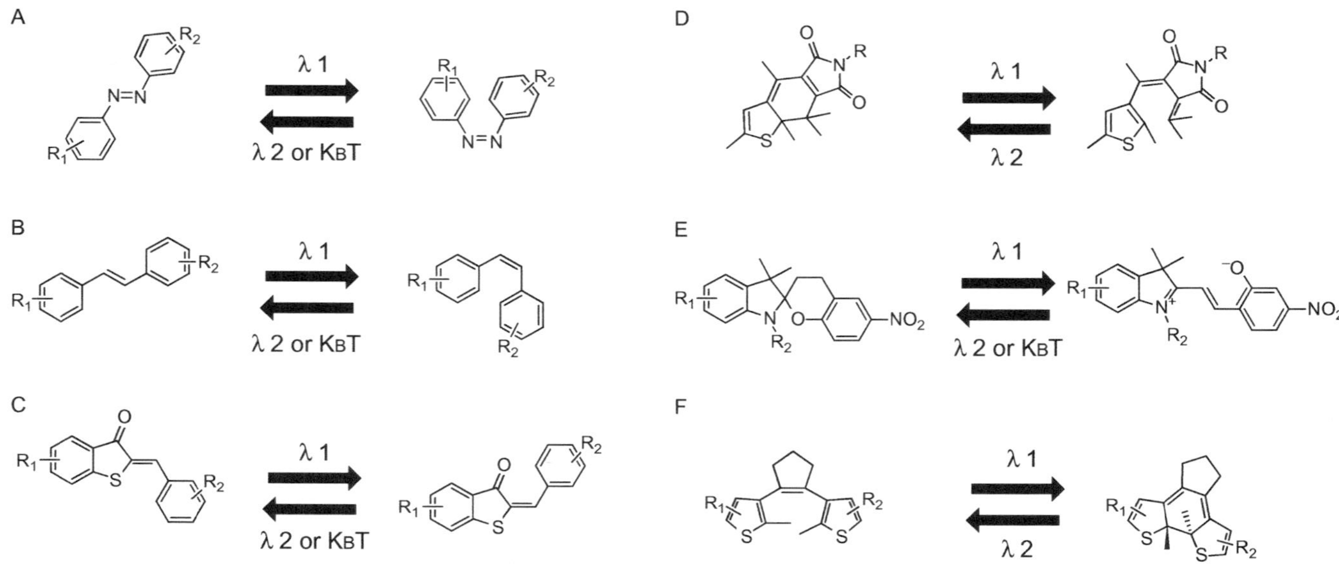

Fig. 4 Photoswitchable cores that can interconvert between *trans* and *cis* or closed and open forms. (A) azobenzenes, (B) stilbenes, (C) hemithioindigos, (D) fulgides, (E) spiropyrans, (F) diarylethenes.

photoswitches can photoisomerize between open and closed formations, tending to result in changes in flexibility and electronic properties (Ricart-Ortega et al., 2019) (Fig. 4D–F). To date, the azobenzene is the most widely used photoswitch; predominantly because it meets the majority of the design criteria for an ideal photoswitch (Agnetta et al., 2017; Broichhagen, Frank, & Trauner, 2015; Gomez-Santacana et al., 2017; Schonberger & Trauner, 2014). Azobenzenes tend to be easy to synthesise, they are small in size, show high quantum yields and have little photobleaching (Beharry & Woolley, 2011). The *trans* isomer tends to be the most stable and following irradiation to the *cis* form the molecule generally relaxes back to the *trans* isomer in darkness. The half-life of the thermodynamically less-stable photoisomer can vary from milliseconds to days, depending on the substituents attached to the molecule. Many of the following examples will relate to azobenzene-based photoswitches.

4. Design criteria for photoswitchable drug-like compounds

When designing a photoswitchable ligand there are a number of criteria determining the pharmacological success of the compound. First, photoswitchable ligands should be able to efficiently switch between their isomers following light irradiation. For most photoswitches it is not possible to completely convert all molecules from the thermodynamically preferred state to the less-stable state with irradiation. Research is progressing toward the development of bistable photoswitches though (Szymanski, Wu, Poloni, Janssen, & Feringa, 2013), and this will be critical to the advancement of photoswitchable ligand development.

Importantly, a molecule may have different photoswitchable efficiencies depending on its local environment. Certainly the solvent system, concentration, temperature, pH, presence of interacting molecules, whether the ligand is bound to its receptor and/or the disease context may affect its ability to photoisomerize (Velema et al., 2014). Taken together, studies should consider measuring isomer concentrations under all experimental conditions used, particularly when a photoswitchable ligand is intended for use in a disease context where physiological conditions are changed. This will ensure pharmacological profiles are attributed to the actions of a specific photoisomer of a ligand.

An important factor for when determining the photoisomer ratio of a ligand is the half-life of the thermodynamically less-stable photoisomer.

Knowledge of the half-life of photoisomers will help to determine the appropriate dosing strategy for photoswitchable ligands and the amount of light required in order for a given pharmacological or therapeutic outcome. For instance, in an in vivo setting, for a candidate drug that is more active in the less-stable isomeric form but that has a short isomeric half-life, it may be preferential to irradiate the molecule at its site of action and not prior to dosing. Using this method, the activity of the ligand will not be lost by the time it reaches its target and it will be less likely to elicit undesirable on-target effects in other tissues. As with the photoisomer ratio of a molecule, it is feasible that the thermal relaxation time may change depending on the local environment of the photoswitchable ligand and as such, care must be taken to fully appreciate the properties of the ligand in changing environmental conditions.

As well as the photoisomer ratio, the metabolism of the photoswitchable ligand and the activity of the resulting metabolites should also be considered. Previous reports show that photoswitchable moieties such as azobenzenes can be subject to either enzymatic degradation or glutathione-mediated reduction depending on their polarity (Boulegue, Loweneck, Renner, & Moroder, 2007; Renner & Moroder, 2006; Zbaida, 1995). Accordingly, the electronic properties of molecules should be examined in the design process of photoswitchable ligands and the synthesized ligands should be tested against glutathione-mediated reduction (Velema et al., 2014). Photoswitchable ligands containing azobenzene cores, nevertheless, have shown in vivo efficacy suggesting that their potential for metabolism may not be a limiting factor (Font et al., 2017; Mehta et al., 2017; Morstein et al., 2019; Taura et al., 2018; Zussy et al., 2018).

The chosen photoswitch should also demonstrate negligible toxicity. Some azobenzenes and their metabolites have reported toxicity (Brown & De Vito, 1993). However, this may not be a restricting factor since drugs containing azobenzenes have been successfully progressed to the clinic for therapeutic use (McGirt, Vasagar, Gober, Saini, & Beck, 2006).

Taken together, as with classical pharmacological approaches, it is clear that adequate knowledge of the overall ADME (absorption, distribution, metabolism, and excretion) properties of a photoswitchable ligand is essential in the design process and is critical to reducing risks associated with their failure toward further optimization and advancement. One of the main advantages that photoswitchable strategies possess over classical pharmacological approaches is that given adequate knowledge of pharmacodynamic and ADME properties, it is possible to fine-tune some aspects of an existing photoswitchable ligand in real-time, and in a spatial and temporal manner with light. For this reason, ensuring that a photoswitchable ligand is designed such that the photoisomerization occurs at very precise wavelengths is paramount. When evaluating the appropriateness of a wavelength for photoswitching, its corresponding photostationary state (a function of the wavelength of light) is important. In theory, the photostationary state is reached when the interconversion between *cis* and *trans* isomers of a molecule proceeds at equilibrium and the isomeric ratio remains constant. Ideally, the absorption spectra of each isomer will be well separated and the isomeric ratio at the photostationary state will be approximately equal to 99:1. This is not always the case though, and the isomeric ratio can be much lower, and as a consequence of the non-linear nature of biological systems a small change in this ratio may have a substantial effect on the biological activity of the photoswitchable ligand.

In general, the isomeric ratio of a photoswitchable ligand's photostationary state, at a given wavelength, can be determined with the use of a ^{1}H NMR spectroscopy assay (Banghart & Trauner, 2013). This assay involves dissolving samples of a photoswitchable ligand into deuterated water and analyzing them firstly by UV–visible spectroscopy to identify which wavelengths produce a photostationary state and then the ratios can be determined by ^{1}H NMR spectroscopy. Since the aromatic protons of azobenzene *trans* and *cis* isomers exhibit different chemical shifts it makes it possible to compare the relative abundance of each isomer for a particular photostationary state of a ligand by peak integration. Regular employment of a technique such as ^{1}H NMR spectroscopy is recommended as it allows for the direct measurement of a photoswitchable ligand's photostationary states.

The wavelengths for photoswitching should also occur outside the UV range to reduce toxicity so that they are appropriate for clinical use. Recently, red-shifted, azobenzenes-based photoswitches have been synthesized, which penetrate tissue more deeply and are more biocompatible (Broichhagen, Frank, Johnston, et al., 2015; Dong, Babalhavaeji, Samanta, Beharry, & Woolley, 2015; Samanta et al., 2013). It should be noted though, that the substitution pattern of a ligand's photoswitchable core cannot only significantly influence the wavelengths required for interconversion between isomers but also can affect photoisomerization rates and photorelaxation times, which should be considered when designing ligands (Dong et al., 2015). Taken together, the design of the ideal photoswitch should enable bi-directional photoisomerization with wavelengths that are well separated in the light spectrum, that are deep-penetrating and show low toxicity to reduce invasiveness.

To determine the most appropriate wavelengths for photoswitching of a ligand, a researcher can determine the photoisomerization score (PIS) and the negative logarithm of the photoinduced potency shift (pPPS) for a small molecule (Gomez-Santacana et al., 2017). The PIS is calculated from the data obtained from the UV–visible absorption spectra of ligands and is given as a score ranging from zero to one; where a score of zero is indicative of a wavelength that results in no isomerization and a score of one refers to complete isomerization following irradiation. Two PIS values are usually determined—one for the interconversion from the *trans* to *cis* isomer ($PIS_{T \rightarrow C}$) and the other for the conversion of the *cis* to *trans* isomer ($PIS_{C \rightarrow T}$). The value for the *trans* to *cis* conversion represents the difference between the absorbance under dark light conditions and illuminated conditions (usually violet light for an azobenzene) over the absorbance for dark light conditions of a ligand (Eq. 1). The resulting value can then be compared against a reference photoswitchable ligand that undergoes complete isomerization (Eq. 1). For determining the $PIS_{C \rightarrow T}$ value the same equation is used, but the maximum absorbance occurring under violet light conditions is compared to a second wavelength, which promotes isomerization back to the *trans* form (usually green light for azobenzenes) (Eq. 2).

$$PIS_{x,t \rightarrow c} = \frac{\frac{A_{x,dark\ maximum} - A_{x,violet}}{A_{x,dark\ maximum}}}{\frac{A_{ref,dark\ maximum} - A_{ref,violet}}{A_{ref,dark\ maximum}}} \quad \text{(Eq.1)}$$

$$PIS_{x,c \rightarrow t} = \frac{\frac{A_{x,violet} - A_{x,green}}{A_{x,dark\ maximum}}}{\frac{A_{ref,dark\ maximum} - A_{ref,violet}}{A_{ref,dark\ maximum}}} \quad \text{(Eq.2)}$$

The pPPS value for a photoswitchable ligand measures the change in potency of a molecule following irradiation with a wavelength of light as compared to its potency under dark light conditions (Gomez-Santacana et al., 2017) (Fig. 5). For example, in the case of an EC_{80} concentration of an agonist interacted with a concentration response curve of a photoswitchable NAM under dark light and illuminated conditions, the pPPS value is determined from the difference between the illuminated curve pIC_{50} value and the dark light curve pIC_{50} value (Fig. 5). The resulting value will aid a researcher in choosing a wavelength of light for future experiments that has the largest activity difference for a photoswitchable ligand between isomerization states. Once the appropriate wavelength has been chosen, it is also possible to determine pPPS values for different light intensities to maximize photoswitching at a particular wavelength.

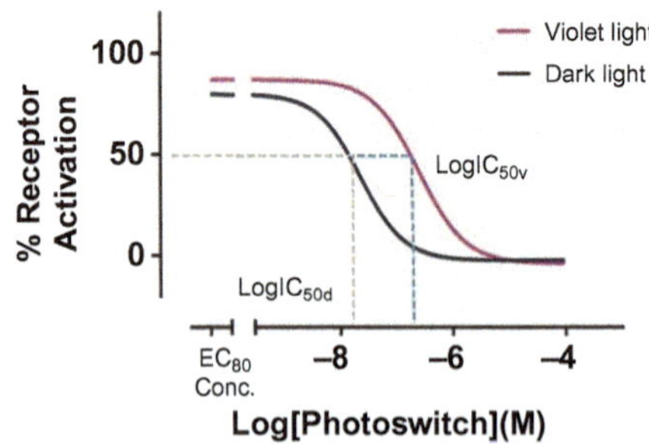

Fig. 5 The photoinduced potency shift (pPPS) measures the change in potency of a photoswitchable ligand following irradiation with a single wavelength of light as compared to its potency under dark light conditions. The above schematic represents the interaction of a photoswitchable NAM with an 80% effective concentration (EC_{80}) of agonist under different light conditions to provide an estimate of the pPPS for the interaction.

5. Advantages and considerations for future applications of photopharmacology to biological systems

As outlined previously, the benefit of using photoswitchable ligands is the ability to control their action externally, in real-time and in a reversible manner. These specific properties may allow photopharmacology approaches to be easily incorporated and applied to a number of research areas toward improving GPCR drug discovery, including in developing our understanding of GPCR signaling and function.

The consideration of the pharmacokinetic and pharmacodynamic properties of drug-like compounds is essential to the success of any GPCR drug discovery program. Since these properties are dictated by the shape, structure and polarity of a drug, being able to rapidly change these aspects of a molecule may allow for dynamic control over the activity, effectiveness and amount of drug that reaches its site of action. Photopharmacology, therefore, offers the potential benefit of designing drug-like molecules with pharmacokinetic and pharmacodynamics properties that can change under different conditions. For instance, a photoswitchable ligand may be designed to be more lipophilic at a particular pH to allow for better absorption at one point of the gastrointestinal system, which may improve the overall effectiveness of the compound. Alternatively, it may be possible to design a photoswitchable ligand to photoisomerize from a low affinity/efficacy state in tissues where its activity is not desired, to a high affinity/efficacy state upon reaching its site of action to minimize off-target effects in undesired tissues. Certainly, strategies of this type would be beneficial when treating many types of cancers that are sub-optimally treated with cytotoxic drugs. This potential benefit has recently been demonstrated with the photocaged mGlu5 NAM; caged-raseglurant, which shows a reduced side-effect profile as compared to its parent compound, raseglurant (Font et al., 2017).

Currently, many of the photoswitchable ligands available that target GPCRs are more active in their more thermodynamically stable form (*trans* isomer), which means they are active under dark light conditions and have to be deactivated with light. For therapeutic purposes, inactive ligands that can be switched on by light are more desirable and to date few GPCR-targeting *cis*-active ligands have been described, including the photoswitchable *cis*-on cannabinoid receptor 1 agonist, azo-THC-4, (Westphal et al., 2017), and the *cis*-on antagonist of the histamine H_3 receptor, VUF14862 (Hauwert et al., 2018). Studies have also emerged that describe alternative photoswitchable ligands that are more thermodynamically stable in their *cis* form, while their *trans* isomer tends to be severely strained and distorted in shape. Ligands of this type generally possess two phenyl rings connected by an ethylene bridge, which creates a locked-azobenzene core. Using this strategy, compounds have been designed that are inactive under dark light conditions and more active following light irradiation (Cabre et al., 2019; Siewertsen et al., 2009; Siewertsen, Schonborn, Hartke, Renth, & Temps, 2011; Thapaliya, Zhao, & Ellis-Davies, 2019; Trads et al., 2019). To date, molecules of this type have only been designed to target non-GPCR proteins so it remains to be seen if GPCR-targeting photoswitchable ligands can be designed in this way.

In the field of GPCR pharmacology and drug discovery, the discovery of biased signaling has been an important development. Biased signaling describes the ability of ligands to act at the same GPCR and preferentially stabilize different conformational states to elicit distinct cellular and pharmacological outcomes (Christopoulos, 2014; Kenakin, 2005; Wootten, Christopoulos, Marti-Solano, Babu, & Sexton, 2018). In the context of GPCR drug discovery, this concept has opened the door for the design of drug-like compounds which are biased toward particular signaling outcomes at the exclusion of others. This will mean that ligands can be tailored to have improved activity and/or reduced risk for adverse effects. In this way, the application of photopharmacology may provide an interesting approach to improve our understanding of biased agonism and modulation at GPCRs in an *in vitro* and *in vivo* setting, and as a tool to implement desired biases in a reversible manner into candidate ligands for preclinical development. For instance, photoswitchable agonists or allosteric modulators may be developed to photoisomerize between forms that stabilize different conformational states of a receptor so that properties, including the kinetics of the ligand-receptor interaction (e.g., ligand-residency time), the signaling efficacy and/or the receptor trafficking can be altered. Following a thorough investigation into the spectrum of photoswitchable ligand effects under different light conditions, it may then be possible to build on structure-activity relationships (SAR) around GPCRs in conjunction with structural and modeling data.

Evidence for biased signaling of photoswitchable ligands at GPCRs is already emerging. Based on the glucagon-like peptide-1 receptor (GLP-1R) agonist liraglutide, Broichhagen, Damijonaitis, et al. (2015), Broichhagen, Frank, Johnston, et al. (2015), Broichhagen, Frank, and Trauner (2015), and Broichhagen, Podewin, et al. (2015) designed a photoswitchable incretin mimetic termed LirAzo (Broichhagen, Podewin, et al., 2015). In the *trans* configuration, LirAzo was suggested to preferentially facilitate calcium influx in pancreatic β-cells, while the *cis* isomer was suggested to preferentially promote cAMP production. The potential for light-sensitive bias of this compound for GLP-1R signaling translated to differential effects on glucose stimulated insulin secretion in pancreatic β-cells and in the ligand's ability to protect β-cells from glucolipotoxic insult (Broichhagen, Podewin, et al., 2015). In a follow-up study, the same group extended on this approach toward rationally designing GLP-1R photoswitchable PAMs, which demonstrated distinct binding kinetic and signaling profiles (Jones et al., 2017). This study provided the first evidence for GLP-1R PAMs to markedly augment agonist-residency times at their receptor, which may contribute to the underlying mechanism driving their potential for signaling bias and modulatory profiles, and it offers a novel therapeutic strategy for achieving sustained responses in vivo (Jones et al., 2017). Taken together, these studies demonstrate the potential for designing biased photoswitchable orthosteric and/or allosteric ligands to reveal the mechanisms underlying GPCR signaling bias and its (patho)physiological consequences.

Although exciting, these studies highlight the complexity of GPCR signaling and the necessity of testing putative photoswitchable ligands of GPCRs against multiple functional based assays, so that orthosteric- and allosteric-targeting ligand efficacy and/or allosteric modulation-induced biases of endogenous ligands can be assessed (Christopoulos, 2014). Furthermore, future studies that intend on assessing and quantifying bias profiles for photoswitchable ligands should ensure that they compare the profile of each ligand against a reference ligand and a reference pathway, since quantitative methods for measuring ligand efficacy can differ greatly depending on the context of the interaction, for example, cell background. For further advice on quantifying and understanding bias the reader is referred to other papers (Rajagopal et al., 2011; Wootten et al., 2018).

Adding further complexity to receptor pharmacology, allosteric interactions at GPCRs can also demonstrate another unique characteristic, which is related to biased agonism and modulation, termed *probe dependence* (Christopoulos, 2014; Kenakin, 2005). This phenomenon refers to how the magnitude and direction of an allosteric effect at a particular GPCR can change depending on the nature of the interacting orthosteric ligand. For instance, the muscarinic acetylcholine receptor (mAChR) allosteric ligand, LY2033298, has been shown to act as a PAM of acetylcholine function at the M_4 mAChR, but as a neutral allosteric ligand (NAL) when interacted with the inverse agonists, [^{3}H]*N*-methylscopolamine ([^{3}H]NMS) or [^{3}H]quinuclidinyl benzilate ([^{3}H]QNB) at the same receptor (Leach et al., 2010). This potential for probe-dependent effects may be of particular importance when attempting to appreciate the pharmacology of photoswitchable allosteric ligands. Since ligands of this type are usually designed to have different levels of activity in each photoisomeric form, it is conceivable that each photoisomer may demonstrate different types and levels of cooperativity with a variety of co-binding orthosteric probes at the same receptor. In this way, a PCL may photoswitch between PAM to NAL activity when co-bound with an endogenous ligand at a receptor, but NAM to PAM activity when interacted with a different orthosteric probe. The potential for probe-dependent effects of different photoisomers will make it possible to investigate multiple pharmacological effects within the same assay. This property also necessitates studies to thoroughly investigate the pharmacological profile of an allosteric PCL if it is intended to be interacted with multiple endogenous or synthetic orthosteric probes in vivo, prior to preclinical advancement.

When considering stimulus bias and probe-dependent effects, it is unsurprising that SAR of allosteric ligands for GPCRs tend to be shallow; with subtle changes in molecular structures resulting in substantial changes in activity (molecular switches) (Conn, Lindsley, Meiler, & Niswender, 2014;

Gregory & Conn, 2015; Lindsley, 2014). For this reason, the development and design of photoswitchable allosteric ligands may be particularly challenging, as the addition of a photoswitchable unit to an existing allosteric ligand may render it inactive or alter its pharmacological profile. Molecular switches of this type have been relatively well-documented, with very slight changes in structure leading to cooperativity switches at the receptor with the same interacting orthosteric probe (Wood, Hopkins, Brogan, Conn, & Lindsley, 2011). Indeed, this has allowed for the design of mGlu PAMs, NAMs and NALs to be generated all from the same parent scaffold (Wood et al., 2011). Similarly, the tendency for molecular switching could also be used for the development of improved photoswitchable modulators. For instance, alloswitch-1 was the first photoswitchable allosteric ligand to be described, which acts as a NAM at the mGlu5 (Pittolo et al., 2014). Intriguingly, alloswitch-1 was based on the scaffold of a potent mGlu4 PAM, but with the strategic addition of an azobenzene core its activity switched to negative cooperativity with glutamate at the mGlu5, and this NAM activity is reversibly controlled by irradiation with different wavelengths of light (Pittolo et al., 2014) (Fig. 3B). Furthermore, in a recent communication by Gomez-Santacana et al. (2018), photoswitchable orthosteric-targeting ligands for the chemokine receptor CXCR3 were rationally designed to have efficacy photoswitches in a [^{35}S]GTPγS binding assay. They showed that depending on the light condition, orthosteric-targeting small molecules could bind to the CXCR3 and demonstrate either full, partial or no agonism at the receptor (Gomez-Santacana et al., 2018). This study illustrates that not only allosteric PCLs, but also orthosteric PCLs can be designed to have subtle structural differences, which result in significant changes in pharmacological activity.

Further intricacy is added to GPCR photopharmacology with the prospect of photoswitchable ligands exhibiting species differences and/or activity differences at splice variants of GPCRs. These effects can occur as a result of changes in affinity for allosteric sites due to differences in receptor homology between species or as a product of changes in cooperativity (Leach et al., 2013; Suratman et al., 2011). Properties like these necessitate PCLs to be screened against receptors of different species and any splice variants that may exist for a receptor under different light conditions. This ensures that the appropriate preclinical model is chosen to test for in vivo efficacy, and informs research of any side-effects that may occur as a result of changed functional activity of a PCL at different polymorphisms of a receptor. It is anticipated that this would reduce the risk of drug failure during clinical progression.

Another interesting consideration for photoswitchable allosteric ligands is the concept of *lateral allostery*. Lateral allostery describes the effects of a ligand that are expressed along the plane of a cell membrane to other GPCRs or membrane proteins, and can lead to receptor dimerization or heterodimerization (Kenakin & Miller, 2010). In this way it is possible that a photoswitchable ligand can demonstrate differences in lateral allosteric effects in different isomeric forms, which could lead to changes in the way proteins interact with each other at the surface of a cell. This becomes particularly important when a target receptor dimerizes with different partners in different cell or tissue types. For example, mGlu2 and mGlu4 receptors are thought to form heterodimers and the interaction of allosteric- and orthosteric-targeting ligands at this heterodimer as compared to the mGlu4 homodimer have shown activity differences (Gonzalez-Maeso et al., 2008; Kammermeier, 2012; Yin et al., 2014). In this regard, it may be possible to design PCLs that have distinct selectivity profiles for dimers in each isomeric form. Certainly, the functional selectivity of some antipsychotics have already been linked with the existence of dimers (Brea et al., 2009; Maroteaux, Bechade, & Roumier, 2019).

Given the challenges that changes in cooperativity present in photoswitchable allosteric drug discovery programs and in the interpretation of SAR, there is a clear need for a multi-disciplinary approach toward identifying active and inactive photoswitchable allosteric ligands. To date, many drug discovery programs rely on the results of modulator potency curves in one signaling pathway and in the presence of a single agonist concentration, which may not be the endogenous ligand or may be one of multiple endogenous ligands for a receptor. As described earlier though, photoswitchable allosteric ligands may demonstrate signaling bias and/or probe dependence, which may lead to active ligands being overlooked in high throughput screens if they are not tested for under appropriate conditions. In the case of GPCRs with multiple endogenous ligands, if an allosteric PCL is selected for its envisioned PAM activity at a receptor but is only tested against one of the endogenous ligands, it may be found to have unexpected effects at the receptor due to uncharacterized cooperativity with a second ligand. Indeed, this is the case for the chemokine receptor type 5 allosteric modulator, aplaviroc, which demonstrates probe-dependent effects with the endogenous ligands of the receptor (Watson, Jenkinson, Kazmierski, & Kenakin, 2005). The use of potency curves in drug screens provides an overall measure of affinity, efficacy and cooperativity of a ligand, so any modifications made to a chemotype in order to understand the influence of a single parameter over the activity of the ligand will not be possible from a single potency readout of a compound. It is clear that more quantitative and qualitative analysis of photoswitchable allosteric ligand effects is necessary to understand how structures of photoswitchable ligands relate to their effects at a receptor under different light conditions.

Taken together, photopharmacological approaches offer the opportunity to better control, modulate and understand GPCR pharmacology in a more spatial and temporal manner than classical pharmacological approaches. However, given the complexity of GPCR pharmacology the development of photopharmacological tools, such as allosteric PCLs, are still subject to many of the same challenges that current approaches face when attempting to target GPCRs.

Despite these challenges, the use of photopharmacology is still in its infancy and many of its applications are yet to be realized. In studies investigating the biophysical properties of receptors the use of photocaged compounds and tethered ligand approaches could allow for the probing of receptor onset kinetics, with PTL and PORTL approaches allowing for the dynamic control of receptor activity without being impeded by issues including ligand diffusion (Leippe et al., 2017). In this way, photopharmacological approaches can mimic the time course of neurotransmitter release from the synaptic cleft and be amenable to studies where access to receptor populations is not as accessible for traditional pharmacological or electrophysical approaches, for example, at pre- or post-synaptic sites or subcellular compartments (Reiner & Levitz, 2018). This may help research to study receptors in a compartment-specific manner to provide information about the receptor trafficking and compartmentalization mechanisms of a receptor. It would also be possible to investigate the signaling of a target receptor in a graded manner by changing the light intensity and/or wavelength used to photoisomerize a PCL; potentially enabling researchers to test multiple pharmacological conditions in one experiment (Fig. 6).

Advantages of photopharmacological approaches to mimic the extent, direction and magnitude of endogenous effects in real-time, may also make them better suited to understanding physiological and behavioral changes in vivo. To date, applying allosteric PCLs to the environment of frog tadpoles or fish larvae modulates the swimming behaviors of these animals in a light-dependent manner (Gomez-Santacana et al., 2017; Pittolo et al., 2014; Rovira et al., 2016). The practicality of controlling neuromodulatory mechanisms in freely-moving rodents has also been demonstrated. As previously mentioned, photo-controllable ligands that target mGlu

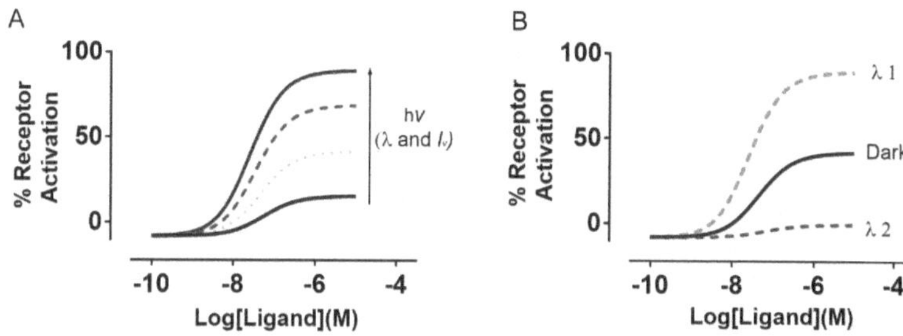

Fig. 6 (A) The signaling of a target receptor can be modulated in a graded manner by changing the light intensity and wavelength used to photoisomerize a PCL. (B) Different wavelengths of light can also result in distinctly different pharmacological effects such that many different conditions can be tested in the one assay in real-time and in a reversible manner.

receptors demonstrate analgesic activity both peripherally and centrally in mice, while photoswitchable analogues of Sphingosine-1-phosphate (S1P) can reversibly control S1P3-dependent hypersensitivity to pain of rodents (Font et al., 2017; Morstein et al., 2019; Zussy et al., 2018). The photocaged A_{2A} adenosine receptor antagonist, MRS7145, was also recently shown to demonstrate efficacy in reversing motor impairment in a preclinical model of Parkinson's disease (Taura et al., 2018).

These studies have demonstrated the potential benefit and feasibility of applying photopharmacological approaches in an in vivo setting and may pave the way for opportunities for innovation in light-regulated therapeutics. One major obstacle that may prevent photopharmacological methods from being translated into the clinic though, will be the ability to deliver light in a precise way to specific regions of the body. At present, preclinical studies have led to the design of devices that can deliver light with minimal damage to neural tissue while also being wireless, small in size, injectable and remotely controlled (Kim et al., 2013; Qazi et al., 2019; Shin et al., 2017). Some designs have also made it possible to control both drug delivery and the activity of light at a particular site of action through the use of optofluidic systems (Jeong et al., 2015). Moreover, the design of photoswitchable ligands that photoisomerize with the application of deep-tissue penetrating wavelengths, such as red or infrared light have now been synthesized, which may remove the need for more invasive approaches that require light emitting implants (Dong et al., 2015). Furthermore, in diseases that affect the skin, eyes and other tissues that are easily accessible by light photopharmacological approaches may find their greatest clinical utility without the need of more invasive approaches (Tochitsky, Trautman, Gallerani,

Malis, & Kramer, 2017). Given these advancements, it is likely that photopharmacological approaches will continue to find novel applications and offer new perspectives in understanding (patho)physiology to ultimately inform future GPCR drug discovery efforts.

6. Conclusion

The current state of the field of photopharmacology is rapidly advancing. The development of novel modalities of photoswitchable ligands and ways to implement them into and modulate biological systems is constantly adapting and improving. It is true that the application of photopharmacology in GPCR research offers the opportunity to better understand receptor pharmacology in a more spatial and temporal manner. However, the complexity of GPCR pharmacology means the development of photopharmacological tools, including allosteric PCLs, is likely to encounter many challenges that traditional pharmacological approaches experience when targeting GPCRs. Once well-understood, some characteristics currently posing challenges for research—such as changes in cooperativity—could be used to fine-tune the activity of photoswitchable allosteric ligands.

Acknowledgments

The authors thank Jack Delaney for critical reading of the manuscript. A.E.B. was supported by the Labex EpiGenMed (program « Investissements d'avenir » , ANR-10-LABX-12-01). C.G. was supported by grants from the Agence Nationale de la Recherche (ANR-16-CE16-0010-01 and ANR-17-NEU3-0001-01 under the frame of Neuron Cofund).

Conflict of interest

Authors declare no conflict of interest.

References

Acosta-Ruiz, A., Broichhagen, J., & Levitz, J. (2019). Optical regulation of class C GPCRs by photoswitchable orthogonal remotely tethered ligands. *Methods in Molecular Biology, 1947*, 103–136. https://doi.org/10.1007/978-1-4939-9121-1_6.

Acosta-Ruiz, A., Gutzeit, V. A., Skelly, M. J., Meadows, S., Lee, J., Parekh, P., et al. (2019). Branched photoswitchable tethered ligands enable ultra-efficient optical control and detection of G protein-coupled receptors in vivo. *Neuron*. https://doi.org/10.1016/j.neuron.2019.10.036.

Agnetta, L., Kauk, M., Canizal, M. C. A., Messerer, R., Holzgrabe, U., Hoffmann, C., et al. (2017). A photoswitchable dualsteric ligand controlling receptor efficacy. *Angewandte Chemie (International Ed. in English), 56*(25), 7282–7287. https://doi.org/10.1002/anie.201701524.

Banghart, M. R., & Trauner, D. (2013). A 1H NMR assay for measuring the photostationary states of photoswitchable ligands. *Methods in Molecular Biology*, *995*, 107–120. https://doi.org/10.1007/978-1-62703-345-9_8.

Beharry, A. A., & Woolley, G. A. (2011). Azobenzene photoswitches for biomolecules. *Chemical Society Reviews*, *40*(8), 4422–4437. https://doi.org/10.1039/c1cs15023e.

Boulegue, C., Loweneck, M., Renner, C., & Moroder, L. (2007). Redox potential of azobenzene as an amino acid residue in peptides. *Chembiochem*, *8*(6), 591–594. https://doi.org/10.1002/cbic.200600495.

Brea, J., Castro, M., Giraldo, J., Lopez-Gimenez, J. F., Padin, J. F., Quintian, F., et al. (2009). Evidence for distinct antagonist-revealed functional states of 5-hydroxytryptamine(2A) receptor homodimers. *Molecular Pharmacology*, *75*(6), 1380–1391. https://doi.org/10.1124/mol.108.054395.

Broichhagen, J., Damijonaitis, A., Levitz, J., Sokol, K. R., Leippe, P., Konrad, D., et al. (2015). Orthogonal optical control of a G protein-coupled receptor with a SNAP-tethered photochromic ligand. *ACS Central Science*, *1*(7), 383–393. https://doi.org/10.1021/acscentsci.5b00260.

Broichhagen, J., Frank, J. A., Johnston, N. R., Mitchell, R. K., Smid, K., Marchetti, P., et al. (2015). A red-shifted photochromic sulfonylurea for the remote control of pancreatic beta cell function. *Chemical Communications (Cambridge, England)*, *51*(27), 6018–6021. https://doi.org/10.1039/c5cc01224d.

Broichhagen, J., Frank, J. A., & Trauner, D. (2015). A roadmap to success in photopharmacology. *Accounts of Chemical Research*, *48*(7), 1947–1960. https://doi.org/10.1021/acs.accounts.5b00129.

Broichhagen, J., Johnston, N. R., von Ohlen, Y., Meyer-Berg, H., Jones, B. J., Bloom, S. R., et al. (2016). Allosteric optical control of a class B G-protein-coupled receptor. *Angewandte Chemie (International Ed. in English)*, *55*(19), 5865–5868. https://doi.org/10.1002/anie.201600957.

Broichhagen, J., Podewin, T., Meyer-Berg, H., von Ohlen, Y., Johnston, N. R., Jones, B. J., et al. (2015). Optical control of insulin secretion using an incretin switch. *Angewandte Chemie (International Ed. in English)*, *54*(51), 15565–15569. https://doi.org/10.1002/anie.201506384.

Broichhagen, J., & Trauner, D. (2014). The in vivo chemistry of photoswitched tethered ligands. *Current Opinion in Chemical Biology*, *21*, 121–127. https://doi.org/10.1016/j.cbpa.2014.07.008.

Brown, M. A., & De Vito, S. C. (1993). Predicting azo dye toxicity. *Critical Reviews in Environmental Science and Technology*, *23*(3), 249–324. https://doi.org/10.1080/10643389309388453.

Cabre, G., Garrido-Charles, A., Gonzalez-Lafont, A., Moormann, W., Langbehn, D., Egea, D., et al. (2019). Synthetic photoswitchable neurotransmitters based on bridged azobenzenes. *Organic Letters*, *21*(10), 3780–3784. https://doi.org/10.1021/acs.orglett.9b01222.

Callaway, E. M., & Katz, L. C. (1993). Photostimulation using caged glutamate reveals functional circuitry in living brain slices. *Proceedings of the National Academy of Sciences of the United States of America*, *90*(16), 7661–7665. https://doi.org/10.1073/pnas.90.16.7661.

Carroll, E. C., Berlin, S., Levitz, J., Kienzler, M. A., Yuan, Z., Madsen, D., et al. (2015). Two-photon brightness of azobenzene photoswitches designed for glutamate receptor optogenetics. *Proceedings of the National Academy of Sciences of the United States of America*, *112*(7), E776–E785. https://doi.org/10.1073/pnas.1416942112.

Cheng, B., Shchepakin, D., Kavanaugh, M. P., & Trauner, D. (2017). Photoswitchable inhibitor of a glutamate transporter. *ACS Chemical Neuroscience*, *8*(8), 1668–1672. https://doi.org/10.1021/acschemneuro.7b00072.

Chilakamarthi, U., & Giribabu, L. (2017). Photodynamic therapy: Past, present and future. *Chemical Record, 17*(8), 775–802. https://doi.org/10.1002/tcr.201600121.

Christopoulos, A. (2014). Advances in G protein-coupled receptor allostery: From function to structure. *Molecular Pharmacology, 86*(5), 463–478. https://doi.org/10.1124/mol.114.094342.

Conn, P. J., Lindsley, C. W., Meiler, J., & Niswender, C. M. (2014). Opportunities and challenges in the discovery of allosteric modulators of GPCRs for treating CNS disorders. *Nature Reviews. Drug Discovery, 13*(9), 692–708. https://doi.org/10.1038/nrd4308.

Damijonaitis, A., Broichhagen, J., Urushima, T., Hull, K., Nagpal, J., Laprell, L., et al. (2015). AzoCholine enables optical control of alpha 7 nicotinic acetylcholine receptors in neural networks. *ACS Chemical Neuroscience, 6*(5), 701–707. https://doi.org/10.1021/acschemneuro.5b00030.

Deiters, A. (2010). Principles and applications of the photochemical control of cellular processes. *Chembiochem, 11*(1), 47–53. https://doi.org/10.1002/cbic.200900529.

Dong, M., Babalhavaeji, A., Samanta, S., Beharry, A. A., & Woolley, G. A. (2015). Red-shifting azobenzene photoswitches for in vivo use. *Accounts of Chemical Research, 48*(10), 2662–2670. https://doi.org/10.1021/acs.accounts.5b00270.

Donthamsetti, P. C., Broichhagen, J., Vyklicky, V., Stanley, C., Fu, Z., Visel, M., et al. (2019). Genetically targeted optical control of an endogenous G protein-coupled receptor. *Journal of the American Chemical Society, 141*(29), 11522–11530. https://doi.org/10.1021/jacs.9b02895.

Donthamsetti, P. C., Winter, N., Schonberger, M., Levitz, J., Stanley, C., Javitch, J. A., et al. (2017). Optical control of dopamine receptors using a photoswitchable tethered inverse agonist. *Journal of the American Chemical Society, 139*(51), 18522–18535. https://doi.org/10.1021/jacs.7b07659.

Farrants, H., Gutzeit, V. A., Acosta-Ruiz, A., Trauner, D., Johnsson, K., Levitz, J., et al. (2018). SNAP-tagged nanobodies enable reversible optical control of a G protein-coupled receptor via a remotely tethered photoswitchable ligand. *ACS Chemical Biology, 13*(9), 2682–2688. https://doi.org/10.1021/acschembio.8b00628.

Font, J., Lopez-Cano, M., Notartomaso, S., Scarselli, P., Di Pietro, P., Bresolí-Obach, R., et al. (2017). Optical control of pain in vivo with a photoactive mGlu5 receptor negative allosteric modulator. *eLife, 6*. https://doi.org/10.7554/eLife.23545.

Gomez-Santacana, X., de Munnik, S. M., Vijayachandran, P., Da Costa Pereira, D., Bebelman, J. P. M., de Esch, I. J. P., et al. (2018). Photoswitching the efficacy of a small-molecule ligand for a peptidergic GPCR: From antagonism to agonism. *Angewandte Chemie (International Ed. in English), 57*(36), 11608–11612. https://doi.org/10.1002/anie.201804875.

Gomez-Santacana, X., Pittolo, S., Rovira, X., Lopez, M., Zussy, C., Dalton, J. A., et al. (2017). Illuminating phenylazopyridines to photoswitch metabotropic glutamate receptors: From the flask to the animals. *ACS Central Science, 3*(1), 81–91. https://doi.org/10.1021/acscentsci.6b00353.

Gonzalez-Maeso, J., Ang, R. L., Yuen, T., Chan, P., Weisstaub, N. V., Lopez-Gimenez, J. F., et al. (2008). Identification of a serotonin/glutamate receptor complex implicated in psychosis. *Nature, 452*(7183), 93–97. https://doi.org/10.1038/nature06612.

Gregory, K. J., & Conn, P. J. (2015). Molecular insights into metabotropic glutamate receptor allosteric modulation. *Molecular Pharmacology, 88*(1), 188–202. https://doi.org/10.1124/mol.114.097220.

Habermacher, C., Martz, A., Calimet, N., Lemoine, D., Peverini, L., Specht, A., et al. (2016). Photo-switchable tweezers illuminate pore-opening motions of an ATP-gated P2X ion channel. *eLife, 5*, e11050. https://doi.org/10.7554/eLife.11050.

Hauser, A. S., Attwood, M. M., Rask-Andersen, M., Schioth, H. B., & Gloriam, D. E. (2017). Trends in GPCR drug discovery: New agents, targets and indications. *Nature Reviews Drug Discovery*, *16*(12), 829–842. https://doi.org/10.1038/nrd.2017.178.

Hauwert, N. J., Mocking, T. A. M., Da Costa Pereira, D., Kooistra, A. J., Wijnen, L. M., Vreeker, G. C. M., et al. (2018). Synthesis and characterization of a bidirectional photoswitchable antagonist toolbox for real-time GPCR photopharmacology. *Journal of the American Chemical Society*, *140*(12), 4232–4243. https://doi.org/10.1021/jacs.7b11422.

Hauwert, N. J., Mocking, T. A. M., Da Costa Pereira, D., Lion, K., Huppelschoten, Y., Vischer, H. F., et al. (2019). A photoswitchable agonist for the histamine H3 receptor, a prototypic family a G-protein-coupled receptor. *Angewandte Chemie (International Ed. in English)*, *58*(14), 4531–4535. https://doi.org/10.1002/anie.201813110.

Hermanson, G. T. (2013). Chapter 1—Introduction to bioconjugation. In G. T. Hermanson (Ed.), *Bioconjugate techniques* (4th ed., pp. 1–125). Boston: Academic Press.

Hull, K., Morstein, J., & Trauner, D. (2018). In vivo photopharmacology. *Chemical Reviews*, *118*(21), 10710–10747. https://doi.org/10.1021/acs.chemrev.8b00037.

Jeong, J. W., McCall, J. G., Shin, G., Zhang, Y., Al-Hasani, R., Kim, M., et al. (2015). Wireless optofluidic systems for programmable in vivo pharmacology and optogenetics. *Cell*, *162*(3), 662–674. https://doi.org/10.1016/j.cell.2015.06.058.

Jones, B. J., Scopelliti, R., Tomas, A., Bloom, S. R., Hodson, D. J., & Broichhagen, J. (2017). Potent prearranged positive allosteric modulators of the glucagon-like peptide-1 receptor. *Chemistry Open*, *6*(4), 501–505. https://doi.org/10.1002/open.201700062.

Kammermeier, P. J. (2012). Functional and pharmacological characteristics of metabotropic glutamate receptors 2/4 heterodimers. *Molecular Pharmacology*, *82*(3), 438–447. https://doi.org/10.1124/mol.112.078501.

Kaplan, J. H., Forbush, B., 3rd, & Hoffman, J. F. (1978). Rapid photolytic release of adenosine 5′-triphosphate from a protected analogue: Utilization by the Na:K pump of human red blood cell ghosts. *Biochemistry*, *17*(10), 1929–1935. https://doi.org/10.1021/bi00603a020.

Kenakin, T. (2005). New concepts in drug discovery: Collateral efficacy and permissive antagonism. *Nature Reviews. Drug Discovery*, *4*(11), 919–927. https://doi.org/10.1038/nrd1875.

Kenakin, T., & Miller, L. J. (2010). Seven transmembrane receptors as shapeshifting proteins: The impact of allosteric modulation and functional selectivity on new drug discovery. *Pharmacological Reviews*, *62*(2), 265–304. https://doi.org/10.1124/pr.108.000992.

Kim, T. I., McCall, J. G., Jung, Y. H., Huang, X., Siuda, E. R., Li, Y., et al. (2013). Injectable, cellular-scale optoelectronics with applications for wireless optogenetics. *Science*, *340*(6129), 211–216. https://doi.org/10.1126/science.1232437.

Klippenstein, V., Ghisi, V., Wietstruk, M., & Plested, A. J. (2014). Photoinactivation of glutamate receptors by genetically encoded unnatural amino acids. *The Journal of Neuroscience*, *34*(3), 980–991. https://doi.org/10.1523/jneurosci.3725-13.2014.

Lagerstrom, M. C., & Schioth, H. B. (2008). Structural diversity of G protein-coupled receptors and significance for drug discovery. *Nature Reviews Drug Discovery*, 7(4), 339–357. https://doi.org/10.1038/nrd2518.

Leach, K., Loiacono, R. E., Felder, C. C., McKinzie, D. L., Mogg, A., Shaw, D. B., et al. (2010). Molecular mechanisms of action and in vivo validation of an M4 muscarinic acetylcholine receptor allosteric modulator with potential antipsychotic properties. *Neuropsychopharmacology*, *35*(4), 855–869. https://doi.org/10.1038/npp.2009.194.

Leach, K., Wen, A., Cook, A. E., Sexton, P. M., Conigrave, A. D., & Christopoulos, A. (2013). Impact of clinically relevant mutations on the pharmacoregulation and signaling bias of the calcium-sensing receptor by positive and negative allosteric modulators. *Endocrinology*, *154*(3), 1105–1116. https://doi.org/10.1210/en.2012-1887.

Leippe, P., Koehler Leman, J., & Trauner, D. (2017). Specificity and speed: Tethered photopharmacology. *ACS Central Science*, *56*(39), 5214–5220. https://doi.org/10.1021/acs.biochem.7b00687.

Levitz, J., Pantoja, C., Gaub, B., Janovjak, H., Reiner, A., Hoagland, A., et al. (2013). Optical control of metabotropic glutamate receptors. *Nature Neuroscience*, *16*(4), 507–516. https://doi.org/10.1038/nn.3346.

Lindsley, C. W. (2014). 2013 Philip S. Portoghese medicinal chemistry lectureship: Drug discovery targeting allosteric sites. *Journal of Medicinal Chemistry*, *57*(18), 7485–7498. https://doi.org/10.1021/jm5011786.

Liu, D., Xie, Y., Shao, H., & Jiang, X. (2009). Using azobenzene-embedded self-assembled monolayers to photochemically control cell adhesion reversibly. *Angewandte Chemie (International Ed. in English)*, *48*(24), 4406–4408. https://doi.org/10.1002/anie.200901130.

Lopez-Cano, M., Font, J., Llebaria, A., Fernandez-Duenas, V., & Ciruela, F. (2019). Optical modulation of metabotropic glutamate receptor type 5 in vivo using a photoactive drug. *Methods in Molecular Biology*, *1947*, 351–359. https://doi.org/10.1007/978-1-4939-9121-1_20.

Maroteaux, L., Bechade, C., & Roumier, A. (2019). Dimers of serotonin receptors: Impact on ligand affinity and signaling. *Biochimie*, *161*, 23–33. https://doi.org/10.1016/j.biochi.2019.01.009.

McGirt, L. Y., Vasagar, K., Gober, L. M., Saini, S. S., & Beck, L. A. (2006). Successful treatment of recalcitrant chronic idiopathic urticaria with sulfasalazine. *Archives of Dermatology*, *142*(10), 1337–1342. https://doi.org/10.1001/archderm.142.10.1337.

Mehta, Z. B., Johnston, N. R., Nguyen-Tu, M. S., Broichhagen, J., Schultz, P., Larner, D. P., et al. (2017). Remote control of glucose homeostasis in vivo using photopharmacology. *Scientific Reports*, 7(1), 291. https://doi.org/10.1038/s41598-017-00397-0.

Morstein, J., Hill, R. Z., Novak, A. J. E., Feng, S., Norman, D. D., Donthamsetti, P. C., et al. (2019). Optical control of sphingosine-1-phosphate formation and function. *Nature Chemical Biology*, *15*(6), 623–631. https://doi.org/10.1038/s41589-019-0269-7.

Noren, C. J., Anthony-Cahill, S. J., Griffith, M. C., & Schultz, P. G. (1989). A general method for site-specific incorporation of unnatural amino acids into proteins. *Science*, *244*(4901), 182–188. https://doi.org/10.1126/science.2649980.

Overington, J. P., Al-Lazikani, B., & Hopkins, A. L. (2006). How many drug targets are there? *Nature Reviews Drug Discovery*, *5*(12), 993–996. https://doi.org/10.1038/nrd2199.

Pittolo, S., Gomez-Santacana, X., Eckelt, K., Rovira, X., Dalton, J., Goudet, C., et al. (2014). An allosteric modulator to control endogenous G protein-coupled receptors with light. *Nature Chemical Biology*, *10*(10), 813–815. https://doi.org/10.1038/nchembio.1612.

Qazi, R., Gomez, A. M., Castro, D. C., Zou, Z., Sim, J. Y., Xiong, Y., et al. (2019). Wireless optofluidic brain probes for chronic neuropharmacology and photostimulation. *Nature Biomedical Engineering*, *3*(8), 655–669. https://doi.org/10.1038/s41551-019-0432-1.

Rajagopal, S., Ahn, S., Rominger, D. H., Gowen-MacDonald, W., Lam, C. M., Dewire, S. M., et al. (2011). Quantifying ligand bias at seven-transmembrane receptors. *Molecular Pharmacology*, *80*(3), 367–377. https://doi.org/10.1124/mol.111.072801.

Rastogi, S. K., Zhao, Z., Barrett, S. L., Shelton, S. D., Zafferani, M., Anderson, H. E., et al. (2018). Photoresponsive azo-combretastatin A-4 analogues. *European Journal of Medicinal Chemistry*, *143*, 1–7. https://doi.org/10.1016/j.ejmech.2017.11.012.

Reiner, A., & Levitz, J. (2018). Glutamatergic signaling in the central nervous system: Ionotropic and metabotropic receptors in concert. *Neuron*, *98*(6), 1080–1098. https://doi.org/10.1016/j.neuron.2018.05.018.

Renner, C., & Moroder, L. (2006). Azobenzene as conformational switch in model peptides. *Chembiochem*, 7(6), 868–878. https://doi.org/10.1002/cbic.200500531.

Ricart-Ortega, M., Font, J., & Llebaria, A. (2019). GPCR photopharmacology. *Molecular and Cellular Endocrinology, 488*, 36–51. https://doi.org/10.1016/j.mce.2019.03.003.

Rovira, X., Trapero, A., Pittolo, S., Zussy, C., Faucherre, A., Jopling, C., et al. (2016). OptoGluNAM4.1, a photoswitchable allosteric antagonist for real-time control of mGlu4 receptor activity. *Cell Chemical Biology, 23*(8), 929–934. https://doi.org/10.1016/j.chembiol.2016.06.013.

Samanta, S., Beharry, A. A., Sadovski, O., McCormick, T. M., Babalhavaeji, A., Tropepe, V., et al. (2013). Photoswitching azo compounds in vivo with red light. *Journal of the American Chemical Society, 135*(26), 9777–9784. https://doi.org/10.1021/ja402220t.

Schonberger, M., & Trauner, D. (2014). A photochromic agonist for mu-opioid receptors. *Angewandte Chemie (International Ed. in English), 53*(12), 3264–3267. https://doi.org/10.1002/anie.201309633.

Shin, G., Gomez, A. M., Al-Hasani, R., Jeong, Y. R., Kim, J., Xie, Z., et al. (2017). Flexible near-field wireless optoelectronics as subdermal implants for broad applications in optogenetics. *Neuron, 93*(3). https://doi.org/10.1016/j.neuron.2016.12.031, 509–521. e503.

Siewertsen, R., Neumann, H., Buchheim-Stehn, B., Herges, R., Nather, C., Renth, F., et al. (2009). Highly efficient reversible Z-E photoisomerization of a bridged azobenzene with visible light through resolved S(1)(n pi*) absorption bands. *Journal of the American Chemical Society, 131*(43), 15594–15595. https://doi.org/10.1021/ja906547d.

Siewertsen, R., Schonborn, J. B., Hartke, B., Renth, F., & Temps, F. (2011). Superior Z--> E and E-->Z photoswitching dynamics of dihydrodibenzodiazocine, a bridged azobenzene, by S1(npi*) excitation at lambda = 387 and 490 nm. *Physical Chemistry Chemical Physics, 13*(3), 1054–1063. https://doi.org/10.1039/c0cp01148g.

Suratman, S., Leach, K., Sexton, P., Felder, C., Loiacono, R., & Christopoulos, A. (2011). Impact of species variability and 'probe-dependence' on the detection and in vivo validation of allosteric modulation at the M4 muscarinic acetylcholine receptor. *British Journal of Pharmacology, 162*(7), 1659–1670. https://doi.org/10.1111/j.1476-5381.2010.01184.x.

Szymanski, W., Wu, B., Poloni, C., Janssen, D. B., & Feringa, B. L. (2013). Azobenzene photoswitches for Staudinger-Bertozzi ligation. *Angewandte Chemie (International Ed. in English), 52*(7), 2068–2072. https://doi.org/10.1002/anie.201208596.

Taura, J., Nolen, E. G., Cabre, G., Hernando, J., Squarcialupi, L., Lopez-Cano, M., et al. (2018). Remote control of movement disorders using a photoactive adenosine A2A receptor antagonist. *Journal of Controlled Release, 283*, 135–142. https://doi.org/10.1016/j.jconrel.2018.05.033.

Thapaliya, E. R., Zhao, J., & Ellis-Davies, G. C. R. (2019). Locked-azobenzene: Testing the scope of a unique photoswitchable scaffold for cell physiology. *ACS Chemical Neuroscience, 10*(5), 2481–2488. https://doi.org/10.1021/acschemneuro.8b00734.

Tochitsky, I., Trautman, J., Gallerani, N., Malis, J. G., & Kramer, R. H. (2017). Restoring visual function to the blind retina with a potent, safe and long-lasting photoswitch. *Scientific Reports*, 7, 45487. https://doi.org/10.1038/srep45487.

Trads, J., Hull, K., Matsuura, B. S., Laprell, L., Fehrentz, T., Gorldt, N., et al. (2019). Sign inversion in photopharmacology: Incorporation of cyclic azobenzenes in photoswitchable potassium channel blockers and openers. *Angewandte Chemie (International ed. in English), 58*(43), 15421–15428. https://doi.org/10.1002/anie.201905790.

Tsai, Y. H., Essig, S., James, J. R., Lang, K., & Chin, J. W. (2015). Selective, rapid and optically switchable regulation of protein function in live mammalian cells. *Nature Chemistry*, 7(7), 554–561. https://doi.org/10.1038/nchem.2253.

Velema, W. A., Szymanski, W., & Feringa, B. L. (2014). Photopharmacology: Beyond proof of principle. *Journal of the American Chemical Society*, *136*(6), 2178–2191. https://doi.org/10.1021/ja413063e.

Wagner, N., Schuhmacher, M., Lohmann, A., & Nadler, A. (2019). A coumarin triflate reagent enables one-step synthesis of photo-caged lipid metabolites for studying cell signaling. *Chemistry—A European Journal*, *25*(68), 15483–15487. https://doi.org/10.1002/chem.201903909.

Warther, D., Gug, S., Specht, A., Bolze, F., Nicoud, J. F., Mourot, A., et al. (2010). Two-photon uncaging: New prospects in neuroscience and cellular biology. *Bioorganic & Medicinal Chemistry*, *18*(22), 7753–7758. https://doi.org/10.1016/j.bmc.2010.04.084.

Watson, C., Jenkinson, S., Kazmierski, W., & Kenakin, T. (2005). The CCR5 receptor-based mechanism of action of 873140, a potent allosteric noncompetitive HIV entry inhibitor. *Molecular Pharmacology*, *67*(4), 1268–1282. https://doi.org/10.1124/mol.104.008565.

Westphal, M. V., Schafroth, M. A., Sarott, R. C., Imhof, M. A., Bold, C. P., Leippe, P., et al. (2017). Synthesis of photoswitchable delta(9)-tetrahydrocannabinol derivatives enables optical control of cannabinoid receptor 1 signaling. *Journal of the American Chemical Society*, *139*(50), 18206–18212. https://doi.org/10.1021/jacs.7b06456.

Wood, M. R., Hopkins, C. R., Brogan, J. T., Conn, P. J., & Lindsley, C. W. (2011). "Molecular switches" on mGluR allosteric ligands that modulate modes of pharmacology. *Biochemistry*, *50*(13), 2403–2410. https://doi.org/10.1021/bi200129s.

Wootten, D., Christopoulos, A., Marti-Solano, M., Babu, M. M., & Sexton, P. M. (2018). Mechanisms of signalling and biased agonism in G protein-coupled receptors. *Nature Reviews. Molecular Cell Biology*, *19*(10), 638–653. https://doi.org/10.1038/s41580-018-0049-3.

Yin, S., Noetzel, M. J., Johnson, K. A., Zamorano, R., Jalan-Sakrikar, N., Gregory, K. J., et al. (2014). Selective actions of novel allosteric modulators reveal functional heteromers of metabotropic glutamate receptors in the CNS. *The Journal of Neuroscience*, *34*(1), 79–94. https://doi.org/10.1523/jneurosci.1129-13.2014.

Zbaida, S. (1995). The mechanism of microsomal azoreduction: Predictions based on electronic aspects of structure-activity relationships. *Drug Metabolism Reviews*, *27*(3), 497–516. https://doi.org/10.3109/03602539508998333.

Zussy, C., Gomez-Santacana, X., Rovira, X., De Bundel, D., Ferrazzo, S., Bosch, D., et al. (2018). Dynamic modulation of inflammatory pain-related affective and sensory symptoms by optical control of amygdala metabotropic glutamate receptor 4. *Molecular Psychiatry*, *23*(3), 509–520. https://doi.org/10.1038/mp.2016.223.

Further reading

Agostinis, P., Berg, K., Cengel, K. A., Foster, T. H., Girotti, A. W., Gollnick, S. O., et al. (2011). Photodynamic therapy of cancer: An update. *CA: A Cancer Journal for Clinicians*, *61*(4), 250–281. https://doi.org/10.3322/caac.20114.

CHAPTER SEVEN

Discovery and pharmacology of the covalent GLP-1 receptor (GLP-1R) allosteric modulator BETP: A novel tool to probe GLP-1R pharmacology

Francis S. Willard[a,*], Joseph D. Ho[b], Kyle W. Sloop[c]
[a]Quantitative Biology, Lilly Research Laboratories, Indianapolis, IN, United States
[b]Lilly Biotechnology Center, San Diego, CA, United States
[c]Diabetes and Complications, Lilly Research Laboratories, Indianapolis, IN, United States
[*]Corresponding author: e-mail address: willardfs@lilly.com

Contents

Abstract

The glucagon-like peptide-1 receptor (GLP-1R) is a significant therapeutic target for small molecule drug discovery given the therapeutic impact of peptide agonists in the diabetes sphere. We review the discovery and subsequent characterization of the small molecule GLP-1R allosteric modulator 4-(3-(Benzyloxy)phenyl)-2-(ethylsulfinyl)-6-(trifluoromethyl)pyrimidine (BETP). BETP is a covalent modulator of the GLP-1R, and we discuss the pharmacological implications and possible structural basis of this novel mode of action. We highlight the insights into class B G-protein coupled receptor pharmacology and biology provided by studies conducted with BETP. These include the descriptions of exquisite allosteric modulator probe dependence and biased signaling *in vitro* and *in vivo*. We conclude with an analysis of the utility of BETP as a chemical probe for the GLP-1R.

Advances in Pharmacology, Volume 88
ISSN 1054-3589
https://doi.org/10.1016/bs.apha.2020.02.001

Abbreviations

α	allosteric affinity cooperativity factor
β	allosteric efficacy cooperativity factor
BETP	4-(3-(benzyloxy)phenyl)-2-(ethylsulfinyl)-6-(trifluoromethyl)pyrimidine
cAMP	3′,5′-cyclic adenosine monophosphate
ECD	extracellular domain
GCGR	glucagon receptor
GLP-1	glucagon-like peptide 1
GLP-1R	glucagon-like peptide 1 receptor
GLP-2R	glucagon-like peptide 2 receptor
GIPR	glucose-dependent insulinotropic peptide receptor
GPCR	G-protein coupled receptor
IVGTT	intravenous glucose tolerance test
SAR	structure activity relationship

1. Introduction

Peptide hormones mediate organ-to-organ communication to help maintain metabolic homeostasis. These factors are released from cells of origin and travel *via* the circulation to distant target sites where they interact with surface membrane receptors to elicit biological responses through signal transduction systems. The class B G-protein coupled receptors (GPCRs) are a major family of receptors that bind peptide hormones to mediate control of many physiological processes, including regulating growth, managing the stress response, and controlling glucose metabolism and energy balance (Hoare, 2005). Similar to other types of GPCRs, these receptors contain seven transmembrane-spanning α-helices connected by intracellular and extracellular loops and a cytoplasmically located C-terminus.

The distinguishing feature of class B receptors is a large N-terminal extracellular ectodomain (ECD) that is at least 100 amino acids in length for all 15 members of the receptor family (Zhao et al., 2016). The ECDs are globular structures forming tri-layer α-β-βα protein folds that are stabilized by three pairs of disulfide bonds formed between six conserved cysteine residues. The disulfide bonds lock the ECD layers into conformations that enable use of these domains as "affinity traps" to recognize and bind cognate peptide ligands for the various receptors. Subsequent interactions between a docked ligand and the helical bundle of the receptor core occur to promote movement of the transmembrane helices that allow interaction with G-protein to induce signaling. Overall, the receptor activation mechanisms for class B GPCRs requires the peptide hormones to make many high-affinity contacts with the receptor over large interaction surfaces (Bortolato et al., 2014).

The glucagon-like peptide-1 receptor (GLP-1R) is one of the preeminent class B GPCRs as both its physiologic control of insulin secretion and its ligand binding-receptor interactions using structural biology have been well-studied, and there are several GLP-1R agonists registered for treating type 2 diabetes mellitus (Jazayeri et al., 2017; Liang et al., 2018; Sloop, Emmerson, Statnick, & Willard, 2018; Song et al., 2017; Zhang et al., 2017). These drugs improve glycemic control, reduce body weight, and some have been shown to provide cardiovascular health benefits (Gerstein et al., 2019; Hernandez et al., 2018; Marso, Bain, et al., 2016; Marso, Daniels, et al., 2016). All of these medicines are peptide-based, therefore requiring subcutaneous injection, but the therapeutic success of GLP-1R agonists justifies investigating additional therapeutic modalities targeting this receptor. These include parenterally administered multi-functional agents (peptide-based GLP-1R agonists that also activate other receptors) and orally bioavailable non-peptide agonists or positive allosteric modulators that may enhance the actions of endogenous GLP-1R ligands (Mendez et al., 2019; Willard, Briere, & Sloop, 2018).

2. The history of small molecule drug discovery at the GLP-1R

The human GLP-1R cDNA was cloned in 1992 leading to the ability to generate cell lines heterologously expressing GLP-1R and allowing the pharmacology of peptide ligands to be determined unambiguously (Graziano, Hey, Borkowski, Chicchi, & Strader, 1993; Thorens, 1992). In this era, the ligand identification strategies used by the pharmaceutical industry were primarily rational design, natural products, and low capacity small molecule screening. At this period of time in the industry, high throughput screening (HTS) was in its infancy (Sittampalam, Kahl, & Janzen, 1997). While not well documented, it is generally accepted that over the two decades following isolation of the GLP-1R DNA sequence, many pharmaceutical companies conducted extensive screening campaigns to find small molecule GLP-1R agonists but met with little success.

The first real indication of pharmacologically useful compounds came with the publication of patent and primary literature by Pfizer and Novo Nordisk (Knudsen et al., 2007) on a series of quinoxalines as exemplified

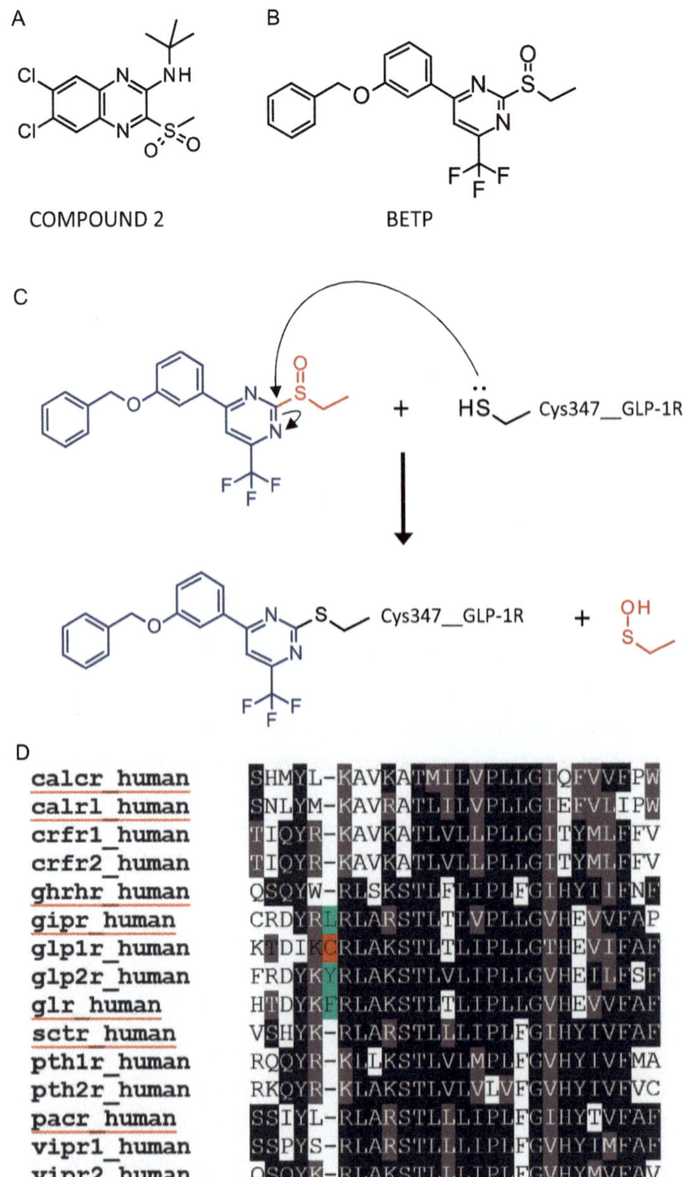

Fig. 1 (A) The chemical structure of the quinoxaline Compound 2. (B) The chemical structure of BETP, 4-(3-(*B*enzyloxy)phenyl)-2-(*e*thylsulfinyl)-6-(*t*rifluoromethyl)*p*yrimidine. (C) A hypothetical reaction mechanism for BETP modification of Cysteine347 on the GLP-1R. This nucleophilic substitution mechanism was proposed for BETP reaction with Glutathione and is supported by mass-spectrometry (Eng et al., 2013). (D) Multiple sequence alignment of the N-terminal portion of transmembrane helix 6 from class B GPCRs. The structure-based multiple sequence alignment was constructed using the GPCRdb (Isberg et al., 2015; Pandy-Szekeres et al., 2018) and then manually optimized and plotted using Clustal and BoxShade (Thompson, Higgins, & Gibson, 1994). A single amino acid insertion has occurred within the glucagon receptor sub-family colored red for GLP-1R and blue for GCGR, GIPR, and GLP-2R sequences.

by Compound 2 (Fig. 1A). Approximately 250,000 compounds were screened for cAMP accumulation in a human GLP-1R expressing cell line to identify the quinazoline scaffold. These molecules demonstrated moderate *in vitro* potency as GLP-1R agonists, with exquisite selectivity against related receptors, and these molecules caused glucose-dependent insulin secretion in mouse islets in a GLP-1R genotype dependent manner (Knudsen et al., 2007). Mechanistic experiments indicated these compounds were allosteric modulators in that they did not compete with peptide ligands for GLP-1R binding (Knudsen et al., 2007). An extensive structure activity relationship (SAR) review was published for these compounds (Teng et al., 2007). It was noted that the compounds were chemically unstable in the presence of nucleophiles and the SAR was strictly dependent on the presence of a sulfone or sulfoxide. Simultaneously, a group at the National Center for Drug Screening in Shanghai discovered the substituted cyclobutane Boc-5 as a non-peptidic GLP-1R agonist after testing 50,000 natural and synthetic compounds in a cAMP response element driven luciferase reporter assay (Chen et al., 2007). The 1076 g/mol Boc-5 compound was formed by *in vitro* dimerization of a smaller molecule in DMSO stocks of compounds. Boc-5 is also a highly GLP-1R selective compound with apparent *in vivo* activity in rodent models. Unfortunately, neither the quinoxalines or Boc-5 appeared to be synthetically tractable or sufficiently drug-like to enable lead optimization and advancement to the clinic (Willard, Bueno, & Sloop, 2012). However, as is common in scientific research, it is likely that these seminal papers on quinoxalines and Boc-5 in concert with the clinical success of the peptide-based GLP-1R agonist exenatide (DeFronzo et al., 2005), in parallel with improved technologies for drug discovery, reinvigorated researchers to search for small molecule GLP-1R ligands (Willard, Bueno, & Sloop, 2012). Therefore, the importance of these initial works cannot be overstated in that they have led to a renewed interest in the discovery of small molecule GLP-1R ligands. We consider novel GLP-1R agonists to be outside the scope of this review and instead will focus on how allosteric GLP-1R probes/tool compounds such as BETP have allowed both industry and academia to generate new pharmacology and biology and advance the field of GLP-1R and class B GPCR allosteric modulator research.

3. Research to probe GLP-1R allosteric modulation

Researchers at the Monash Institute of Pharmaceutical Sciences paved the way for using tool compounds such as Compound 2 to probe the allosteric pharmacology of the GLP-1R, illuminating the novel pharmacology of class B GPCRs (Koole et al., 2010; Wootten et al., 2011). Using Compound 2 and a series of flavonoids, key aspects of the class B allosteric ligand pharmacology were elucidated (Koole et al., 2010). Compound 2 was shown to be highly probe-dependent in that it modulated signaling of some GLP-1R peptidergic ligands but not others. For instance, Compound 2 demonstrated high levels of functional cooperativity with oxyntomodulin but essentially neutral cooperativity with exendin-4 for $G\alpha_s$ signaling to cAMP generation. Similarly, the flavonoid quercetin displayed positive cooperativity for GLP-1(7-36) and exendin-4 stimulation of intracellular Ca^{2+} mobilization with no effect on oxyntomodulin. These studies were essential in translating analytical pharmacological methods previously used with class A and class C GPCRs into use for Class B GPCRs (Koole et al., 2010; Leach, Sexton, & Christopoulos, 2007).

4. The discovery of BETP

Using a knowledge-based pharmacophore approach, our group at Eli Lilly and Company identified a small molecular weight series of sulfones and sulfoxides analogous to the Novo quinoxalines (Sloop et al., 2010). Compound B (now known as BETP), 4-(3-(*B*enzyloxy)phenyl)-2-(*e*thylsulfinyl)-6-(*t*rifluoromethyl)*p*yrimidine, was identified as a low micromolar potency agonist of the GLP-1R (Fig. 1B). BETP exhibited partial agonist activity in functional cAMP accumulation and CRE reporter assays for GLP-1R and was highly selective against related receptors (Sloop et al., 2010). Notably, BETP did not require the GLP-1R extracellular domain for activity as distinct from peptidergic GLP-1R ligands and did not displace [^{125}I]-GLP-1(7-36) binding from the GLP-1R, indicative of an allosteric mode of action. Moreover, BETP generated a robust insulinotropic response in cultures of isolated rat islets and had substantial insulinotropic activity following intravenous dosing in a glucose tolerance test (Sloop et al., 2010). Scientists at Pfizer conducted a panoply of studies on the metabolism and disposition of BETP (Eng et al., 2013). They showed that BETP rapidly conjugates to glutathione *in vitro* ($t_{1/2} < 0.5$ min), and *in vivo* exposure by intravenous administration was low (200 nM), sporadic, and transient. Analogous to these studies, we observed that BETP was rapidly metabolized *in vivo* ($t_{1/2} < 5$ min), quickly conjugated to glutathione *in vitro*, and that electrophilicity of BETP analogues was required for bioactivity. These findings and analogous published SAR data on the quinoxalines led to the hypothesis that BETP may covalently modify the GLP-1R (Teng et al., 2007).

5. Covalent mechanism of action of BETP

Nolte and colleagues at Pfizer conducted an elegant set of chemoproteomic experiments to elucidate the specific mechanism of action of BETP (Nolte et al., 2014). They synthesized an alkyne analogue of BETP and utilized click-chemistry, affinity purification and mass-spectrometry detection to identify cysteine 347 at the beginning of transmembrane helix 6 as the site of functional adduction to the GLP-1R (Fig. 1C and D). Both loss- and gain-of-function mutation data proved this is the site of BETP action on the GLP-1R. BETP and Compound 2 were functionally inactive on GLP-1R containing a Cys347Ala substitution; moreover, substitution of the analogous residue in the glucagon receptor (Phe345 to Cys) engendered sensitivity to BETP. These data entirely explain the actions of BETP in terms of receptor selectivity within class B GPCRs, as this cysteine is unique to GLP-1R (Fig. 1D). In parallel, our group investigated the mechanism of BETP, and we showed by immunoprecipitation and autoradiography that [^{3}H]-labeled BETP irreversibly binds the GLP-1R. A thiol analogue of BETP did not interact with GLP-1R, consistent with the need for a leaving group as provided by the sulfone or sulfoxide moiety. The mechanism is likely nucleophilic displacement of BETP with ethyl sulfoxide as the leaving group (Fig. 1C), as was postulated based on experiments with BETP and reduced glutathione (Eng et al., 2013). Utilizing the BETP-insensitivity Cys347Ala mutation, we pharmacologically characterized an array of small molecule ligands identified from our allosteric modulator HTS campaigns (Bueno et al., 2016). We observed that many compounds identified as positive allosteric modulators in HTS campaigns against the GLP-1R were covalent modifiers of the GLP-1R, albeit with *bona fide* allosteric activity. These compounds were idiosyncratic covalent modifiers of the GLP-1R and not necessarily well predicted by medicinal chemists or computational filters and were not generally known promiscuous compounds (Bueno et al., 2016).

6. The *in vitro* pharmacology of BETP

The pharmacological profile of BETP at the GLP-1R has been quantified by Sexton and colleagues in CHO cell lines heterologously expressing GLP-1R. This represents a convenient and consistent method of obtaining pharmacological parameters for allosteric modulators by quantifying potency and efficacy alone and in combination with orthosteric or other allosteric ligands. Fitting these data to operational models of allosteric agonism can produce parameters (*e.g.*, affinity (α) and efficacy (β) cooperativity) that can be used to interpret experimental data in endogenous systems (Leach et al., 2007). In collaboration with Wootten and colleagues, we performed a detailed pharmacological analysis of the interactions of BETP with other pharmacological ligands of the GLP-1R, including peptides and recently described agonist compounds such as Boc-5 and TT-15 (Wootten et al., 2013). An unanticipated set of results were generated, that are summarized in Table 1. BETP displayed positive, negative, or neutral cooperativity with small molecule and peptide ligands dependent on the signaling pathway being measured and the cognate ligand being combined with. The key point from these studies is that BETP exemplified two of the most exciting facets attributed to allosteric modulators: probe dependence and biased signaling. These provide a theoretical opportunity for fine tuning therapeutic strategies that perhaps are not feasible or are more difficult with orthosteric molecules. For instance, identifying a compound that modulates angiotensin type 1 arrestin recruitment but not G-protein

Table 1 Summary of the allosteric pharmacology of BETP in cell-based signal transduction assays.

Ligand cooperativity (αβ)	**Ligand tested in combination with BETP**						
Signaling pathway	**Exendin-4**	**GLP-1 (7-36)**	**Oxyntomodulin**	**GLP-1 (9-36)**	**TTP15**	**BMS21**	**Boc-5**
cAMP	2.8	2	16	>10	46	560	20
Ca^{2+} mobilization	10	3.8	1.7	1.0	NT	NT	NT
pERK1/2	0.1	0.1	2.8	ND	NT	NT	NT
β-Arrestin	1.5	4.7	3.5	ND	NT	NT	NT

Data are summarized from experiments presented in Willard, Wootten, et al. (2012), Wootten et al. (2012, 2013) where ligands were tested in combination with BETP in different signal transduction readouts. Pharmacological parameters were derived by model fitting and cooperativity values were calculated for the BETP-ligand interaction using an operational model of agonism (Leach et al., 2007; Willard, Wootten, et al., 2012; Wootten et al., 2012, 2013). The cooperativity value αβ represents combined effects of BETP on affinity (α) and efficacy (β). ND, allosteric parameters could not be determined. NT, combination was not tested.

activation was postulated to be useful for heart failure, and similar hypotheses exist around the GLP-1R (Kenakin, 2019; Pabreja, Mohd, Koole, Wootten, & Furness, 2014; Violin et al., 2010).

7. BETP as a cAMP biased GLP-1(9-36) and oxyntomodulin positive allosteric modulator

BETP alone is a low efficacy, low potency partial agonist for cAMP modulation with close to no observable effects on other signaling pathways (Wootten et al., 2012). GLP-1(7-36)NH_2 by virtue of being the *bona fide* endogenous agonist of the GLP-1R is used to benchmark 100% efficacy for different signaling pathways. We observed that BETP is especially effective in the potentiation of GLP-1(9-36) and the proglucagon-derivative oxyntomodulin: both circulating peptides with possible physiological utility (Drucker, Habener, & Holst, 2017). GLP-1(9-36)NH_2 is the primary metabolite of the endogenous GLP-1R agonist: GLP-1(7-36). In fact, one class of anti-diabetic drugs, the gliptins, are inhibitors that block the DPP-IV mediated proteolysis of GLP-1(7-36) and enhance the endogenous incretin effect (Thornberry & Gallwitz, 2009). *In vitro*, BETP is a highly effective positive allosteric modulator of GLP-1(9-36). For cAMP accumulation responses, BETP enhances functional potency of GLP-1(9-36) by at least 10-fold at saturating doses and converts GLP-1(9-36) from a low efficacy partial agonist into a full agonist, relative to GLP-1 (7-36) (Wootten et al., 2012). BETP was able to cause pathway-specific modulation of GLP-1R signal transduction in that it had neutral cooperativity for Ca^{2+} mobilization, ERK phosphorylation and β-arrestin recruitment (Wootten et al., 2012). In parallel, several other groups reported confirmation of some aspects of these *in vitro* findings (Li, Lu, & Willars, 2012) in similar model systems (Cheong, Kim, Son, & Kaang, 2012; Li et al., 2012).

Using BETP as a tool to selectively modulate GLP-1R mediated cyclase activation, we conducted *ex vivo* experiments in isolated rat islets (Wootten et al., 2012). In the absence of BETP, GLP-1(9-36) did not exert an insulinotropic effect, consistent with its pharmacology as a low efficacy partial agonist. At a minimally efficacious dose of BETP, GLP-1(9-36) became highly active (approximately threefold increase in insulin secretion with a potency of 40 nM). This response was glucose dependent and abolished in *Glp1r* knockout mice, indicating that it was mediated by the GLP-1R and not *via* off-target effects (Bueno et al., 2016). This effect could be translated to the intravenous glucose tolerance test (IVGTT) in animals, wherein the administration of BETP alone and GLP-1(9-36) alone had marginal effects on insulin secretion, but when co-dosed, they exhibited a substantial insulin secretion response (Wootten et al., 2012). This is consistent with the known pharmacology of BETP, and it generated the first data indicating that the cAMP response may be the principal mediator of insulinotropic action by the GLP-1R. In this acute setting, these data fit the known aspects of islet biology with respect to Gα_s-coupled receptor mediated insulin secretion (Tomas, Jones, & Leech, 2019).

We developed this paradigm by performing similar *in vitro* and *in vivo* experiments with BETP and glucagon-derived peptide oxyntomodulin. Oxyntomodulin, relative to GLP-1(7-36), is a lower affinity full agonist that increases cAMP formation *via* Gα_s, recruits β-arrestin, mobilizes intracellular calcium, and activates ERK1/2 in CHO cells expressing the GLP-1R (Willard, Wootten, et al., 2012). BETP exhibits highly biased modulation of oxyntomodulin signal transduction with 16-fold αβ cooperativity for the cAMP pathway in comparison with two- to threefold for other tested signaling readouts (Table 1). IVGTT experiments with oxyntomodulin clearly demonstrated an *in vivo* allosteric interaction (Fig. 2). At low doses of oxyntomodulin (0.3 and 3 nmol/kg), limited and approximately additive effects of BETP and oxyntomodulin were observed. In the presence of a robust, but not biologically saturating concentration of oxyntomodulin (30 nmol/kg), impressive synergy was observed. The calculated area under the curve for predicted additivity is 124 ng/mL · min insulin whereas it is 210 ng/mL · min insulin for the BETP + oxyntomodulin treatment. These data add further support to the hypothesis that cAMP accumulation is the principal component responsible for GLP-1R mediated insulin secretion. There are some data with novel cAMP biased GLP-1 analogs that supports this hypothesis; we await further studies with more drug-like allosteric modulators or peptides to delineate the roles of different signaling pathways in acute and chronic GLP-1 action (Jones et al., 2018; Willard & Sloop, 2012). Insights into the structural basis of G-protein biased signaling at the GLP-1R are apparent from the CryoEM structure of the ligand ExP5 in complex with GLP-1R and the Gαs heterotrimer (Liang et al., 2018). In this case, subtle changes in the conformation of extracellular loop 3 and proximal transmembrane regions may propagate to induce enhanced rates of G-protein conformational change for this G-protein biased ligand. Determining the mechanistic structural basis for allosteric and orthosteric ligand bias at the GLP-1R is a key question for the GLP-1R field.

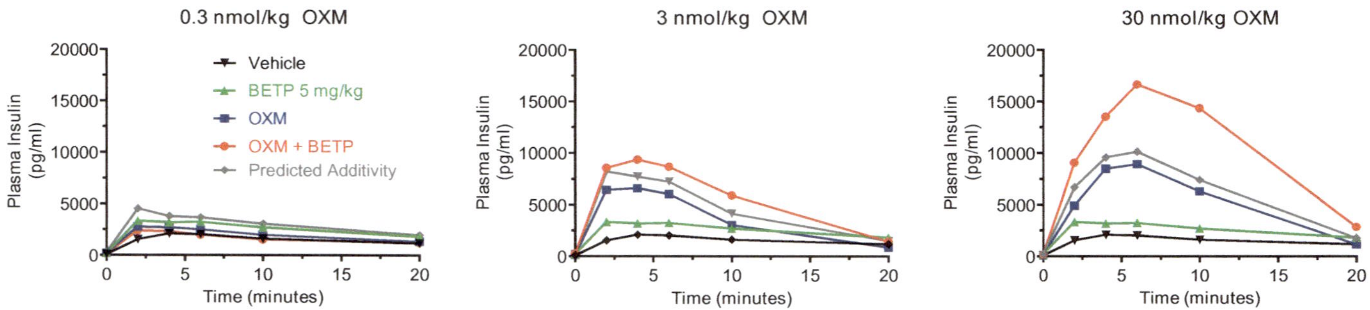

Fig. 2 BETP synergistically enhances oxyntomodulin-induced insulin secretion. Data represent a time course of plasma insulin concentrations in fasted, anesthetized Wistar rats following treatment with either vehicle, BETP (5 mg/kg), oxyntomodulin (OXM, one of three different concentrations). Immediately following compound dosing, an intravenous glucose bolus (0.5 g/kg) was administered. The predicted additive response of BETP and oxyntomodulin was calculated by vehicle correction and is plotted. Data are from a single experiment, but oxyntomodulin doses are plotted on separate graphs for clarity (Willard, Wootten, et al., 2012).

8. The structural basis of BETP action

During the last decade, GPCR structural biology has rapidly evolved, and multiple X-ray crystallographic and cryo-electron microscopy structures of the GLP-1R bound to ligands are available (Jazayeri et al., 2017; Liang et al., 2018; Song et al., 2017; Zhang et al., 2017). During receptor activation, the cytoplasmic side of GLP-1R undergoes a dramatic conformation change. Notably, transmembrane helix 6 (TM6) adopts a 90° kink, forming the binding pocket for engaging the trimeric G-protein complex (Fig. 3A) (Liang et al., 2018; Zhang et al., 2017). Cysteine347 in the GLP-1R is positioned at the bottom of TM6, near intracellular loop 3 (ICL3) (Fig. 3). Using molecular modeling, we generated a hypothesis as to how BETP induces allosteric modulation of the GLP-1R. Upon covalent

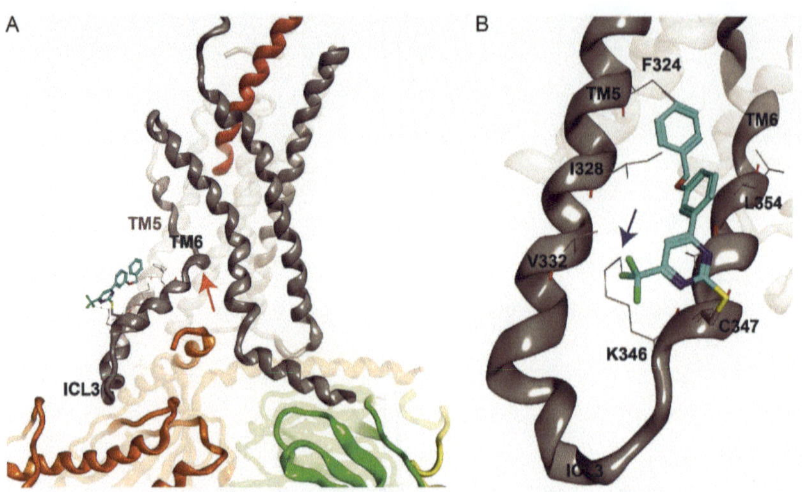

Fig. 3 Modeling the covalent modification of Cys347 by BETP using the GLP-1R:GLP1: G-protein ternary complex (PDB code: 5VAI) as template (Zhang et al., 2017). Transmembrane 5 (TM5) and 6 (TM6) and the intracellular loop 3 (ICL3) are labeled. (A) The GLP-1R-G-protein active ternary complex. Binding to the G-protein complex is stabilized by the kink in TM6 (indicated by the red arrow). BETP is shown as cyan sticks. The ternary complex is shown as ribbons: GLP-1R in gray, $G\alpha_s$ subunit in orange, Gβ subunit in green, Gγ subunit in yellow, and the GLP-1 peptide in red. (B) Detailed view of the BETP binding site. BETP was modeled in the groove formed by TM5 and TM6 with a covalent bond to Cys347. A preferred halogen interaction between the positively charged ε-amino group of Lys346 and the trifluoromethyl of BETP was modeled (indicated by the blue arrow).

modification of residue Cys347, the trifluoromethyl group of BETP is positioned to form a halogen interaction with Lys346 while the remainder of the BETP molecule maintain Van der Waals contacts along the groove between transmembrane helix 5 and 6 (Fig. 3B). It is likely that these proposed interactions contribute to stabilizing TM6 in the kinked conformation, thereby enhancing G-protein coupling. At this point, there is not enough experimental data to explain how BETP induces biased modulation. This would await further biochemical or structural insights. In this regard, one group has engineered GLP-1R variants with enhanced constitutive activity and sensitivity to agonists. To do this, they substituted Cys347 of GLP-1R with a tetrapeptide Glu-Glu-Tyr-Arg (Kopin & Beinborn, 2004) and it is likely that the mechanism of enhanced receptor activity is due to TM6 perturbation. Analysis of multiple sequence alignments of class B GPCRs indicates that the glucagon receptor family contains a single amino acid insertion at the position equivalent to Cys347 in GLP-1R (Fig. 1D). They are Leu in GIPR, Tyr in GLP-2R and Phe in GCGR (Fig. 1D). In light of this, the covalent allosteric mechanism of BETP is most likely a fortuitous result given the placement of this apparently free and nucleophilic cysteine residue in this conformationally important part of the GLP-1R.

9. Is BETP a useful tool for understanding GLP-1R pharmacology?

Arguments can be made for and against the use of BETP to probe GLP-1R pharmacology. At the time BETP was discovered and characterized, there was a very limited set of GLP-1R small molecule ligands available (Willard, Bueno, & Sloop, 2012). Undeniably, studies on BETP facilitated the discovery of high level pharmacology concepts, new methods, and new compounds to probe GLP-1R biology (Buenaventura et al., 2019; Jones et al., 2017; Mendez et al., 2019; Morris et al., 2014; Wootten et al., 2012; Yin et al., 2016). Moreover, the history of chemical probes suggests that availability of tool compounds spurs innovative research (Edwards, Bountra, Kerr, & Willson, 2009). These are all arguments that support the use of BETP as a tool for preclinical GLP-1R biology work. The counter argument is that BETP is a strong electrophile and clearly not-selective as it had appreciable activity in several assays in a selectivity panel for off-target effects (Nolte et al., 2014). Chemoproteomic studies also indicated that BETP modified several uncharacterized cellular proteins (Nolte et al., 2014).

If BETP were an orthosteric agonist of GLP-1R, it would be hard to isolate on-target from off-target effects. Fortunately, the allosteric mode of action provided by BETP helps in this regard. Based on allosteric pharmacology principles, co-treatment with an orthosteric ligand (*e.g.*, GLP-1 or oxyntomodulin) reveals the cellular effects of BETP, and based on orthosteric pharmacology principles, the potency of BETP is enhanced by cooperativity. Although it must be noted that the various allosteric pharmacology models in use do not account for covalent interactions (May et al., 2007). We note that relevant tissue-based *in vivo* and *ex vivo* studies display a strong dependence on allosteric pharmacology (the need for both an allosteric and orthosteric component) and in all instances we have investigated, the response is entirely dependent on the presence of the *Glp1r* gene (Bueno et al., 2016). One advantage of a covalent ligand is a high receptor occupancy, and this may explain the ability to observe *in vivo* activity of BETP despite the poor pharmacokinetics. If parent BETP is rapidly metabolized and eliminated (*e.g.*, conjugation to glutathione) but has covalently adducted to Cys347 of the GLP-1R, then in principle, BETP action is determined by the rate of synthesis and degradation of the GLP-1R (Strelow, 2017). Thus, a single bolus of BETP can have pharmacological activity despite low exposure. A benefit of this mechanism is that off-target and non-specific effects of BETP may be minimized due to the low exposure achieved *in vivo*.

Our overall opinion is that while BETP is a highly imperfect chemical probe by current standards (Arrowsmith et al., 2015), it has been immensely impactful with respect to generating new research on GLP-1R. Unfortunately, a BETP-type covalent mechanism cannot be used as a discovery strategy for novel allosteric modulators of other Class B GPCRs as this residue is Cys in only GLP-1R (Fig. 1D). However, introduction of Cys into this position of the GCGR can induce a BETP-sensitive GCGR (Nolte et al., 2014), indicating that synthetic receptors that respond to BETP can be created. Indeed, a recent disclosure from Pfizer indicates BETP was used as a tool to screen and identify a new class of small molecule GLP-1R agonists (Edmonds et al., 2019) and it may be that this approach can be translated to other Class B GPCRs with drug discovery applications. We anticipate that several such advances in GLP-1R biology are imminent and note the recent reports of new GLP-1R allosteric modulators in the literature (Cheng, Ho, Huang, Chou, & King, 2015; King, Lin, Cheng, Chen, & Chein, 2015; Mendez et al., 2019; Morris et al., 2014).

Acknowledgments

The authors thank their numerous past and present collaborators in Diabetes Research, Quantitative Biology, Medicinal Chemistry, Structural Biology and ADME groups at Eli Lilly and Company. The authors also thank their collaborators in the Sexton-Wootten lab at MIPS.

Conflict of interest

All authors are employees of Eli Lilly and Company and may own company stock or possess stock options.

References

Arrowsmith, C. H., Audia, J. E., Austin, C., Baell, J., Bennett, J., Blagg, J., et al. (2015). The promise and peril of chemical probes. *Nature Chemical Biology*, *11*(8), 536–541. https://doi.org/10.1038/nchembio.1867.

Bortolato, A., Dore, A. S., Hollenstein, K., Tehan, B. G., Mason, J. S., & Marshall, F. H. (2014). Structure of class B GPCRs: New horizons for drug discovery. *British Journal of Pharmacology*, *171*(13), 3132–3145. https://doi.org/10.1111/bph.12689.

Buenaventura, T., Bitsi, S., Laughlin, W. E., Burgoyne, T., Lyu, Z., Oqua, A. I., et al. (2019). Agonist-induced membrane nanodomain clustering drives GLP-1 receptor responses in pancreatic beta cells. *PLoS Biology*, *17*(8), e3000097. https://doi.org/10.1371/journal.pbio.3000097.

Bueno, A. B., Showalter, A. D., Wainscott, D. B., Stutsman, C., Marin, A., Ficorilli, J., et al. (2016). Positive allosteric modulation of the glucagon-like Peptide-1 receptor by diverse electrophiles. *The Journal of Biological Chemistry*, *291*(20), 10700–10715. https://doi.org/10.1074/jbc.M115.696039.

Chen, D., Liao, J., Li, N., Zhou, C., Liu, Q., Wang, G., et al. (2007). A nonpeptidic agonist of glucagon-like peptide 1 receptors with efficacy in diabetic db/db mice. *Proceedings of the National Academy of Sciences of the United States of America*, *104*(3), 943–948. https://doi.org/10.1073/pnas.0610173104.

Cheng, Y. H., Ho, M. S., Huang, W. T., Chou, Y. T., & King, K. (2015). Modulation of glucagon-like Peptide-1 (GLP-1) potency by endocannabinoid-like lipids represents a novel mode of regulating GLP-1 receptor signaling. *The Journal of Biological Chemistry*, *290*(23), 14302–14313. https://doi.org/10.1074/jbc.M115.655662.

Cheong, Y. H., Kim, M. K., Son, M. H., & Kaang, B. K. (2012). Two small molecule agonists of glucagon-like peptide-1 receptor modulate the receptor activation response differently. *Biochemical and Biophysical Research Communications*, *417*(1), 558–563. https://doi.org/10.1016/j.bbrc.2011.12.004.

DeFronzo, R. A., Ratner, R. E., Han, J., Kim, D. D., Fineman, M. S., & Baron, A. D. (2005). Effects of exenatide (exendin-4) on glycemic control and weight over 30 weeks in metformin-treated patients with type 2 diabetes. *Diabetes Care*, *28*(5), 1092–1100. https://doi.org/10.2337/diacare.28.5.1092.

Drucker, D. J., Habener, J. F., & Holst, J. J. (2017). Discovery, characterization, and clinical development of the glucagon-like peptides. *The Journal of Clinical Investigation*, *127*(12), 4217–4227. https://doi.org/10.1172/JCI97233.

Edmonds, D. J., Griffith, D. A., Bagley, S. W., Buckeridge, C., Curto, J. M., Derksen, D. R., et al. (2019). Discovery of PF06882961: A potent, orally bioavailable small molecule agonist of the GLP-1 receptor. In *Paper presented at the proceedings of the 20th SCI/RSC medicinal chemistry symposium*. Cambridge, UK: SCI/RSC. Sep 8 – 11, 2019.

Edwards, A. M., Bountra, C., Kerr, D. J., & Willson, T. M. (2009). Open access chemical and clinical probes to support drug discovery. *Nature Chemical Biology*, *5*(7), 436–440. https://doi.org/10.1038/nchembio0709-436.

Eng, H., Sharma, R., McDonald, T. S., Edmonds, D. J., Fortin, J. P., Li, X., et al. (2013). Demonstration of the innate electrophilicity of 4-(3-(benzyloxy)phenyl)-2-(ethylsulfinyl)-6-(trifluoromethyl)pyrimidine (BETP), a small-molecule positive allosteric modulator of the glucagon-like peptide-1 receptor. *Drug Metabolism and Disposition*, *41*(8), 1470–1479. https://doi.org/10.1124/dmd.113.052183.

Gerstein, H. C., Colhoun, H. M., Dagenais, G. R., Diaz, R., Lakshmanan, M., Pais, P., et al. (2019). Dulaglutide and cardiovascular outcomes in type 2 diabetes (REWIND): A double-blind, randomised placebo-controlled trial. *Lancet*, *394*, 121–130. https://doi.org/10.1016/S0140-6736(19)31149-3.

Graziano, M. P., Hey, P. J., Borkowski, D., Chicchi, G. G., & Strader, C. D. (1993). Cloning and functional expression of a human glucagon-like peptide-1 receptor. *Biochemical and Biophysical Research Communications*, *196*(1), 141–146. https://doi.org/10.1006/bbrc.1993.2226.

Hernandez, A. F., Green, J. B., Janmohamed, S., D'Agostino, R. B., Sr., Granger, C. B., Jones, N. P., et al. (2018). Albiglutide and cardiovascular outcomes in patients with type 2 diabetes and cardiovascular disease (harmony outcomes): A double-blind, randomised placebo-controlled trial. *Lancet*, *392*(10157), 1519–1529. https://doi.org/10.1016/S0140-6736(18)32261-X.

Hoare, S. R. (2005). Mechanisms of peptide and nonpeptide ligand binding to class B G-protein-coupled receptors. *Drug Discovery Today*, *10*(6), 417–427. https://doi.org/10.1016/S1359-6446(05)03370-2.

Isberg, V., de Graaf, C., Bortolato, A., Cherezov, V., Katritch, V., Marshall, F. H., et al. (2015). Generic GPCR residue numbers—Aligning topology maps while minding the gaps. *Trends in Pharmacological Sciences*, *36*(1), 22–31. https://doi.org/10.1016/j.tips.2014.11.001.

Jazayeri, A., Rappas, M., Brown, A. J. H., Kean, J., Errey, J. C., Robertson, N. J., et al. (2017). Crystal structure of the GLP-1 receptor bound to a peptide agonist. *Nature*, *546*(7657), 254–258. https://doi.org/10.1038/nature22800.

Jones, B., Buenaventura, T., Kanda, N., Chabosseau, P., Owen, B. M., Scott, R., et al. (2018). Targeting GLP-1 receptor trafficking to improve agonist efficacy. *Nature Communications*, *9*(1), 1602. https://doi.org/10.1038/s41467-018-03941-2.

Jones, B. J., Scopelliti, R., Tomas, A., Bloom, S. R., Hodson, D. J., & Broichhagen, J. (2017). Potent prearranged positive allosteric modulators of the glucagon-like peptide-1 receptor. *ChemistryOpen*, *6*(4), 501–505. https://doi.org/10.1002/open.201700062.

Kenakin, T. (2019). Biased receptor signaling in drug discovery. *Pharmacological Reviews*, *71*(2), 267–315. https://doi.org/10.1124/pr.118.016790.

King, K., Lin, N. P., Cheng, Y. H., Chen, G. H., & Chein, R. J. (2015). Isolation of positive modulator of glucagon-like Peptide-1 signaling from Trigonella foenum-graecum (fenugreek) seed. *The Journal of Biological Chemistry*, *290*(43), 26235–26248. https://doi.org/10.1074/jbc.M115.672097.

Knudsen, L. B., Kiel, D., Teng, M., Behrens, C., Bhumralkar, D., Kodra, J. T., et al. (2007). Small-molecule agonists for the glucagon-like peptide 1 receptor. *Proceedings of the National Academy of Sciences of the United States of America*, *104*(3), 937–942. https://doi.org/10.1073/pnas.0605701104.

Koole, C., Wootten, D., Simms, J., Valant, C., Sridhar, R., Woodman, O. L., et al. (2010). Allosteric ligands of the glucagon-like peptide 1 receptor (GLP-1R) differentially modulate endogenous and exogenous peptide responses in a pathway-selective manner: Implications for drug screening. *Molecular Pharmacology*, *78*(3), 456–465. https://doi.org/10.1124/mol.110.065664.

Kopin, A. S., & Beinborn, M. (2004). Methods and compositions for the treatment of metabolic disorders. WO 2004/103310A2.

Leach, K., Sexton, P. M., & Christopoulos, A. (2007). Allosteric GPCR modulators: Taking advantage of permissive receptor pharmacology. *Trends in Pharmacological Sciences*, *28*(8), 382–389. https://doi.org/10.1016/j.tips.2007.06.004.

Li, N., Lu, J., & Willars, G. B. (2012). Allosteric modulation of the activity of the glucagon-like peptide-1 (GLP-1) metabolite GLP-1 9-36 amide at the GLP-1 receptor. *PLoS One*, 7(10), e47936. https://doi.org/10.1371/journal.pone.0047936.

Liang, Y. L., Khoshouei, M., Glukhova, A., Furness, S. G. B., Zhao, P., Clydesdale, L., et al. (2018). Phase-plate cryo-EM structure of a biased agonist-bound human GLP-1 receptor-Gs complex. *Nature*, *555*(7694), 121–125. https://doi.org/10.1038/nature25773.

Marso, S. P., Bain, S. C., Consoli, A., Eliaschewitz, F. G., Jodar, E., Leiter, L. A., et al. (2016). Semaglutide and cardiovascular outcomes in patients with type 2 diabetes. *The New England Journal of Medicine*, *375*(19), 1834–1844. https://doi.org/10.1056/NEJMoa1607141.

Marso, S. P., Daniels, G. H., Brown-Frandsen, K., Kristensen, P., Mann, J. F., Nauck, M. A., et al. (2016). Liraglutide and cardiovascular outcomes in type 2 diabetes. *The New England Journal of Medicine*, *375*(4), 311–322. https://doi.org/10.1056/NEJMoa1603827.

May, L. T., Leach, K., Sexton, P. M., & Christopoulos, A. (2007). Allosteric modulation of G protein-coupled receptors. *Annual Review of Pharmacology and Toxicology*, *47*, 1–51. https://doi.org/10.1146/annurev.pharmtox.47.120505.105159.

Mendez, M., Matter, H., Defossa, E., Kurz, M., Lebreton, S., Li, Z., et al. (2019). Design, synthesis, and pharmacological evaluation of potent positive allosteric modulators of the glucagon-like peptide-1 receptor (GLP-1R). *Journal of Medicinal Chemistry*. https://doi.org/10.1021/acs.jmedchem.9b01071.

Morris, L. C., Nance, K. D., Gentry, P. R., Days, E. L., Weaver, C. D., Niswender, C. M., et al. (2014). Discovery of (S)-2-cyclopentyl-N-(1-isopropylpyrrolidin2-yl)-9-methyl-1-oxo-2,9-dihydro-1H-py rrido[3,4-b]indole-4-carboxamide (VU0453379): A novel, CNS penetrant glucagon-like peptide 1 receptor (GLP-1R) positive allosteric modulator (PAM). *Journal of Medicinal Chemistry*, *57*(23), 10192–10197. https://doi.org/10.1021/jm501375c.

Nolte, W. M., Fortin, J. P., Stevens, B. D., Aspnes, G. E., Griffith, D. A., Hoth, L. R., et al. (2014). A potentiator of orthosteric ligand activity at GLP-1R acts via covalent modification. *Nature Chemical Biology*, *10*(8), 629–631. https://doi.org/10.1038/nchembio.1581.

Pabreja, K., Mohd, M. A., Koole, C., Wootten, D., & Furness, S. G. (2014). Molecular mechanisms underlying physiological and receptor pleiotropic effects mediated by GLP-1R activation. *British Journal of Pharmacology*, *171*(5), 1114–1128. https://doi.org/10.1111/bph.12313.

Pandy-Szekeres, G., Munk, C., Tsonkov, T. M., Mordalski, S., Harpsoe, K., Hauser, A. S., et al. (2018). GPCRdb in 2018: Adding GPCR structure models and ligands. *Nucleic Acids Research*, *46*(D1), D440–D446. https://doi.org/10.1093/nar/gkx1109.

Sittampalam, G. S., Kahl, S. D., & Janzen, W. P. (1997). High-throughput screening: Advances in assay technologies. *Current Opinion in Chemical Biology*, *1*(3), 384–391. https://doi.org/10.1016/s1367-5931(97)80078-6.

Sloop, K. W., Emmerson, P. J., Statnick, M. A., & Willard, F. S. (2018). The current state of GPCR-based drug discovery to treat metabolic disease. *British Journal of Pharmacology*, *175*(21), 4060–4071. https://doi.org/10.1111/bph.14157.

Sloop, K. W., Willard, F. S., Brenner, M. B., Ficorilli, J., Valasek, K., Showalter, A. D., et al. (2010). Novel small molecule glucagon-like peptide-1 receptor agonist stimulates insulin secretion in rodents and from human islets. *Diabetes*, *59*(12), 3099–3107. https://doi.org/10.2337/db10-0689.

Song, G., Yang, D., Wang, Y., de Graaf, C., Zhou, Q., Jiang, S., et al. (2017). Human GLP-1 receptor transmembrane domain structure in complex with allosteric modulators. *Nature*, *546*(7657), 312–315. https://doi.org/10.1038/nature22378.

Strelow, J. M. (2017). A perspective on the kinetics of covalent and irreversible inhibition. *SLAS discovery : Advancing Life Sciences R & D*, *22*(1), 3–20. https://doi.org/10.1177/1087057116671509.

Teng, M., Johnson, M. D., Thomas, C., Kiel, D., Lakis, J. N., Kercher, T., et al. (2007). Small molecule ago-allosteric modulators of the human glucagon-like peptide-1 (hGLP-1) receptor. *Bioorganic & Medicinal Chemistry Letters*, *17*(19), 5472–5478. https://doi.org/10.1016/j.bmcl.2007.06.086.

Thompson, J. D., Higgins, D. G., & Gibson, T. J. (1994). CLUSTAL W: Improving the sensitivity of progressive multiple sequence alignment through sequence weighting, position-specific gap penalties and weight matrix choice. *Nucleic Acids Research*, *22*(22), 4673–4680. https://doi.org/10.1093/nar/22.22.4673.

Thorens, B. (1992). Expression cloning of the pancreatic beta cell receptor for the gluco-incretin hormone glucagon-like peptide 1. *Proceedings of the National Academy of Sciences of the United States of America*, *89*(18), 8641–8645. https://doi.org/10.1073/pnas.89.18.8641.

Thornberry, N. A., & Gallwitz, B. (2009). Mechanism of action of inhibitors of dipeptidyl-peptidase-4 (DPP-4). *Best Practice & Research Clinical Endocrinology & Metabolism*, *23*(4), 479–486. https://doi.org/10.1016/j.beem.2009.03.004.

Tomas, A., Jones, B., & Leech, C. (2019). New insights into Beta-cell GLP-1 receptor and cAMP signaling. *Journal of Molecular Biology*. https://doi.org/10.1016/j.jmb.2019.08.009.

Violin, J. D., DeWire, S. M., Yamashita, D., Rominger, D. H., Nguyen, L., Schiller, K., et al. (2010). Selectively engaging beta-arrestins at the angiotensin II type 1 receptor reduces blood pressure and increases cardiac performance. *The Journal of Pharmacology and Experimental Therapeutics*, *335*(3), 572–579. https://doi.org/10.1124/jpet.110.173005.

Willard, F. S., Briere, D. A., & Sloop, K. W. (2018). Beyond glucagon-like peptide-1: Is G-protein coupled receptor Polypharmacology the path forward to treating metabolic diseases? *ACS Pharmacology & Translational Science*, *1*(1), 3–11.

Willard, F. S., Bueno, A. B., & Sloop, K. W. (2012). Small molecule drug discovery at the glucagon-like peptide-1 receptor. *Experimental Diabetes Research*, *2012*, 709893. https://doi.org/10.1155/2012/709893.

Willard, F. S., & Sloop, K. W. (2012). Physiology and emerging biochemistry of the glucagon-like peptide-1 receptor. *Experimental Diabetes Research*, *2012*, 470851. https://doi.org/10.1155/2012/470851.

Willard, F. S., Wootten, D., Showalter, A. D., Savage, E. E., Ficorilli, J., Farb, T. B., et al. (2012). Small molecule allosteric modulation of the glucagon-like Peptide-1 receptor enhances the insulinotropic effect of oxyntomodulin. *Molecular Pharmacology*, *82*(6), 1066–1073. https://doi.org/10.1124/mol.112.080432.

Wootten, D., Savage, E. E., Valant, C., May, L. T., Sloop, K. W., Ficorilli, J., et al. (2012). Allosteric modulation of endogenous metabolites as an avenue for drug discovery. *Molecular Pharmacology*, *82*(2), 281–290. https://doi.org/10.1124/mol.112.079319.

Wootten, D., Savage, E. E., Willard, F. S., Bueno, A. B., Sloop, K. W., Christopoulos, A., et al. (2013). Differential activation and modulation of the glucagon-like peptide-1 receptor by small molecule ligands. *Molecular Pharmacology*, *83*(4), 822–834. https://doi.org/10.1124/mol.112.084525.

Wootten, D., Simms, J., Koole, C., Woodman, O. L., Summers, R. J., Christopoulos, A., et al. (2011). Modulation of the glucagon-like peptide-1 receptor signaling by naturally occurring and synthetic flavonoids. *The Journal of Pharmacology and Experimental Therapeutics*, *336*(2), 540–550. https://doi.org/10.1124/jpet.110.176362.

Yin, Y., Zhou, X. E., Hou, L., Zhao, L. H., Liu, B., Wang, G., et al. (2016). An intrinsic agonist mechanism for activation of glucagon-like peptide-1 receptor by its extracellular domain. *Cell discovery*, *2*, 16042. https://doi.org/10.1038/celldisc.2016.42.

Zhang, Y., Sun, B., Feng, D., Hu, H., Chu, M., Qu, Q., et al. (2017). Cryo-EM structure of the activated GLP-1 receptor in complex with a G protein. *Nature*, *546*(7657), 248–253. https://doi.org/10.1038/nature22394.

Zhao, L. H., Yin, Y., Yang, D., Liu, B., Hou, L., Wang, X., et al. (2016). Differential requirement of the extracellular domain in activation of class B G protein-coupled receptors. *The Journal of Biological Chemistry*, *291*(29), 15119–15130. https://doi.org/10.1074/jbc.M116.726620.

CHAPTER EIGHT

Allosteric modulation of metabotropic glutamate receptors in alcohol use disorder: Insights from preclinical investigations

Kari A. Johnson[a,*], David M. Lovinger[b]

[a]Department of Pharmacology, Uniformed Services University of the Health Sciences, Bethesda, MD, United States

[b]Laboratory for Integrative Neuroscience, National Institute on Alcohol Abuse and Alcoholism, US National Institutes of Health, Rockville, MD, United States

[*]Corresponding author: e-mail address: kari.johnson@usuhs.edu

Contents

Advances in Pharmacology, Volume 88
ISSN 1054-3589
https://doi.org/10.1016/bs.apha.2020.02.002

Abstract

Metabotropic glutamate (mGlu) receptors are family C G protein-coupled receptors (GPCRs) that modulate neuronal excitability and synaptic transmission throughout the nervous system. Owing to recent advances in development of subtype-selective allosteric modulators of mGlu receptors, individual members of the mGlu receptor family have been proposed as targets for treating a variety of neurological and psychiatric disorders, including substance use disorders. In this chapter, we highlight preclinical evidence that allosteric modulators of mGlu receptors could be useful for reducing alcohol consumption and preventing relapse in alcohol use disorder (AUD). We begin with an overview of the preclinical models that are used to study mGlu receptor involvement in alcohol-related behaviors. Alcohol exposure causes adaptations in both expression and function of various mGlu receptor subtypes, and pharmacotherapies aimed at reversing these adaptations have the potential to reduce alcohol consumption and seeking. Positive allosteric modulators (PAMs) of $mGlu_2$ and negative allosteric modulators of $mGlu_5$ show particular promise for reducing alcohol intake and/or preventing relapse. Finally, this chapter discusses important considerations for translating preclinical findings toward the development of clinically useful drugs, including the potential for PAMs to avoid tolerance issues that are frequently observed with repeated administration of GPCR agonists.

Nonstandard abbreviations

AUD alcohol use disorder
CIE chronic intermittent ethanol exposure
CPP conditioned place preference
DID drinking in the dark
GPCR G protein-coupled receptor
mGlu metabotropic glutamate receptor
NAM negative allosteric modulator
PAM positive allosteric modulator
PET positron emission tomography
SUD substance use disorder

1. Introduction

Chronic alcohol exposure is associated with widespread adaptations in brain function from the cellular to circuit level. Alcohol use disorder (AUD) affects millions of individuals worldwide, and is implicated in 3.3 million deaths per year along with substantial economic and medical consequences (Sacks, Gonzales, Bouchery, Tomedi, & Brewer, 2015; World Health Organization, 2014). A variety of therapeutic strategies have been developed to treat AUD including counseling, community-based and pharmacological approaches (Jonas et al., 2014; Koob, Kenneth Lloyd, & Mason, 2009; Miller & Wilbourne, 2002). While some of these treatments are efficacious in reducing alcohol drinking and relapse in individuals with AUD, the success rates, while encouraging, are less than ideal for any given therapy (Jonas et al., 2014; Maisel, Blodgett, Wilbourne, Humphreys, & Finney, 2013; Miller & Wilbourne, 2002). Indeed, the most effective pharmacotherapeutics, acamprosate and naltrexone, appear to be somewhat less effective than other medications used for other mental health indications (Maisel et al., 2013). Furthermore, information about therapeutic options is not disseminated as widely as it could be (Carvalho, Heilig, Perez, Probst, & Rehm, 2019), although the NIAAA Alcohol Treatment Navigator provides a new web-based tool to address this need (https://alcoholtreatment.niaaa.nih.gov/). Thus, there is an ongoing need for more effective AUD-targeted therapies and better information about potential treatments.

To effectively develop new pharmacological treatments for AUD, an improved understanding of the neurotransmitter systems and circuits involved in alcohol-related behaviors is required. In recent years, alcohol-induced adaptations in glutamatergic circuits of the cerebral cortex, basal ganglia, and extended amygdala have been the subject of increased investigations (reviewed in Bell et al., 2016; Gremel & Lovinger, 2017; Hwa, Besheer, & Kash, 2017). Adaptations in glutamatergic systems in these regions are associated with many maladaptive aspects of behavior that likely contribute to problematic alcohol use, including impaired behavioral flexibility, enhanced habit formation, emergence of negative affect during withdrawal, and susceptibility to relapse. Thus, targeting glutamatergic systems involved in alcohol-related maladaptive behaviors represents an important strategy for identifying novel therapeutic mechanisms.

The metabotropic glutamate (mGlu) receptor family of G protein-coupled receptors (GPCRs) modulate glutamatergic transmission throughout the CNS and have received substantial attention as therapeutic targets in a wide variety of CNS disorders. The eight subtypes of mGlu receptors, which are class C GPCRs, are classified into three subgroups based on sequence homology, ligand-binding profiles, and shared downstream signaling pathways (Fig. 1) (Niswender & Conn, 2010). Group I mGlu receptors include $mGlu_1$ and $mGlu_5$. These receptors typically couple to $G_{q/11}$ family

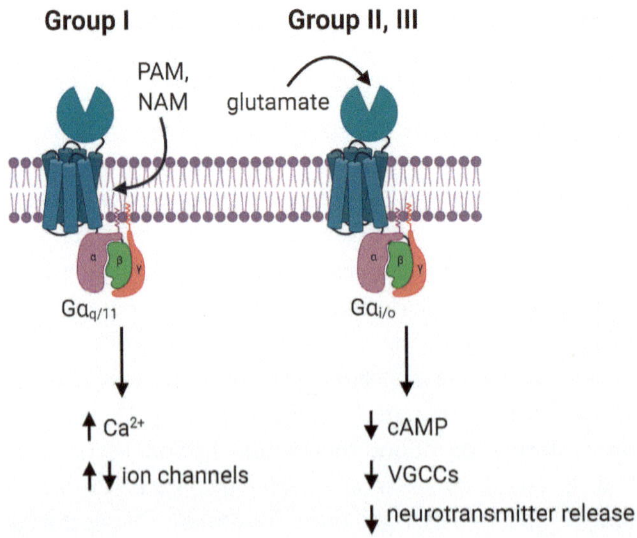

Fig. 1 Ligand binding sites and signaling downstream of mGlu receptors. mGlu receptors have a large N-terminal venus fly trap domain that contains the glutamate binding site, whereas known PAM and NAM binding sites are typically in the transmembrane domain. Group I mGlu receptors ($mGlu_1$ and $mGlu_5$) couple to $G_{q/11}$ family G proteins and activate phospholipase C pathways to increase intracellular calcium levels. These receptors can also modulate activity of ion channels to impact neuronal excitability and synaptic transmission (i.e., via effects on ionotropic glutamate receptors). Groups II ($mGlu_2$, $mGlu_3$) and III ($mGlu_4$, $mGlu_7$, and $mGlu_8$) couple to $G_{i/o}$ family G proteins, which leads to inhibition of adenylyl cyclase and decreases in cyclic AMP production, but also impacts neurotransmitter release by inhibiting voltage-gated calcium channels (VGCCs) and directly modulating vesicle fusion machinery.

G proteins and are typically found postsynaptically, where they generate second messenger signals, modulate neuronal excitability and synaptic transmission via effects on ion channels, and play important roles in synaptic plasticity. Group II mGlu receptors ($mGlu_2$ and $mGlu_3$) typically signal through $G_{i/o}$ family G proteins, and are often found to inhibit glutamatergic transmission by acting at presynaptic sites. The group III mGlu receptors include $mGlu_4$, $mGlu_6$, $mGlu_7$, and $mGlu_8$, all of which typically signal through $G_{i/o}$ family G proteins. Of these receptors, $mGlu_4$, $mGlu_7$, and $mGlu_8$ are known to presynaptically regulate glutamatergic transmission, but also modulate release of other neurotransmitters as well. Conversely, expression of $mGlu_6$ is historically considered to be restricted to the retina, and this receptor has not been of interest in the context of AUD. Each mGlu receptor subtype has a unique distribution in the CNS, and the physiological effects of activating each receptor subtype can vary widely depending on the specific neuron population in which it is expressed. In addition, mGlu receptors form obligatory dimers that can be either homo- or heterodimers, further expanding the diversity of CNS functions (Doumazane et al., 2011; Ferre et al., 2014).

The mGlu receptor family has proven highly amenable to drug discovery efforts geared toward identification of allosteric ligands, as selective positive and/or negative allosteric modulators (PAMs, NAMs) suitable for use in vivo have been identified for most mGlu receptor subtypes (Hellyer, Leach, & Gregory, 2017; Nickols & Conn, 2014). Notably, a number of recently developed drugs targeting mGlu receptors (particularly $mGlu_5$ and $mGlu_2$) have had properties suitable for advancement to clinical trials, allowing critical assessments of the translational validity of targets identified in preclinical studies. Allosteric ligands of mGlu receptors bind to sites on the receptor that are distinct from the *N*-terminal glutamate binding domain, often in the transmembrane domain (Dore et al., 2014; Koehl et al., 2019; Wu et al., 2014). Because these allosteric sites are less conserved among receptor subtypes, targeting these sites has proven a fruitful approach to developing drugs selective for individual mGlu receptor subtypes (Conn, Lindsley, Meiler, & Niswender, 2014; Foster & Conn, 2017; Leach & Gregory, 2017). The success of mGlu receptor drug discovery efforts has provided preclinical tools that are indispensable for studying the roles of mGlu receptors in a variety of CNS disorders, and this progress has been accompanied by extensive efforts to develop mGlu receptor allosteric modulators that have suitable pharmacodynamic, pharmacokinetic, and safety profiles for use in human neurological and psychiatric disorders (e.g., mavoglurant, basimglurant, AZD8529).

Substantial research efforts have focused on identifying roles for mGlu receptors in the etiology and treatment of AUD. On the genetic level, variants of at least one mGlu receptor are associated with high levels of drinking, and deletion of several mGlu receptor subtypes in rats or mice alters levels of alcohol reward and consumption. Chronic alcohol exposure can change both expression and function of various mGlu receptor subtypes in ways that support the emergence of maladaptive alcohol self-administration. This chapter will review evidence that mGlu receptors influence alcohol reward, consumption, and seeking in preclinical experimental systems, and that allosteric modulators of mGlu receptors, particularly $mGlu_5$ and $mGlu_2$, have effects on alcohol seeking and taking in animals that could translate to treatments for AUD. A list of allosteric modulators used in preclinical investigations of AUD and other substance use disorders (SUDs) can be found in Table 1. Although it is outside the scope of this chapter, there is

Table 1 mGlu receptor PAMs and NAMs used in alcohol-related experiments.

Receptor	PAM	NAM	Selected references
Group I			
$mGlu_1$		CPCCOEt	Schroeder, Overstreet, and Hodge (2005), Hodge et al. (2006), and Lominac et al. (2006)
		JNJ16259685	Besheer et al. (2008a), Cozzoli, Courson, et al. (2014), and Lum, Campbell, Rostock, and Szumlinski (2014)
$mGlu_5$	CDPPB		Gass, Glen, et al. (2014), Gass, Trantham-Davidson, et al. (2014), and Gass, McGonigal, and Chandler (2017)
		MPEP	McGeehan and Olive (2003), Backstrom, Bachteler, Koch, Hyytia, and Spanagel (2004), McMillen, Crawford, Kulers, and Williams (2005), Hodge et al. (2006), Lominac et al. (2006), Besheer et al. (2008b), Gupta et al. (2008), Schroeder et al. (2008), and Lee, Choe, et al. (2016)
		MTEP	Cowen, Djouma, and Lawrence (2005), Cowen, Krstew, and Lawrence (2007), Adams, Cowen, Short, and Lawrence (2008), Adams, Short, and Lawrence (2010), Cozzoli, Courson, et al. (2014), Lee, Coelho, Class, Sern, et al. (2018), Lee, Coelho, Class, and Szumlinski (2018), and Gobin and Schwendt (2019)
Group II			
$mGlu_2$	AZD8529		Augier et al. (2016), Li et al. (2016), and Sidhpura, Weiss, and Martin-Fardon (2010)
	BINA		Windisch and Czachowski (2018)
	JNJ-42153605		Ahnaou et al. (2015) and Ahnaou, de Boer, et al. (2016)
	AZD8418		Li et al. (2016)
	LY487379		Nikiforuk et al. (2010)
Group III			
$mGlu_7$	AMN082 (agonist)		Bahi (2012) and Kotlinska et al. (2019)

extensive literature detailing preclinical investigations of mGlu receptor orthosteric and allosteric ligands on reward, consumption, and seeking of other psychoactive drugs, and we refer readers to several recent reviews that address these topics (Barnes, Sheffler, Semenova, Cosford, & Bespalov, 2018; Caprioli, Justinova, Venniro, & Shaham, 2018; Cross, Anthenelli, & Li, 2018; Joffe, Centanni, Jaramillo, Winder, & Conn, 2018; Johnson & Lovinger, 2016; Li & Markou, 2015; Scofield et al., 2016).

2. Experimental systems for studying mGlu receptor relevance to AUD

A variety of organisms and behavioral paradigms have been used to examine the actions of acute and chronic ethanol that are thought to contribute to drinking. The majority of studies have used rodent models (e.g., rat and mouse), and these models have been used in almost all experiments examining mGlu roles in ethanol-induced neuroadaptations and drinking. Thus, we will focus on rodent models in the current discussion. We will not describe all the techniques used for these purposes, but will instead focus on those that have been used to examine mGlu roles in alcohol actions and alcohol drinking.

2.1 Evaluation of ethanol-mediated reward

To assess if ethanol has rewarding effects (i.e., if intoxication is a desired outcome), researchers often use the conditioned place preference (CPP) test (Huston, Silva, Topic, & Muller, 2013; Valyear, Villaruel, & Chaudhri, 2017). This involves ethanol exposure in one compartment of a chamber containing two or more total compartments. In other compartments the animal normally receives vehicle. Following training with the treatment/compartment combinations, the animal is given a test trial in which it can freely choose which compartment it prefers, and the percentage of time spent in the ethanol-paired compartment signals the animal's ethanol preference. This paradigm has been used extensively in mice, and C57BL/6J mice (as well as transgenic mice with this genetic background) show preference for a compartment in which they received low-moderate ethanol doses. Interestingly, DBA/2J mice show stronger CPP for ethanol (Cunningham, Niehus, Malott, & Prather, 1992), perhaps indicating more rewarding subjective ethanol effects in this strain. The ethanol CPP test is not administered often in rat for the odd reason that commonly used rat strains do not exhibit CPP, but rather conditioned place aversion, after ethanol injection or intragastric infusion (Cunningham, 1981; Fidler, Bakner, & Cunningham, 2004; Stewart & Grupp, 1981). While CPP is useful for assessing subjective reward, this is not the only factor that controls ethanol intake, and thus more direct measures of drinking or operant self-administration often show outcomes that appear to differ from CPP in the same animal or treatment conditions.

Locomotor activation and sensitization (i.e., increased locomotion following repeated drug administration) were originally touted as measures of rewarding drug actions (Wise & Bozarth, 1987). Sensitization to ethanol-induced locomotor activation can be seen in some rodent strains, but is highly dependent on dose, and some strains show little locomotor activation following acute ethanol administration. Several studies have now revealed discrepancies between findings with sensitization and CPP or other measures of drug reward, raising concerns as to whether this behavioral change provides information about reward.

2.2 Models of voluntary ethanol drinking

Investigators have also employed a variety of more direct measures of ethanol intake to determine animals' willingness to consume the drug. The most straightforward technique is to provide the animal with a choice between two or more bottles (i.e., two-bottle choice), one containing ethanol dissolved in water and the other water alone (Griffin, 2014). The amount of ethanol consumed and the preference for ethanol compared to water are measured. Ethanol content is often increased from low (e.g., 5%) to high (20%) levels as the animals become more familiar with the solution. More sophisticated versions include "lickometers" or other devices to measure consumption rate and patterns. Different rat and mouse strains show varying ethanol intake and preference in two-bottle choice experiments, with C57BL/6J mice consistently observed to prefer alcohol (Belknap, Crabbe, & Young, 1993; Yoneyama, Crabbe, Ford, Murillo, & Finn, 2008). In addition to strain differences, sex also influences levels of voluntary ethanol consumption, and female mice are routinely reported to consume larger amounts of ethanol and show higher ethanol preference than male mice (Hilderbrand & Lasek, 2018). While this approach provides a ready index of how much ethanol an animal is willing to drink, all factors that control drinking, such as taste preference, contribute to the experimental outcome. Thus, two-bottle choice drinking and preference does not always provide a good index of how much a particular rodent likes the subjective effects of ethanol.

Researchers have also developed other relatively simple ethanol drinking paradigms based on more naturalistic patterns of activity and feeding/drinking in rodents. The drinking-in-the-dark paradigm is the most popular of these paradigms, as it is designed to assay drinking during the circadian period when mice, a nocturnal species, are most active (Crabbe, Phillips, & Belknap, 2010; Thiele & Navarro, 2014). Mice are given access to ethanol in water for 2–4 h starting a few hours into the dark period. They will generally drink more alcohol and achieve higher blood alcohol concentrations during this period in comparison to all-day drinking or drinking in the light period (Thiele & Navarro, 2014). It must be noted that placement of the ethanol-containing bottle in the cage is one trigger for the enhanced drinking (Wilcox et al., 2014). Two-bottle choice variants of the paradigm have also been developed, but drinking is generally not as robust as in the original single-bottle version.

Early studies from the Wise laboratory found that rats would consume more ethanol in a two-bottle choice paradigm if the ethanol was only available every other day, as opposed to every day (Carnicella, Ron, & Barak, 2014; Wise, 1973). This "intermittent access" paradigm has now been used in mice as well (Hwa et al., 2011; Melendez, 2011). In both species, ethanol intake and preference increases across access sessions, and this escalation can lead to consumption of levels generally associated with intoxication. The factors that drive increased consumption in this paradigm are not clear, but may involve unique neural effects of cycles of intoxication and sobriety as well as the general finding that rodents increase rate of intake of commodities when access is tightly scheduled. The intermittent access paradigm affords a good test of how much animals are willing to escalate ethanol intake and effects of treatments on this intake. In some strains the schedule results in what might be considered binge or excessive drinking. However, it should be noted that drinking and preference levels usually fall back to the original level if continuous access is provided following intermittent access. This indicates that the animals do not show permanent enhancement of their desire to consume ethanol, and thus consume excessively only under conditions of intermittent access.

Rodents do not generally prefer the taste of ethanol, and thus paradigms have been developed to foster ethanol drinking by adding desired tastants during the initial phases of drinking. The most common procedure is "sucrose fading," in which the sweetened ethanol solution is available when the animal first starts drinking, and then the sucrose is gradually removed, and ethanol content often increased, as the animal becomes more familiar with the ethanol taste (Tolliver, Sadeghi, & Samson, 1988). This procedure generally increases ethanol intake relative to unadulterated ethanol solution once the fading is complete. A similar paradigm has also been developed with monosodium glutamate (an umami tastant) (McCool & Chappell, 2012). This procedure is especially effective in DBA mice that have a strong aversion to ethanol taste and a poor preference for sweet taste, but a strong preference for umami. The major concern with tastant fading procedures is that neural associations will develop to the tastant or tastant-alcohol combination that are different from those produced by ethanol alone. However, humans often consume ethanol with tastants, so this procedure has some naturalistic appeal.

2.3 Operant self-administration of ethanol

Different paradigms for operant ethanol self-administration have been developed to determine what actions rodents will perform to obtain the drug. This can be viewed as a measure of alcohol seeking or wanting (Samson & Czachowski, 2003). Operant ethanol self-administration models have been used extensively to preclinically evaluate interventions that reduce ethanol seeking or taking. Indeed, there is some predictive validity observed using these models, as some drugs used to treat human AUD (e.g., acamprosate, naltrexone, nalmefene) reduce ethanol self-administration in rodents (Bachteler, Economidou, Danysz, Ciccocioppo, & Spanagel, 2005; Czachowski, Legg, & Samson, 2001; Herz, 1997; Spanagel, 2017). The most commonly used self-administration technique involves rodents pressing a lever to receive access to an ethanol drinking opportunity. The ethanol is usually delivered to a receptacle or a "dipper" that becomes accessible following the required number of presses. Versions of ethanol self-administration involving intragastric, intravenous and intracerebral injection have also been developed. These approaches are understandably more difficult than the drinking-based design due to the need for surgery, patency of delivery lines, and irritation of blood vessels or stomach by ethanol. Nonetheless, useful information has been obtained with these techniques, as they eliminate taste effects on preference. In the case of intracerebral injection investigators can also locate brain regions involved in alcohol consumption (McBride, Murphy, & Ikemoto, 1999).

As with all instrumental conditioning paradigms, different schedules of reinforcement can be used to control operant self-administration.

Simple fixed ratio (FR) schedules are most often employed to maximize pressing rates. The progressive ratio (PR) schedule in which increased numbers of presses must be made for each consecutive reinforcer is a favorite paradigm for assessing how hard animals will work for the drug. Random interval schedules have also been used to produce lever pressing that is independent of outcome (so-called stimulus-response behavior) (Corbit & Janak, 2016). Ethanol self-administration paradigms designed to separate "seeking" and taking have also been devised (Samson & Czachowski, 2003). In these paradigms animals are usually taught to perform one action (e.g., lever press) to obtain access to perform a second action (e.g., chain pull) that results in ethanol delivery.

Investigators often using predictive stimuli or conditioned reinforcers (e.g., brief light or tone presentations) in their self-administration training and testing paradigms. The predictive "cues" are thought to mimic environmental stimuli that lead to enhanced ethanol seeking or reinstatement of behavior (Venniro, Caprioli, & Shaham, 2016). Indeed, cue-induced reinstatement is readily measured in most ethanol self-administration paradigms. Operant responding for ethanol might also be invigorated by prior presentation of the predictive stimulus through Pavlovian-to-Instrumental transfer (PIT) conditioning, although whether this translates to a meaningful increase in ethanol intake has been called into question (Lamb, Schindler, & Pinkston, 2016). Conditioned reinforcers can support operant actions in the absence of the primary reinforcer. It should be noted that there is evidence for differential engagement of different neural circuits in self-paced (e.g., cue-free) versus PIT-driven operant responding (Cartoni, Balleine, & Baldassarre, 2016; Yin & Knowlton, 2006). Thus, it is important to consider the choice of experimental design when evaluating neurobiological underpinnings of ethanol self-administration. The general features of the environmental context also alter ethanol self-administration (Valyear et al., 2017), and context-induced reinstatement has also been demonstrated for this drug. Experimenter administration of low doses of ethanol can also induce relapse to ethanol self-administration, perhaps mimicking the first drink in relapse (Venniro et al., 2016).

There is extensive literature from both humans and laboratory animal studies indicating interactions between stress and drug use disorders (Blaine & Sinha, 2017; Koob, 2015). A prominent hypothesis is that stressful life events can drive individuals toward relapse to drug seeking and taking that provides temporary relief from the effects of stress. This has been modeled in rodents using approaches for stress-induced reinstatement of drinking and self-administration (Becker, 2017; Cozzoli, Tanchuck-Nipper, Kaufman, Horowitz, & Finn, 2014; Spanagel, Noori, & Heilig, 2014). With respect to ethanol, the majority of studies have been performed in rat, although there is increasing evidence that mice will also show stress-induced reinstatement (Mantsch, Baker, Funk, Le, & Shaham, 2016).

2.4 Compulsive ethanol seeking

Various measures of persistent drug seeking and taking in the absence of drug or the presence of adverse events have been developed with the aim of assessing if seeking/taking are compulsive (Hopf & Lesscher, 2014). These include measuring responses when the drug is not delivered and examining effects of foot shock or other painful and stress-inducing stimuli on seeking/taking. With ethanol drinking, investigators have also developed techniques for taste adulteration, particularly by adding quinine to the ethanol solution to discourage drinking. Animals that continue to drink in spite of the addition of quinine are considered to show compulsive drinking. In this paradigm it is important to demonstrate that experience with the ethanol/quinine mixture does not alter the aversion to quinine taste.

2.5 Ethanol effects on cognition

Other experimental approaches have been used to determine consequences of chronic ethanol exposure or drinking that could affect decision-making. Performance in set-shifting tasks is disrupted following chronic ethanol exposure in rats and mice (Gass, Glen, et al., 2014; Spear, 2018). This cognitive impairment may be related to ethanol effects that impair prefrontal cortex and its connections to the hippocampus. Spatial learning that involves the hippocampus is also disrupted by ethanol (Van Skike, Goodlett, & Matthews, 2019). Chronic ethanol exposure and drinking also promote stimulus-response (habit) learning in mice and rats (Barker et al., 2015; Corbit & Janak, 2016; Everitt & Robbins, 2016; Renteria, Baltz, & Gremel, 2018). This is generally thought to involve effects on cortico-basal ganglia circuitry. Indeed, there is evidence that chronic ethanol exposure enhances behaviors that involve the sensorimotor striatum, which is part of this circuitry (DePoy et al., 2013). The combination of disrupted cognition and increased habitual responding following chronic ethanol exposure may foster poor decision-making, especially in the presence of the drug.

2.6 Passive ethanol exposure models

It should be noted that effects of chronic ethanol in rodents are examined using a variety of drug exposure methods. In addition to the drinking and self-administration paradigms mentioned above, several methods for involuntary ethanol administration have been used over the years. These include intragastric gavage, intraperitoneal injection, liquid diet consumption in which no alternative liquid is provided, and vapor inhalation-based exposure (Crabbe, Harris, & Koob, 2011). These "forced administration" paradigms are very useful, as rodents generally will not voluntarily consume doses of ethanol that produce blood and brain levels commonly observed in humans. These procedures also ensure predictable blood and brain concentrations on a regular schedule, free from the variability observed with drinking or ethanol self-administration. Passive ethanol administration is often employed in conjunction with voluntary drinking or self-administration paradigms to produce escalation of drinking and to allow investigators to study volitional alcohol consumption during dependence (Griffin, 2014; Lopez & Becker, 2014; Vendruscolo & Roberts, 2014). As we will see, some effects of mGlu receptor ligands on alcohol-related behaviors are particularly robust in animals that have been exposed to both passive and voluntary forms of alcohol exposure. Thus, experimenter-administered ethanol provides information that complements results obtained from drinking and self-administration paradigms.

3. Group I mGlu receptors in preclinical models of alcohol exposure

The group I mGlu receptors, particularly $mGlu_5$, have received considerable attention as therapeutic targets for the treatment of AUD and other SUDs due to their ability to modulate glutamatergic transmission in brain regions associated with psychoactive drug misuse (Caprioli et al., 2018; Joffe et al., 2018; Kasten, Holmgren, & Wills, 2019). Alcohol exposure affects expression and function of $mGlu_1$ and $mGlu_5$, and pharmacological reversal of adaptations that support alcohol taking and seeking could therefore modify maladaptive behaviors. Alcohol exposure causes upregulation of $mGlu_1$ mRNA in several brain regions, whereas $mGlu_5$ regulation by alcohol appears to be more complex. Voluntary alcohol drinking or passive alcohol exposure can increase $mGlu_1$ expression in the nucleus accumbens, central amygdala, and hippocampus depending on the model used (Alasmari, Bell, Rao, Hammad, & Sari, 2018; Cozzoli et al., 2009; Cozzoli, Courson, et al., 2014; Goulding et al., 2011; Lee, Coelho, et al., 2016; Obara et al., 2009; Szumlinski, Ary, Lominac, Klugmann, & Kippin, 2008), and mice selectively bred for high levels of binge-like drinking show higher expression levels of $mGlu_1$ and the associated scaffolding protein Homer2 in the nucleus accumbens (Cozzoli et al., 2012, 2009). Alcohol effects on $mGlu_5$ expression are more complex and depend on the alcohol exposure paradigm, species, and time since last alcohol exposure. Voluntary drinking and passive forms of alcohol exposure are associated with increased $mGlu_5$ mRNA in rodents (Lee, Coelho, et al., 2016), although a longitudinal study of $mGlu_5$ availability measured using positron emission tomography (PET) showed that voluntary alcohol consumption decreases $mGlu_5$ availability in the amygdala and hippocampus (de Laat et al., 2019). In humans, lower $mGlu_5$ receptor availability in cortical and striatal regions is associated with alcohol dependence (Ceccarini et al., 2019; Leurquin-Sterk, Ceccarini, Crunelle, de Laat, Verbeek, et al., 2018), whereas in moderate social drinkers, $mGlu_5$ availability in cortical, striatal, and thalamic regions is positively correlated with euphoric effects of alcohol (Leurquin-Sterk, Ceccarini, Crunelle, Weerasekera, et al., 2018). Higher $mGlu_5$ availability in the striatum at onset of alcohol abstinence is associated with risk of relapse (Ceccarini et al., 2019). Conversely, after $\sim$1 month of alcohol abstinence, higher $mGlu_5$ levels in the amygdala are associated with lower temptation to drink (Akkus et al., 2018), indicating that there are complex, region-specific dynamics of $mGlu_5$ expression in humans with a history of heavy alcohol use.

In addition to effects on expression, alcohol impacts the modulatory effects of $mGlu_1$ and $mGlu_5$ in multiple brain regions. For example, acute application of alcohol to nucleus accumbens slices disrupts group I mGlu receptor-mediated potentiation of NMDA receptors (Mishra, Zhang, & Chergui, 2012). Group I mGlu receptor-mediated mobilization of retrograde endocannabinoid signaling in the nucleus accumbens and cerebellum are also disrupted by acute alcohol exposure (Carta, Mameli, & Valenzuela, 2006; Renteria, Jeanes, & Morrisett, 2014; Su, Sun, & Shen, 2010), and chronic intermittent ethanol vapor exposure (CIE) disrupts $mGlu_{1/5}$-mediated long-term depression in the CA1 region of the hippocampus (Wills et al., 2017).

Although NAMs of $mGlu_1$ have been evaluated in preclinical models of AUDs, the vast majority of studies have focused on $mGlu_5$. Thus, this section will primarily explore the effects of $mGlu_5$ NAMs in models of alcohol reward, drinking, and seeking, and will briefly consider the potential for $mGlu_5$ NAMs to impact negative affective states induced by alcohol withdrawal.

3.1 mGlu$_5$ NAM effects on alcohol reward

Blockade of mGlu$_5$ reduces expression of ethanol CPP in both rats and mice (Kotlinska, Bochenski, & Danysz, 2011; Lominac et al., 2006). In CPP studies that were designed to dissociate effects of mGlu$_5$ blockade on acquisition, expression, and reinstatement following extinction training in mice, the mGlu$_5$ NAM MPEP (2-Methyl-6-(phenylethynyl)pyridine) was found to differentially modulate discrete phases involved in reward conditioning in mice. Specifically, when MPEP was administered during conditioning, it did not affect place preference post-conditioning (Lee, Choe, et al., 2016; McGeehan & Olive, 2003). This finding aligns with intact low-dose ethanol CPP observed in mice with global mGlu$_5$ deletion (Bird, Kirchhoff, Djouma, & Lawrence, 2008). Conversely, MPEP administration prior to a post-conditioning test or a reinstatement challenge reduces both expression and reinstatement of ethanol CPP (Lee, Choe, et al., 2016). Effects of mGlu$_5$ NAMs on ethanol-induced changes in neurotransmission could contribute to the observation that these drugs reduce ethanol reward. Notably, MPEP pretreatment prevents ethanol-induced changes in dopamine, glutamate and GABA levels in the nucleus accumbens of mice (Lominac et al., 2006).

3.2 mGlu$_5$ NAM effects on alcohol consumption and seeking

Findings that mGlu$_5$ is involved in alcohol reward suggest that mGlu$_5$ blockade could interfere with the primary reinforcing effects of alcohol, and thus reduce voluntary alcohol consumption. mGlu$_5$ NAM effects have been evaluated in a variety of models of volitional alcohol consumption, including two-bottle choice and DID tasks as well as operant ethanol self-administration models. Across rat and mouse strains and models, there has been remarkable consistency in the reported ability of mGlu$_5$ NAMs to reduce alcohol consumption. Chronic administration of the mGlu$_5$ NAM MTEP (3-((2-Methyl-1,3-thiazol-4-yl)ethynyl)pyridine) reduces voluntary drinking in Fawn-Hooded and alcohol-preferring rats (Cowen et al., 2005), and MPEP administration reduces alcohol intake in a mouse DID model (Gupta et al., 2008) and in Myers high ethanol-preferring rats (McMillen et al., 2005). Similarly, MTEP administration prior to binge drinking sessions reduces drinking in adolescent and adult mice of both sexes (Cozzoli, Courson, et al., 2014). Interestingly, adolescent female mice that are treated with MTEP during binge drinking show reduced alcohol consumption when re-introduced to alcohol after a period of abstinence. Conversely, MTEP treatment during binge drinking leads to higher levels of alcohol consumption upon re-exposure in adult female mice (Cozzoli, Courson, et al., 2014). Despite decreasing alcohol consumption during binge drinking sessions, MTEP does not significantly alter subsequent alcohol consumption in adolescent or adult male mice (Cozzoli, Courson, et al., 2014). Studies in mice lacking $mGlu_5$ expression specifically in D_1 dopamine receptor-expressing neurons suggest that $mGlu_5$ activity in D_1-expressing neurons is critical for escalation of alcohol drinking following forced abstinence (Parkitna et al., 2013). MPEP fails to reduce ethanol consumption or preference in mice with genetic deletion of the ε isoform of protein kinase C (PKCε) (Olive et al., 2005). Further, PKCε-null mice show lower levels of voluntary alcohol consumption, suggesting that signaling through this pathway, perhaps downstream of $mGlu_5$, supports alcohol consumption under normal conditions (Olive et al., 2005).

In addition to effects in voluntary drinking models, $mGlu_5$ NAMs also reduce alcohol consumption in operant ethanol self-administration models. For example, in an operant ethanol self-administration paradigm designed to distinguish between appetitive and consummatory phases of self-administration in mice, MTEP reduced both appetitive responding and consumption (Cowen et al., 2007), and this finding is supported by earlier studies showing reduced operant ethanol self-administration in mice after MPEP administration (Hodge et al., 2006; Lominac et al., 2006) and in alcohol-preferring rats following MPEP or MTEP administration (Cowen et al., 2005; Schroeder et al., 2005). These effects likely involve $mGlu_5$ in the nucleus accumbens, as direct infusion of MPEP or MTEP into the accumbens (but not into the dorsomedial striatum or medial prefrontal cortex) of alcohol-preferring rats also reduces alcohol self-administration (Besheer et al., 2010; Gass & Olive, 2009). In addition to reduced alcohol self-administration, MPEP also reduces the breakpoint in alcohol-preferring rats during a progressive ratio task, suggesting a specific modulation of motivation to take ethanol (Besheer, Faccidomo, Grondin, & Hodge, 2008b). Moreover, $mGlu_5$ NAM administration reduces the subjective (discriminative stimulus) effects of ethanol in rats, which could contribute to reduced alcohol self-administration (Besheer & Hodge, 2005; Besheer, Stevenson, & Hodge, 2006).

Reducing $mGlu_5$ activity is also associated with inhibition of cue-induced reinstatement of ethanol seeking following extinction training. Systemic administration of MPEP reduces cue-induced reinstatement in Long Evans rats (Backstrom et al., 2004), and MPEP also attenuates cue-induced reinstatement in selectively bred alcohol-preferring rats (Schroeder et al., 2008). Interestingly, robust reductions of cue-induced reinstatement of ethanol seeking have been observed when MTEP is co-administered with either an antagonist of CB1 cannabinoid receptors (Adams et al., 2010) or an adenosine A_{2A} receptor antagonist (Adams et al., 2008) in alcohol-preferring rats, suggesting that simultaneous targeting of $mGlu_5$ and other receptor systems could be an effective strategy for prevention of relapse in AUD. Studies evaluating the effects of direct infusion of MTEP into the basolateral amygdala or nucleus accumbens prior to cue-induced reinstatement of ethanol seeking suggest that both regions contribute to effects on reinstatement following systemic MTEP administration (Sinclair, Cleva, Hood, Olive, & Gass, 2012). In addition, systemic administration of MPEP attenuates reinstatement-induced increases in ERK phosphorylation in the basolateral amygdala and nucleus accumbens (Schroeder et al., 2008). The ability of $mGlu_5$ NAMs to reduce relapse-like behavior is particularly interesting in light of recent findings in humans diagnosed with AUD that high striatal $mGlu_5$ availability at the onset of alcohol abstinence is associated with a higher risk of relapse (Ceccarini et al., 2019). Although we have focused on findings specifically related to alcohol here, $mGlu_5$ NAMs reduce taking and seeking of other psychoactive drugs as well (Caprioli et al., 2018), suggesting that these drugs affect circuitry that is commonly recruited during self-administration of many drugs.

Although preclinical investigations have focused on using $mGlu_5$ NAMs to reduce ethanol taking and seeking, enhancement of $mGlu_5$ activity using PAMs has also been explored for effects on drug seeking behavior. Interestingly, the $mGlu_5$ PAM CDPPB (3-Cyano-*N*-(1,3-diphenyl-1*H*-pyrazol-5-yl)benzamide), which (along with other $mGlu_5$ PAMs) has been shown to enhance learning in a variety of models, facilitates extinction of ethanol seeking in rat self-administration studies (Gass, Trantham-Davidson, et al., 2014). Further, CDPBB administration during extinction reduces subsequent sensitivity to cue-induced reinstatement. Rats exhibit impaired extinction of ethanol seeking following CIE, and this resistance to extinction can be alleviated by CDPPB administration (Gass et al., 2017). Thus, while preclinical studies have largely focused on $mGlu_5$ blockade for treatment of AUD, both positive and negative modulation of $mGlu_5$ impact drug taking and seeking by modulating unique aspects of behavior.

3.3 mGlu$_5$ NAM effects on negative affective states following alcohol withdrawal

Alcohol withdrawal after voluntary drinking or passive forms of exposure is associated with behaviors characteristic of negative affect including increased measures of anhedonia, avoidance, and anxiety-like behavior (Centanni, Bedse, Patel, & Winder, 2019; Cover, Kerkhoff, & Mathur, 2018; Holleran et al., 2016; Holleran & Winder, 2017; Koob, 2009; Lee, Coehlo, McGregor, Waltermire, & Szumlinski, 2015; Lee, Coehlo, Solton, & Szumlinski, 2017; Metten et al., 2018; Vranjkovic, Winkler, & Winder, 2018), and negative affective states are viewed as a critical component of the addiction cycle in humans (Koob & Volkow, 2016). There is extensive preclinical evidence that mGlu$_5$ NAMs reduce behavioral despair and avoidance behavior in rodents (Barnes et al., 2018; Nickols & Conn, 2014; Terbeck, Akkus, Chesterman, & Hasler, 2015), and the mGlu$_5$ NAM fenobam (*N*-(3-Chlorophenyl)-*N′*-(4,5-dihydro-1-methyl-4-oxo-1*H*-imidazol-2-yl)urea) reduced anxiety (or anxiety-like behavior) in both preclinical assessments and in a clinical trial (Pecknold, McClure, Appeltauer, Wrzesinski, & Allan, 1982; Porter et al., 2005). These findings spurred investigation of mGlu$_5$ NAM effects in rodent models of negative affect associated with alcohol withdrawal (reviewed in Kasten et al., 2019). In rats and mice with a history of alcohol exposure, mGlu$_5$ NAMs (MPEP and MTEP) reverse avoidance/anxiety-like measures in elevated plus maze, light-dark box, and marble burying tests (Kotlinska & Bochenski, 2008; Kumar, Hapidin, Bee, & Ismail, 2013; Lee, Coelho, Class, Sern, et al., 2018; Lee, Coelho, Class, & Szumlinski, 2018; Lee, Coelho, Sern, et al., 2017). Direct infusion of MTEP into the nucleus accumbens shell in mice replicates some, but not all, effects of systemic MTEP administration on alcohol withdrawal-induced negative affective behaviors (Lee, Coelho, Class, Sern, et al., 2018), suggesting that mGlu$_5$ modulation in other circuitry is also involved.

3.4 Additional considerations regarding exploration of mGlu$_5$ as a therapeutic target in AUD

Despite the extensive preclinical evidence that mGlu$_5$ NAMs have potential for treating SUDs, to date there has been little progress translating these findings in clinical trials. Trials for smoking cessation conducted with the mGlu$_5$ NAM mavoglurant (AFQ-056; Methyl (3aR,4S,7aR)-4-hydroxy-4-[(3-methylphenyl)ethynyl]octahydro-1*H*-indole-1-carboxylate) were completed (ClinicalTrials.gov ID: NCT00414752), but results of this trial have not been disclosed. A clinical trial evaluating the efficacy of mavoglurant in cocaine use disorder is also in progress (NCT03242928), and disclosure of results from this trial will be eagerly anticipated.

Concerns related to on- or off-target adverse effects of $mGlu_5$ NAMs could hinder translation of this class of compounds to clinical use (Barnes et al., 2018). For example, $mGlu_5$ NAMs including fenobam and AZD9272 (3-Fluoro-5-[3-(5-fluoro-2-pyridinyl)-1,2,4-oxadiazol-5-yl]benzonitrile) have produced pro-psychotic effects in clinical trials for other indications (Pecknold et al., 1982; Stahle, Jonzon, Eriksson, & Kagedal, 2012), although recent evidence of off-target binding of these drugs suggests that the pro-psychotic effects of these drugs could occur independent of $mGlu_5$ inhibition (Varnas et al., 2019). Additional concerns stem from findings that enhancing $mGlu_5$ activity with PAMs has pro-cognitive effects, raising the possibility that $mGlu_5$ NAM administration could cause undesired cognitive impairments when used to decrease drug taking or relapse. Supporting this concern, when rats that have been trained to self-administer cocaine are assessed in a working memory task (delayed match-to-sample) during abstinence, they show markedly impaired performance with repeated MTEP administration (Gobin & Schwendt, 2019). As mentioned previously, the $mGlu_5$ PAM CDPPB facilitates extinction of ethanol self-administration (Gass, Trantham-Davidson, et al., 2014). In addition, CDPPB reduces impairments in behavioral flexibility during adulthood in rats exposed to alcohol during adolescence (Gass, Glen, et al., 2014). These findings raise the possibility that $mGlu_5$ activation rather than inhibition might be useful as a therapeutic strategy in conjunction with behavioral interventions for AUD treatment. If $mGlu_5$-selective compounds advance toward evaluation for AUD, It will be important to consider how these pharmacotherapies might interact with behavioral interventions that reduce drug use or relapse in humans.

A final consideration is that many people diagnosed with AUD also use other psychoactive drugs. Thus, consideration of $mGlu_5$ effects on alcohol taking and seeking must be considered in the context of polysubstance use. This concern is particularly relevant to nicotine, as roughly three quarters of individuals diagnosed with AUD also smoke cigarettes (Guydish et al., 2016). Notably, nicotine use is associated with reduced $mGlu_5$ availability (Akkus et al., 2013; Hulka et al., 2014; Muller Herde et al., 2019), which is likely to alter the efficacy of $mGlu_5$ NAM treatment. As pharmacotherapies for AUDs progress to clinical trials, it will be critical to consider additional factors such as concurrent or former use of other drugs to identify subpopulations that are most amenable to the treatment in question.

3.5 Effects of $mGlu_1$ modulation in models of alcohol exposure

Relative to $mGlu_5$, $mGlu_1$ modulation has received far less attention as a therapeutic strategy in AUD. Among the few reports that exist, there are several conflicting results. Multiple studies reported that the $mGlu_1$ NAM CPCCOEt (7-(Hydroxyimino)cyclopropa[*b*]chromen-1a-carboxylate ethyl ester) does not significantly reduce alcohol self-administration in male P rats or male C57BL/6J mice (Hodge et al., 2006; Schroeder et al., 2005). However, in another study, CPCCOEt decreased alcohol self-administration, voluntary drinking, and CPP in male C57BL/6J mice (Lominac et al., 2006). Interestingly, CPCCOEt facilitates reduction of spontaneous locomotor activity following ethanol administration, which suggests that $mGlu_1$ blockade increases sensitivity to the sedating effects of alcohol (Lominac et al., 2006). However, another study failed to observe this effect on locomotor activity (Sharko & Hodge, 2008). Another $mGlu_1$ NAM, JNJ16259685 ((3,4-Dihydro-2*H*-pyrano[2,3-*b*]quinolin-7-yl)-(*cis*-4-methoxycyclohexyl)-methanone), decreases operant responding for alcohol in male P rats under both a fixed ratio 1 (FR1) schedule and in a progressive ratio task, but also decreases locomotor activity and responding for sucrose, indicating a possible non-specific motor effect (Besheer, Faccidomo, Grondin, & Hodge, 2008a; Besheer et al., 2008b). Direct infusion of JNJ16259685 into the nucleus accumbens shell or central amygdala of C57BL/6J mice reduces alcohol drinking in a DID paradigm at doses that do not decrease sucrose intake (Cozzoli, Courson, et al., 2014; Lum et al., 2014), suggestive of a specific effect of $mGlu_1$ blockade when this circuitry is targeted. However, intra-accumbens infusion of CPCCOEt does not significantly reduce voluntary drinking, which could reflect differences in the models used or the pharmacodynamic properties of different $mGlu_1$ NAMs (Cozzoli et al., 2012, 2009). Effects of $mGlu_1$ NAMs on reinstatement of alcohol seeking after extinction or abstinence have not been reported. Although the preclinical data are inconclusive with regards to the potential for targeting $mGlu_1$ in AUDs, a recent finding that genetic variants of the gene encoding $mGlu_1$ (GRM1) predict higher levels of alcohol consumption and are associated with adverse events in a human population suggests that further investigation of this target may be warranted (Meyers et al., 2015).

4. Group II mGlu receptors in preclinical models of alcohol exposure

A number of recent studies evaluating the relationship between group II mGlu receptor expression and function and alcohol consumption have provided substantial support for the involvement of group II mGlu receptors, particularly $mGlu_2$, in AUD. Selectively bred alcohol-preferring (P) rats are homozygous for a *Grm2* variant containing a premature stop codon (*Grm2* *407), and mice with global $mGlu_2$ deletion show higher alcohol consumption and preference in a two-bottle choice test (Zhou et al., 2013). Genetic analysis of other alcohol-preferring rat strains has identified a high prevalence of the *Grm2* *407 allele in other selectively bred lines as well (Wood et al., 2016). Rats lacking $mGlu_2$ also self-administer cocaine and heroin at higher rates (Gao et al., 2018; Yang et al., 2017), suggesting a broad tendency for loss of $mGlu_2$ function to predict high levels of drug consumption.

In addition to the discovery that $mGlu_2$ deletion predisposes rats to high rates of drug and alcohol self-administration, several studies have considered the effects of alcohol exposure on $mGlu_2$ expression and function. Rats trained to self-administer alcohol and made alcohol-"dependent" by CIE show lower $mGlu_2$ mRNA levels in the infralimbic cortex, and this correlates with impaired ability of the $mGlu_{2/3}$ agonist LY379268 to reduce extracellular glutamate levels in the nucleus accumbens (Meinhardt et al., 2013). Notably, the same study reported downregulation of $mGlu_2$ mRNA in the anterior cingulate cortex in postmortem brain samples obtained from humans diagnosed with AUD (Meinhardt et al., 2013), supporting the translational relevance of these findings. Our recent work demonstrated that CIE also disrupts $mGlu_2$-mediated inhibition of glutamatergic transmission in the dorsolateral and dorsomedial striatum, but this effect is limited to alcohol exposure during adolescence (Johnson, Liput, Homanics, & Lovinger, 2019). Importantly, $mGlu_2$ function could be rescued with an $mGlu_2$ PAM, suggesting that pharmacological targeting of $mGlu_2$ could be a viable strategy for reversing alcohol-induced behavioral adaptations associated with altered synaptic modulation. Upregulation of $mGlu_3$ mRNA has also been reported in postmortem brain tissue from humans with AUD (Enoch et al., 2014), but because preclinical studies have not identified a specific role for allosteric modulation of $mGlu_3$ in relation to alcohol, the section will primarily focus on $mGlu_2$. We will then briefly consider evidence that $mGlu_3$ may also warrant attention as a target for AUD.

4.1 $mGlu_2$ PAM effects on alcohol consumption and seeking

Preclinical studies using nonselective group II mGlu receptor agonists such as LY379268 ((1*R*,4*R*,5*S*,6*R*)-4-Amino-2-oxabicyclo[3.1.0]hexane-4,6-dicarboxylic acid) have identified these receptors as targets for reducing alcohol consumption and seeking. $mGlu_{2/3}$ agonist administration reduces alcohol self-administration (Backstrom & Hyytia, 2005; Sidhpura et al., 2010; Windisch & Czachowski, 2018). This regulation of alcohol self-administration is bidirectional, as $mGlu_{2/3}$ blockade with the orthosteric antagonist LY341495 ((2*S*)-2-Amino-2-[(1*S*,2*S*)-2-carboxycycloprop-1-yl]-3-(xanth-9-yl) propanoic acid) increases alcohol self-administration in rats (Zhou et al., 2013). Systemic or intra-amygdala administration of the agonist LY379268 disrupts the discriminative stimulus properties of alcohol in rats (Cannady, Grondin, Fisher, Hodge, & Besheer, 2011), which could contribute to the ability of this drug to reduce alcohol self-administration. In a limited access two-bottle choice model, intra-accumbal infusion of LY379268 reduces voluntary drinking (Griffin, Haun, Hazelbaker, Ramachandra, & Becker, 2014), suggesting that regulation of glutamatergic transmission in the nucleus accumbens could also support agonist effects on alcohol self-administration. Activation of $mGlu_{2/3}$ is also effective at reducing both cue-induced and stress-induced reinstatement of alcohol seeking following extinction training (Backstrom & Hyytia, 2005; Kufahl, Martin-Fardon, & Weiss, 2011; Sidhpura et al., 2010; Zhao et al., 2006). The effect of LY379268 on stress-induced reinstatement is enhanced in "dependent" rats that had a history of investigator-administered alcohol exposure (Sidhpura et al., 2010). These effects of $mGlu_{2/3}$ activation extend to other psychoactive drugs including nicotine, methamphetamine, and cocaine (Johnson & Lovinger, 2016). Moreover, pharmacological inhibition of reinstatement is consistent with findings that viral overexpression of $mGlu_2$ in the medial prefrontal cortex prevents reinstatement of alcohol seeking in dependent rats (Meinhardt et al., 2013).

Development of $mGlu_2$ PAMs suitable for in vivo behavioral testing has allowed more specific assessment of $mGlu_2$ as a target for treating AUD. For example, the $mGlu_2$-selective PAM AZD8529 (7-methyl-5-[3-(piperazin-1-ylmethyl)-1,2,4-oxadiazol-5-yl]-2-[[4-(trifluoromethoxy)phenyl]methyl]-3H-isoindol-1-one), which has advanced to clinical trials for smoking cessation in female subjects (ClinicalTrials.gov ID: NCT02401022), modestly reduces alcohol self-administration in rats (Augier et al., 2016). The ability of AZD8529 to modify relapse-like behavior is more robust, as cue-induced reinstatement of alcohol seeking was prevented by this drug (Augier et al., 2016). Interestingly, AZD8529 failed to prevent stress-induced reinstatement, despite earlier findings that $mGlu_{2/3}$ agonists effectively reduce stress-induced reinstatement (Sidhpura et al., 2010). Conversely, a recent study using the $mGlu_2$-selective PAM BINA (biphenyl-indanone A) failed to replicate the effects of AZD8529 on alcohol taking and seeking (Windisch & Czachowski, 2018), suggesting that these effects may be dependent on the specific PAM used. Differences in self-administration paradigms between groups could also contribute to discordant findings. Given the effects of agonists and AZD8529 on alcohol self-administration and seeking, as well as promising effects in preclinical models of other substance use disorders (Caprioli et al., 2015; Dhanya et al., 2014; Justinova et al., 2015; Li et al., 2016) and substantial progress in developing drug candidates that have suitable properties and promising safety profiles in humans, further assessment of $mGlu_2$ as a target for reducing alcohol consumption and relapse is warranted.

4.2 Avoiding tolerance with $mGlu_2$ PAMs

Chronic dosing of GPCR agonists is commonly associated with development of tolerance to therapeutic effects. Because PAMs enhance the effects of endogenous agonists when they are naturally released rather than persistently activating the receptor, one potential advantage of PAMs is that tolerance to the therapeutic effects of these drugs due to receptor desensitization could be less likely (Conn et al., 2014). Although tolerance to the effects of $mGlu_2$ ligands has not been explicitly assessed in alcohol self-administration paradigms, important insight comes from preclinical assessments of $mGlu_2$ ligands in other behavioral measures, including nicotine self-administration and effects on sleep architecture. For example, in rats trained to self-administer nicotine, treatment with the $mGlu_{2/3}$ agonist LY379268 for 14 days reduces nicotine infusions earned early in the treatment course, but nicotine infusion rates gradually return to baseline levels by the end of the treatment period, an observation which is suggestive of tolerance to LY379268 effects (Liechti, Lhuillier, Kaupmann, & Markou, 2007). Similarly, repeated dosing of LY379268 produces tolerance to analgesic effects (Jones, Eberle, Peters, Monn, & Shannon, 2005; Zammataro et al., 2011), and repeated dosing of the $mGlu_{2/3}$ agonist LY354740

((1*S*,2*S*,5*R*,6*S*)-2-Aminobicyclo[3.1.0]hexane-2,6-dicarboxylic acid) causes tolerance to effects on sleep architecture (Ahnaou et al., 2015). Promisingly, several preclinical studies employing $mGlu_2$ PAMs lend support to the idea that use of PAMs could circumvent the problem of tolerance. Notably, the $mGlu_2$ PAM AZD8529 retains its ability to reduce nicotine self-administration in both rats and squirrel monkeys following repeated dosing (Justinova et al., 2015; Li et al., 2016). Another $mGlu_2$ PAM, JNJ-42153605 (3-(cyclopropylmethyl)-7-(4-phenyl-1-piperidinyl)-8-(trifluoromethyl)-1,2,4-triazolo[4,3-*a*]pyridine), shows similar resistance to development of tolerance when measuring effects on sleep architecture in rats (Ahnaou, de Boer, et al., 2016; Ahnaou et al., 2015). Interestingly, tolerance does develop to inhibition of nicotine self-administration by another $mGlu_2$ PAM, AZD8418 (5-{7-chloro-2-[(1*S*)-1-cyclopropylethyl]-1-oxo-2,3-dihydro-1*H*-isoindol-5-yl}-*N*,*N*-dimethyl-1,2-oxazole-3-carboxamide) (Li et al., 2016), indicating that resistance to tolerance is not common to all $mGlu_2$ PAMs, and needs to be evaluated for each drug. Some PAMs possess intrinsic efficacy and thus could be more likely to desensitize the receptor than PAMs that exclusively act to enhance the affinity or coupling of a GPCR when it is activated by its endogenous agonist. Thus, attention to the unique properties of individual PAMs will be critical as efforts to develop $mGlu_2$ PAMs for clinical use continue. Further, careful attention should be paid to drug efficacy over time when evaluating results of clinical trials.

4.3 Additional considerations regarding exploration of $mGlu_2$ as a therapeutic target in AUD

Identification of *Grm2* mutations that lead to global loss of $mGlu_2$ protein in Wistar rats and selectively-bred lines derived from this strain provided a serendipitous opportunity to identify a role for $mGlu_2$ in psychoactive drug consumption (Ceolin et al., 2011; Wood et al., 2016; Zhou et al., 2013). However, it is important to note that some commercial suppliers of rats commonly used in SUD research still maintain colonies in which some rats are heterozygous or homozygous for the mutant allele, and thus it is important to consider the source and strain of rats used and their *Grm2* genotype when studying the effects of $mGlu_2$ in preclinical models of SUDs. Rats lacking $mGlu_2$ have proven useful, however, for verifying the specificity of pharmacological manipulations targeting $mGlu_2$. For example, Augier et al. employed $mGlu_2$-lacking P rats to verify that the inhibition of cue-induced reinstatement of alcohol seeking by AZD8529 was indeed dependent on $mGlu_2$ (Augier et al., 2016).

While most studies have focused on roles for $mGlu_2$ in seeking and consumption of alcohol and other psychoactive drugs, it will be interesting to consider what other behavioral effects of $mGlu_2$ PAMs could be advantageous in the context of AUD. For example, enhancement of $mGlu_2$ activity using the PAM LY487379 (2,2,2-Trifluoro-*N*-[4-(2-methoxyphenoxy)phenyl]-*N*-(3-pyridinylmethyl)ethanesulfonamide) has been shown to improve behavioral flexibility in rats (Nikiforuk et al., 2010). This finding is of particular interest because history of alcohol exposure is commonly associated with impaired behavioral flexibility, which could contribute to maladaptive decision-making related to alcohol use. To date, the effects of $mGlu_2$ PAMs in tasks requiring cognitive flexibility (e.g., reversal learning, attentional set-shifting) have not been evaluated in alcohol-exposed animals, but this question merits future investigation.

Progress in establishing safety profiles of multiple $mGlu_2$ PAMs that have entered clinical trials provides hope that efforts to target this receptor will not be hampered by safety or tolerability issues. Multiple PAMs that have undergone Phase I or II clinical trials have been reported to be well-tolerated (Kent et al., 2016; Litman et al., 2016; Salih et al., 2015). Results of clinical trials of $mGlu_2$ PAMs for AUD and other SUDs are eagerly anticipated, and development of new clinical candidates with improved profiles for use in humans continues.

4.4 Potential involvement of $mGlu_3$ AUD

In addition to changes in $mGlu_3$ expression associated with AUD (Enoch et al., 2014), several additional lines of evidence suggest that $mGlu_3$ involvement in alcohol-related behaviors warrants future investigation. For example, variants of *Grm3* have been associated with alcohol use in humans (Levey et al., 2014; O'Brien et al., 2014; Xia et al., 2012, 2014). Further, global deletion of $mGlu_3$ in mice abolishes ethanol CPP, suggesting a role for $mGlu_3$ in contextual reward (Lainiola, Hietala, Linden, & Aitta-Aho, 2019). Although studies of $mGlu_3$-selective allosteric modulators in animal models of alcohol-related behaviors have not been reported, other known roles of $mGlu_3$ in behavior could provide clues regarding the potential involvement of $mGlu_3$ in AUD. Notably, $mGlu_3$ NAM administration decreases passive coping and measures of anhedonia in models of chronic stress (Joffe et al., 2020); these findings suggest that inhibition of $mGlu_3$ could also be evaluated as a strategy to alleviate negative affect associated with alcohol withdrawal.

5. Group III mGlu receptors in preclinical models of alcohol exposure

Group III mGlu receptors modulate neurotransmission in many regions associated with alcohol reward, consumption, and seeking. Alcohol exposure has been associated with changes in expression of various group III mGlu receptor subtypes, suggesting that evaluation of each of these receptors for effects on alcohol-related behavioral measures is warranted. In rats fed an ethanol-containing diet, lower levels of $mGlu_7$ expression in the hippocampus have been reported (Simonyi, Christian, Sun, & Sun, 2004). Conversely, in human postmortem hippocampal tissue, upregulation of $mGlu_4$ expression is observed in association with AUD diagnosis (Enoch et al., 2014).

On the behavioral level, there is evidence that $mGlu_4$ regulates stimulatory effects of ethanol, as mice lacking $mGlu_4$ are resistant to ethanol-induced increases in locomotion (Blednov, Walker, Osterndorf-Kahanek, & Harris, 2004); interestingly, the same study failed to observe $mGlu_4$-mediated differences in ethanol consumption or sedation. Intracerebroventricular infusion of the dual orthosteric $mGlu_4/mGlu_7$ agonist LSP2-9166 ((2*S*)-2-amino-4-(((4-(carboxymethoxy)-3-(trifluoromethoxy)phenyl)(hydroxy)methyl)(hydroxy)phosphoryl)butanoic acid) reduces alcohol self-administration as well as motivation to obtain alcohol in a progressive ratio test in rats (Lebourgeois et al., 2018). Despite recent advances in identification of subtype-selective orthosteric and allosteric ligands targeting these receptors, few results of studies employing these compounds have been reported. This is partially owing to a relative paucity of subtype-selective allosteric ligands that target these receptors and are well-suited for in vivo studies. However, the somewhat surprising lack of reports of effects of known drugs that selectively target these receptors might also be due to negative results remaining unpublished.

The $mGlu_7$-selective allosteric agonist AMN082 (*N*,*N'*-Bis(diphenylmethyl)-1,2-ethanediamine) has been evaluated for modulation of ethanol reward and self-administration. Further studies evaluating the effects of $mGlu_7$ activation on alcohol withdrawal-induced negative affect found that AMN082 decreases alcohol-enhanced avoidance of open arms in the elevated plus maze test in rats (Kotlinska et al., 2019). AMN082 administered during CPP extinction training does not modify the rate at which ethanol CPP is extinguished (Bahi, 2012). However, following extinction, AMN082 attenuates ethanol priming-induced reinstatement of CPP

(Bahi, 2012). In operant ethanol self-administration experiments in mice, AMN082 reduces levels of responding for ethanol reinforcement, but also reduces responding for sucrose reinforcement and decreases locomotor activity in an open field test, suggestive of nonspecific suppression of behavior (Salling, Faccidomo, & Hodge, 2008). We note that significant off-target effects of AMN082 on monoamine transporters and physiological measures have been reported (Ahnaou, Raeyemaekers, Huysmans, & Drinkenburg, 2016; Sukoff Rizzo et al., 2011), highlighting the need for control experiments in $mGlu_7$ knockout mice or attenuation of AMN082 effects with an $mGlu_7$ NAM. In addition, AMN082 promotes rapid internalization of $mGlu_7$ in dissociated hippocampal neurons (Pelkey, Yuan, Lavezzari, Roche, & McBain, 2007), thus whether the effects of this drug can be attributed to enhanced receptor activation or reduced receptor availability is unclear, and may be context-dependent.

Although selective allosteric modulators of $mGlu_8$ suitable for in vivo investigations have not been reported, studies using the $mGlu_8$-selective agonist DCPG ((*S*)-3,4-Dicarboxyphenylglycine) suggest that $mGlu_8$ activation can modulate ethanol reward and consumption. Systemic injection of DCPG in mice reduces alcohol consumption and preference in a two-bottle choice test and attenuates acquisition of ethanol CPP (Bahi, 2017). DCPG also attenuates alcohol self-administration and cue-induced reinstatement of alcohol seeking, but concerns about nonspecific effects on locomotor activity limit the impact of these findings (Backstrom & Hyytia, 2005). As more selective allosteric modulators of group III mGlu receptors that are suitable for long-term in vivo studies become available, evaluation of these receptors in preclinical models of AUD will likely continue to be of interest.

6. Conclusion

The ability of mGlu receptor allosteric modulators to modify maladaptive behaviors in experimental systems used to identify potential AUD treatments has produced substantial interest in targeting these receptors in the clinic. Although clinical evaluation of an $mGlu_2$ PAM and an $mGlu_5$ NAM for nicotine use disorder have been performed, no data resulting from these trials has been disclosed. mGlu receptor allosteric modulators have not yet entered trials specifically for treatment of AUD, but recent success in development of clinical candidates suggests that such trials could commence in the near future. As novel pharmacotherapies for AUD and other SUDs continue to be developed, attention to complex details will be required to ensure that clinical trials are designed optimally and that analyses take into account all relevant factors. High rates of comorbidity between AUD and other SUDs highlight the need for more preclinical investigations of therapeutic target evaluation in animals exposed to multiple psychoactive drugs. Interestingly, a recent study demonstrated that sequential self-administration of cocaine followed by alcohol altered glutamate homeostasis in the nucleus accumbens core, and these changes were accompanied by impaired anti-reinstatement effects of a drug known to target glutamate dysregulation (Stennett, Padovan-Hernandez, & Knackstedt, 2019). As noted above, current or recent nicotine exposure alters $mGlu_5$ expression, which will likely impact how drugs targeting this receptor modulate behavior. Currently, the majority of potential interactions between use of multiple drugs and mGlu receptor expression and function remain untested. Looking forward, polysubstance use will be an important consideration in both preclinical and clinical investigations of mGlu receptor allosteric modulators.

There is still much to be learned about the circuitry affected by mGlu receptor ligands that reduce alcohol consumption and seeking, and an increased understanding of how these receptors modulate circuitry to drive behavioral effects should improve our ability to predict the translational potential of these effects. Direct-site infusion of $mGlu_5$ NAMs into the nucleus accumbens and basolateral amygdala have demonstrated roles for these regions in the behavioral effects of $mGlu_5$ NAMs, but most cellular and/or circuit-level mechanisms by which these drugs modify maladaptive behaviors have not been identified. Even less is known about the circuitry modulated by $mGlu_2$ PAMs to inhibit reinstatement of alcohol seeking. The increased availability of PET tracers and other imaging techniques that allow evaluation of mGlu receptor localization in relevant circuitry in the human brain (Xu & Li, 2019), as well as occupancy of these receptors by drug candidates, will likely improve translation of mGlu receptor allosteric modulators to success in clinical trials.

Acknowledgments

This work was supported by NIAAA Division of Intramural Clinical and Biological Research ZIA AA000416 (D.M.L.) and NIH Grant R00 AA025403 (K.A.J.). The authors are employees of the US Government, and this work was prepared as part of their official duties. Title 17 U.S.C. §105 provides that "Copyright protection under this title is not available for any work of the US Government." Title 17 U.S.C §101 defined a US Government work as a work prepared by a military service member or employees of the US Government as part of that person's official duties. The views in this article are those of the authors and do not necessarily reflect the views, official policy, or position of the Uniformed Services University of the Health Sciences, the Armed Forces Radiobiology Research Institute, Department of the Navy, Department of Defense or the US Federal Government. Fig. 1 was created using Biorender.com.

Conflicts of interest statement

The authors declare no conflicts of interest.

References

Adams, C. L., Cowen, M. S., Short, J. L., & Lawrence, A. J. (2008). Combined antagonism of glutamate mGlu5 and adenosine A2A receptors interact to regulate alcohol-seeking in rats. *The International Journal of Neuropsychopharmacology*, *11*, 229–241.

Adams, C. L., Short, J. L., & Lawrence, A. J. (2010). Cue-conditioned alcohol seeking in rats following abstinence: Involvement of metabotropic glutamate 5 receptors. *British Journal of Pharmacology*, *159*, 534–542.

Ahnaou, A., de Boer, P., Lavreysen, H., Huysmans, H., Sinha, V., Raeymaekers, L., et al. (2016). Translational neurophysiological markers for activity of the metabotropic glutamate receptor (mGluR2) modulator JNJ-40411813: Sleep EEG correlates in rodents and healthy men. *Neuropharmacology*, *103*, 290–305.

Ahnaou, A., Lavreysen, H., Tresadern, G., Cid, J. M., & Drinkenburg, W. H. (2015). mGlu2 receptor Agonism, but not positive allosteric modulation, elicits rapid tolerance towards their primary efficacy on sleep measures in rats. *PLoS One*, *10*, e0144017.

Ahnaou, A., Raeyemaekers, L., Huysmans, H., & Drinkenburg, W. (2016). Off-target potential of AMN082 on sleep EEG and related physiological variables: Evidence from mGluR7 (−/−) mice. *Behavioural Brain Research*, *311*, 287–297.

Akkus, F., Ametamey, S. M., Treyer, V., Burger, C., Johayem, A., Umbricht, D., et al. (2013). Marked global reduction in mGluR5 receptor binding in smokers and ex-smokers determined by [11C]ABP688 positron emission tomography. *Proceedings of the National Academy of Sciences of the United States of America*, *110*, 737–742.

Akkus, F., Mihov, Y., Treyer, V., Ametamey, S. M., Johayem, A., Senn, S., et al. (2018). Metabotropic glutamate receptor 5 binding in male patients with alcohol use disorder. *Translational Psychiatry*, *8*, 17.

Alasmari, F., Bell, R. L., Rao, P. S. S., Hammad, A. M., & Sari, Y. (2018). Peri-adolescent drinking of ethanol and/or nicotine modulates astroglial glutamate transporters and metabotropic glutamate receptor-1 in female alcohol-preferring rats. *Pharmacology, Biochemistry, and Behavior*, *170*, 44–55.

Augier, E., Dulman, R. S., Rauffenbart, C., Augier, G., Cross, A. J., & Heilig, M. (2016). The mGluR2 positive allosteric modulator, AZD8529, and Cue-induced relapse to alcohol seeking in rats. *Neuropsychopharmacology*, *41*, 2932–2940.

Bachteler, D., Economidou, D., Danysz, W., Ciccocioppo, R., & Spanagel, R. (2005). The effects of acamprosate and neramexane on cue-induced reinstatement of ethanol-seeking behavior in rat. *Neuropsychopharmacology*, *30*, 1104–1110.

Backstrom, P., Bachteler, D., Koch, S., Hyytia, P., & Spanagel, R. (2004). mGluR5 antagonist MPEP reduces ethanol-seeking and relapse behavior. *Neuropsychopharmacology*, *29*, 921–928.

Backstrom, P., & Hyytia, P. (2005). Suppression of alcohol self-administration and cue-induced reinstatement of alcohol seeking by the mGlu2/3 receptor agonist LY379268 and the mGlu8 receptor agonist (S)-3,4-DCPG. *European Journal of Pharmacology*, *528*, 110–118.

Bahi, A. (2012). The selective metabotropic glutamate receptor 7 allosteric agonist AMN082 prevents reinstatement of extinguished ethanol-induced conditioned place preference in mice. *Pharmacology, Biochemistry, and Behavior*, *101*, 193–200.

Bahi, A. (2017). Decreased anxiety, voluntary ethanol intake and ethanol-induced CPP acquisition following activation of the metabotropic glutamate receptor 8 "mGluR8". *Pharmacology, Biochemistry, and Behavior*, *155*, 32–42.

Barker, J. M., Corbit, L. H., Robinson, D. L., Gremel, C. M., Gonzales, R. A., & Chandler, L. J. (2015). Corticostriatal circuitry and habitual ethanol seeking. *Alcohol*, *49*, 817–824.

Barnes, S. A., Sheffler, D. J., Semenova, S., Cosford, N. D. P., & Bespalov, A. (2018). Metabotropic glutamate receptor 5 as a target for the treatment of depression and smoking: Robust preclinical data but inconclusive clinical efficacy. *Biological Psychiatry*, *83*, 955–962.

Becker, H. C. (2017). Influence of stress associated with chronic alcohol exposure on drinking. *Neuropharmacology*, *122*, 115–126.

Belknap, J. K., Crabbe, J. C., & Young, E. R. (1993). Voluntary consumption of ethanol in 15 inbred mouse strains. *Psychopharmacology*, *112*, 503–510.

Bell, R. L., Hauser, S. R., McClintick, J., Rahman, S., Edenberg, H. J., Szumlinski, K. K., et al. (2016). Ethanol-associated changes in glutamate reward Neurocircuitry: A Minireview of clinical and preclinical genetic findings. *Progress in Molecular Biology and Translational Science*, *137*, 41–85.

Besheer, J., Faccidomo, S., Grondin, J. J., & Hodge, C. W. (2008a). Effects of mGlu1-receptor blockade on ethanol self-administration in inbred alcohol-preferring rats. *Alcohol*, *42*, 13–20.

Besheer, J., Faccidomo, S., Grondin, J. J., & Hodge, C. W. (2008b). Regulation of motivation to self-administer ethanol by mGluR5 in alcohol-preferring (P) rats. *Alcoholism, Clinical and Experimental Research*, *32*, 209–221.

Besheer, J., Grondin, J. J., Cannady, R., Sharko, A. C., Faccidomo, S., & Hodge, C. W. (2010). Metabotropic glutamate receptor 5 activity in the nucleus accumbens is required for the maintenance of ethanol self-administration in a rat genetic model of high alcohol intake. *Biological Psychiatry*, *67*, 812–822.

Besheer, J., & Hodge, C. W. (2005). Pharmacological and anatomical evidence for an interaction between mGluR5- and GABA(A) alpha1-containing receptors in the discriminative stimulus effects of ethanol. *Neuropsychopharmacology*, *30*, 747–757.

Besheer, J., Stevenson, R. A., & Hodge, C. W. (2006). mGlu5 receptors are involved in the discriminative stimulus effects of self-administered ethanol in rats. *European Journal of Pharmacology*, *551*, 71–75.

Bird, M. K., Kirchhoff, J., Djouma, E., & Lawrence, A. J. (2008). Metabotropic glutamate 5 receptors regulate sensitivity to ethanol in mice. *The International Journal of Neuropsychopharmacology*, *11*, 765–774.

Blaine, S. K., & Sinha, R. (2017). Alcohol, stress, and glucocorticoids: From risk to dependence and relapse in alcohol use disorders. *Neuropharmacology*, *122*, 136–147.

Blednov, Y. A., Walker, D., Osterndorf-Kahanek, E., & Harris, R. A. (2004). Mice lacking metabotropic glutamate receptor 4 do not show the motor stimulatory effect of ethanol. *Alcohol*, *34*, 251–259.

Cannady, R., Grondin, J. J., Fisher, K. R., Hodge, C. W., & Besheer, J. (2011). Activation of group II metabotropic glutamate receptors inhibits the discriminative stimulus effects of alcohol via selective activity within the amygdala. *Neuropsychopharmacology*, *36*, 2328–2338.

Caprioli, D., Justinova, Z., Venniro, M., & Shaham, Y. (2018). Effect of novel allosteric modulators of metabotropic glutamate receptors on drug self-administration and relapse: A review of preclinical studies and their clinical implications. *Biological Psychiatry*, *84*, 180–192.

Caprioli, D., Venniro, M., Zeric, T., Li, X., Adhikary, S., Madangopal, R., et al. (2015). Effect of the novel positive allosteric modulator of metabotropic glutamate receptor 2 AZD8529 on incubation of methamphetamine craving after prolonged voluntary abstinence in a rat model. *Biological Psychiatry*, *78*, 463–473.
Carnicella, S., Ron, D., & Barak, S. (2014). Intermittent ethanol access schedule in rats as a preclinical model of alcohol abuse. *Alcohol*, *48*, 243–252.
Carta, M., Mameli, M., & Valenzuela, C. F. (2006). Alcohol potently modulates climbing fiber→Purkinje neuron synapses: Role of metabotropic glutamate receptors. *The Journal of Neuroscience*, *26*, 1906–1912.
Cartoni, E., Balleine, B., & Baldassarre, G. (2016). Appetitive Pavlovian-instrumental transfer: A review. *Neuroscience and Biobehavioral Reviews*, *71*, 829–848.
Carvalho, A. F., Heilig, M., Perez, A., Probst, C., & Rehm, J. (2019). Alcohol use disorders. *Lancet*, *394*, 781–792.
Ceccarini, J., Leurquin-Sterk, G., Crunelle, C., de Laat, B., Bormans, G., Peuskens, H., et al. (2019). Recovery of decreased metabotropic glutamate receptor 5 availability in abstinent alcohol-dependent patients. *Journal of Nuclear Medicine*, *61*, 256–262.
Centanni, S. W., Bedse, G., Patel, S., & Winder, D. G. (2019). Driving the downward spiral: Alcohol-induced dysregulation of extended amygdala circuits and negative affect. *Alcoholism, Clinical and Experimental Research*, *43*, 2000–2013.
Ceolin, L., Kantamneni, S., Barker, G. R., Hanna, L., Murray, L., Warburton, E. C., et al. (2011). Study of novel selective mGlu2 agonist in the temporo-ammonic input to CA1 neurons reveals reduced mGlu2 receptor expression in a Wistar substrain with an anxiety-like phenotype. *The Journal of Neuroscience*, *31*, 6721–6731.
Conn, P. J., Lindsley, C. W., Meiler, J., & Niswender, C. M. (2014). Opportunities and challenges in the discovery of allosteric modulators of GPCRs for treating CNS disorders. *Nature Reviews. Drug Discovery*, *13*, 692–708.
Corbit, L. H., & Janak, P. H. (2016). Habitual alcohol seeking: Neural bases and possible relations to alcohol use disorders. *Alcoholism, Clinical and Experimental Research*, *40*, 1380–1389.
Cover, K. K., Kerkhoff, W. G., & Mathur, B. N. (2018). The best defense is a strong offense: Preventing alcohol abstinence-induced depression. *Neuropsychopharmacology*, *43*, 2331–2332.
Cowen, M. S., Djouma, E., & Lawrence, A. J. (2005). The metabotropic glutamate 5 receptor antagonist 3-[(2-methyl-1,3-thiazol-4-yl)ethynyl]-pyridine reduces ethanol self-administration in multiple strains of alcohol-preferring rats and regulates olfactory glutamatergic systems. *The Journal of Pharmacology and Experimental Therapeutics*, *315*, 590–600.
Cowen, M. S., Krstew, E., & Lawrence, A. J. (2007). Assessing appetitive and consummatory phases of ethanol self-administration in C57BL/6J mice under operant conditions: Regulation by mGlu5 receptor antagonism. *Psychopharmacology*, *190*, 21–29.
Cozzoli, D. K., Courson, J., Caruana, A. L., Miller, B. W., Greentree, D. I., Thompson, A. B., et al. (2012). Nucleus accumbens mGluR5-associated signaling regulates binge alcohol drinking under drinking-in-the-dark procedures. *Alcoholism, Clinical and Experimental Research*, *36*, 1623–1633.
Cozzoli, D. K., Courson, J., Wroten, M. G., Greentree, D. I., Lum, E. N., Campbell, R. R., et al. (2014). Binge alcohol drinking by mice requires intact group 1 metabotropic glutamate receptor signaling within the central nucleus of the amygdala. *Neuropsychopharmacology*, *39*, 435–444.
Cozzoli, D. K., Goulding, S. P., Zhang, P. W., Xiao, B., Hu, J. H., Ary, A. W., et al. (2009). Binge drinking upregulates accumbens mGluR5-Homer2-PI3K signaling: Functional implications for alcoholism. *The Journal of Neuroscience*, *29*, 8655–8668.

Cozzoli, D. K., Tanchuck-Nipper, M. A., Kaufman, M. N., Horowitz, C. B., & Finn, D. A. (2014). Environmental stressors influence limited-access ethanol consumption by C57BL/6J mice in a sex-dependent manner. *Alcohol, 48*, 741–754.

Crabbe, J. C., Harris, R. A., & Koob, G. F. (2011). Preclinical studies of alcohol binge drinking. *Annals of the New York Academy of Sciences, 1216*, 24–40.

Crabbe, J. C., Phillips, T. J., & Belknap, J. K. (2010). The complexity of alcohol drinking: Studies in rodent genetic models. *Behavior Genetics, 40*, 737–750.

Cross, A. J., Anthenelli, R., & Li, X. (2018). Metabotropic glutamate receptors 2 and 3 as targets for treating nicotine addiction. *Biological Psychiatry, 83*, 947–954.

Cunningham, C. L. (1981). Spatial aversion conditioning with ethanol. *Pharmacology, Biochemistry, and Behavior, 14*, 263–264.

Cunningham, C. L., Niehus, D. R., Malott, D. H., & Prather, L. K. (1992). Genetic differences in the rewarding and activating effects of morphine and ethanol. *Psychopharmacology, 107*, 385–393.

Czachowski, C. L., Legg, B. H., & Samson, H. H. (2001). Effects of acamprosate on ethanol-seeking and self-administration in the rat. *Alcoholism, Clinical and Experimental Research, 25*, 344–350.

de Laat, B., Weerasekera, A., Leurquin-Sterk, G., Gsell, W., Bormans, G., Himmelreich, U., et al. (2019). Effects of alcohol exposure on the glutamatergic system: A combined longitudinal (18) F-FPEB and (1) H-MRS study in rats. *Addiction Biology, 24*, 696–706.

DePoy, L., Daut, R., Brigman, J. L., MacPherson, K., Crowley, N., Gunduz-Cinar, O., et al. (2013). Chronic alcohol produces neuroadaptations to prime dorsal striatal learning. *Proceedings of the National Academy of Sciences of the United States of America, 110*, 14783–14788.

Dhanya, R. P., Sheffler, D. J., Dahl, R., Davis, M., Lee, P. S., Yang, L., et al. (2014). Design and synthesis of systemically active metabotropic glutamate subtype-2 and -3 (mGlu2/3) receptor positive allosteric modulators (PAMs): Pharmacological characterization and assessment in a rat model of cocaine dependence. *Journal of Medicinal Chemistry, 57*, 4154–4172.

Dore, A. S., Okrasa, K., Patel, J. C., Serrano-Vega, M., Bennett, K., Cooke, R. M., et al. (2014). Structure of class C GPCR metabotropic glutamate receptor 5 transmembrane domain. *Nature, 511*, 557–562.

Doumazane, E., Scholler, P., Zwier, J. M., Trinquet, E., Rondard, P., & Pin, J. P. (2011). A new approach to analyze cell surface protein complexes reveals specific heterodimeric metabotropic glutamate receptors. *The FASEB Journal, 25*, 66–77.

Enoch, M. A., Rosser, A. A., Zhou, Z., Mash, D. C., Yuan, Q., & Goldman, D. (2014). Expression of glutamatergic genes in healthy humans across 16 brain regions; altered expression in the hippocampus after chronic exposure to alcohol or cocaine. *Genes, Brain, and Behavior, 13*, 758–768.

Everitt, B. J., & Robbins, T. W. (2016). Drug addiction: Updating actions to habits to compulsions ten years on. *Annual Review of Psychology, 67*, 23–50.

Ferre, S., Casado, V., Devi, L. A., Filizola, M., Jockers, R., Lohse, M. J., et al. (2014). G protein-coupled receptor oligomerization revisited: Functional and pharmacological perspectives. *Pharmacological Reviews, 66*, 413–434.

Fidler, T. L., Bakner, L., & Cunningham, C. L. (2004). Conditioned place aversion induced by intragastric administration of ethanol in rats. *Pharmacology, Biochemistry, and Behavior, 77*, 731–743.

Foster, D. J., & Conn, P. J. (2017). Allosteric modulation of GPCRs: New insights and potential utility for treatment of schizophrenia and other CNS disorders. *Neuron, 94*, 431–446.

Gao, J. T., Jordan, C. J., Bi, G. H., He, Y., Yang, H. J., Gardner, E. L., et al. (2018). Deletion of the type 2 metabotropic glutamate receptor increases heroin abuse vulnerability in transgenic rats. *Neuropsychopharmacology*, *43*, 2615–2626.

Gass, J. T., Glen, W. B., Jr., McGonigal, J. T., Trantham-Davidson, H., Lopez, M. F., Randall, P. K., et al. (2014). Adolescent alcohol exposure reduces behavioral flexibility, promotes disinhibition, and increases resistance to extinction of ethanol self-administration in adulthood. *Neuropsychopharmacology*, *39*, 2570–2583.

Gass, J. T., McGonigal, J. T., & Chandler, L. J. (2017). Deficits in the extinction of ethanol-seeking behavior following chronic intermittent ethanol exposure are attenuated with positive allosteric modulation of mGlu5. *Neuropharmacology*, *113*, 198–205.

Gass, J. T., & Olive, M. F. (2009). Role of protein kinase C epsilon (PKCvarepsilon) in the reduction of ethanol reinforcement due to mGluR5 antagonism in the nucleus accumbens shell. *Psychopharmacology*, *204*, 587–597.

Gass, J. T., Trantham-Davidson, H., Kassab, A. S., Glen, W. B., Jr., Olive, M. F., & Chandler, L. J. (2014). Enhancement of extinction learning attenuates ethanol-seeking behavior and alters plasticity in the prefrontal cortex. *The Journal of Neuroscience*, *34*, 7562–7574.

Gobin, C., & Schwendt, M. (2019). The cognitive cost of reducing relapse to cocaine-seeking with mGlu5 allosteric modulators. *Psychopharmacology*, *237*, 115–125.

Goulding, S. P., Obara, I., Lominac, K. D., Gould, A. T., Miller, B. W., Klugmann, M., et al. (2011). Accumbens Homer2-mediated signaling: A factor contributing to mouse strain differences in alcohol drinking? *Genes, Brain, and Behavior*, *10*, 111–126.

Gremel, C. M., & Lovinger, D. M. (2017). Associative and sensorimotor cortico-basal ganglia circuit roles in effects of abused drugs. *Genes, Brain, and Behavior*, *16*, 71–85.

Griffin, W. C., 3rd (2014). Alcohol dependence and free-choice drinking in mice. *Alcohol*, *48*, 287–293.

Griffin, W. C., 3rd, Haun, H. L., Hazelbaker, C. L., Ramachandra, V. S., & Becker, H. C. (2014). Increased extracellular glutamate in the nucleus accumbens promotes excessive ethanol drinking in ethanol dependent mice. *Neuropsychopharmacology*, *39*, 707–717.

Gupta, T., Syed, Y. M., Revis, A. A., Miller, S. A., Martinez, M., Cohn, K. A., et al. (2008). Acute effects of acamprosate and MPEP on ethanol drinking-in-the-dark in male C57BL/6J mice. *Alcoholism, Clinical and Experimental Research*, *32*, 1992–1998.

Guydish, J., Passalacqua, E., Pagano, A., Martinez, C., Le, T., Chun, J., et al. (2016). An international systematic review of smoking prevalence in addiction treatment. *Addiction*, *111*, 220–230.

Hellyer, S., Leach, K., & Gregory, K. J. (2017). Neurobiological insights and novel therapeutic opportunities for CNS disorders from mGlu receptor allosteric and biased modulation. *Current Opinion in Pharmacology*, *32*, 49–55.

Herz, A. (1997). Endogenous opioid systems and alcohol addiction. *Psychopharmacology*, *129*, 99–111.

Hilderbrand, E. R., & Lasek, A. W. (2018). Studying sex differences in animal models of addiction: An emphasis on alcohol-related behaviors. *ACS Chemical Neuroscience*, *9*, 1907–1916.

Hodge, C. W., Miles, M. F., Sharko, A. C., Stevenson, R. A., Hillmann, J. R., Lepoutre, V., et al. (2006). The mGluR5 antagonist MPEP selectively inhibits the onset and maintenance of ethanol self-administration in C57BL/6J mice. *Psychopharmacology*, *183*, 429–438.

Holleran, K. M., Wilson, H. H., Fetterly, T. L., Bluett, R. J., Centanni, S. W., Gilfarb, R. A., et al. (2016). Ketamine and MAG lipase inhibitor-dependent reversal of evolving depressive-like behavior during forced abstinence from alcohol drinking. *Neuropsychopharmacology*, *41*, 2062–2071.

Holleran, K. M., & Winder, D. G. (2017). Preclinical voluntary drinking models for alcohol abstinence-induced affective disturbances in mice. *Genes, Brain, and Behavior*, *16*, 8–14.

Hopf, F. W., & Lesscher, H. M. (2014). Rodent models for compulsive alcohol intake. *Alcohol*, *48*, 253–264.

Hulka, L. M., Treyer, V., Scheidegger, M., Preller, K. H., Vonmoos, M., Baumgartner, M. R., et al. (2014). Smoking but not cocaine use is associated with lower cerebral metabotropic glutamate receptor 5 density in humans. *Molecular Psychiatry*, *19*, 625–632.

Huston, J. P., Silva, M. A., Topic, B., & Muller, C. P. (2013). What's conditioned in conditioned place preference? *Trends in Pharmacological Sciences*, *34*, 162–166.

Hwa, L., Besheer, J., & Kash, T. (2017). Glutamate plasticity woven through the progression to alcohol use disorder: A multi-circuit perspective. *F1000Res*, *6*, 298.

Hwa, L. S., Chu, A., Levinson, S. A., Kayyali, T. M., DeBold, J. F., & Miczek, K. A. (2011). Persistent escalation of alcohol drinking in C57BL/6J mice with intermittent access to 20% ethanol. *Alcoholism, Clinical and Experimental Research*, *35*, 1938–1947.

Joffe, M. E., Centanni, S. W., Jaramillo, A. A., Winder, D. G., & Conn, P. J. (2018). Metabotropic glutamate receptors in alcohol use disorder: Physiology, plasticity, and promising pharmacotherapies. *ACS Chemical Neuroscience*, *9*, 2188–2204.

Joffe, M. E., Santiago, C. I., Oliver, K. H., Maksymetz, J., Harris, N. A., Engers, J. L., et al. (2020). mGlu2 and mGlu3 negative allosteric modulators divergently enhance Thalamocortical transmission and exert rapid antidepressant-like effects. *Neuron*, *105*, 46–59.e43.

Johnson, K. A., Liput, D. J., Homanics, G. E., & Lovinger, D. M. (2019). Age-dependent impairment of metabotropic glutamate receptor 2-dependent long-term depression in the mouse striatum by chronic ethanol exposure. *Alcohol*, *82*, 11–21.

Johnson, K. A., & Lovinger, D. M. (2016). Presynaptic G protein-coupled receptors: Gatekeepers of addiction? *Frontiers in Cellular Neuroscience*, *10*, 264.

Jonas, D. E., Amick, H. R., Feltner, C., Bobashev, G., Thomas, K., Wines, R., et al. (2014). Pharmacotherapy for adults with alcohol use disorders in outpatient settings: A systematic review and meta-analysis. *JAMA*, *311*, 1889–1900.

Jones, C. K., Eberle, E. L., Peters, S. C., Monn, J. A., & Shannon, H. E. (2005). Analgesic effects of the selective group II (mGlu2/3) metabotropic glutamate receptor agonists LY379268 and LY389795 in persistent and inflammatory pain models after acute and repeated dosing. *Neuropharmacology*, *49*(Suppl. 1), 206–218.

Justinova, Z., Panlilio, L. V., Secci, M. E., Redhi, G. H., Schindler, C. W., Cross, A. J., et al. (2015). The novel metabotropic glutamate receptor 2 positive allosteric modulator, AZD8529, decreases nicotine self-administration and relapse in squirrel Monkeys. *Biological Psychiatry*, *78*, 452–462.

Kasten, C. R., Holmgren, E. B., & Wills, T. A. (2019). Metabotropic glutamate receptor subtype 5 in alcohol-induced negative affect. *Brain Sciences*, *9*, 183.

Kent, J. M., Daly, E., Kezic, I., Lane, R., Lim, P., De Smedt, H., et al. (2016). Efficacy and safety of an adjunctive mGlu2 receptor positive allosteric modulator to a SSRI/SNRI in anxious depression. *Progress in Neuro-Psychopharmacology & Biological Psychiatry*, *67*, 66–73.

Koehl, A., Hu, H., Feng, D., Sun, B., Zhang, Y., Robertson, M. J., et al. (2019). Structural insights into the activation of metabotropic glutamate receptors. *Nature*, *566*, 79–84.

Koob, G. F. (2009). Neurobiological substrates for the dark side of compulsivity in addiction. *Neuropharmacology*, *56*(Suppl. 1), 18–31.

Koob, G. F. (2015). The dark side of emotion: The addiction perspective. *European Journal of Pharmacology*, *753*, 73–87.

Koob, G. F., Kenneth Lloyd, G., & Mason, B. J. (2009). Development of pharmacotherapies for drug addiction: A Rosetta stone approach. *Nature Reviews. Drug Discovery*, *8*, 500–515.

Koob, G. F., & Volkow, N. D. (2016). Neurobiology of addiction: A neurocircuitry analysis. *Lancet Psychiatry*, *3*, 760–773.
Kotlinska, J., & Bochenski, M. (2008). The influence of various glutamate receptors antagonists on anxiety-like effect of ethanol withdrawal in a plus-maze test in rats. *European Journal of Pharmacology*, *598*, 57–63.
Kotlinska, J. H., Bochenski, M., & Danysz, W. (2011). The role of group I mGlu receptors in the expression of ethanol-induced conditioned place preference and ethanol withdrawal seizures in rats. *European Journal of Pharmacology*, *670*, 154–161.
Kotlinska, J. H., Lopatynska-Mazurek, M., Gawel, K., Gabka, P., Jenda-Wojtanowska, M., Kruk-Slomka, M., et al. (2019). Impact of the metabotropic glutamate receptor7 (mGlu7) allosteric agonist, AMN082, on fear learning and memory and anxiety-like behavior. *European Journal of Pharmacology*, *858*, 172512.
Kufahl, P. R., Martin-Fardon, R., & Weiss, F. (2011). Enhanced sensitivity to attenuation of conditioned reinstatement by the mGluR 2/3 agonist LY379268 and increased functional activity of mGluR 2/3 in rats with a history of ethanol dependence. *Neuropsychopharmacology*, *36*, 2762–2773.
Kumar, J., Hapidin, H., Bee, Y. T., & Ismail, Z. (2013). Effects of the mGluR5 antagonist MPEP on ethanol withdrawal induced anxiety-like syndrome in rats. *Behavioral and Brain Functions*, *9*, 43.
Lainiola, M., Hietala, L., Linden, A. M., & Aitta-Aho, T. (2019). The lack of conditioned place preference, but unaltered stimulatory and ataxic effects of alcohol in mGluR3-KO mice. *Journal of Psychopharmacology*, *33*, 855–864.
Lamb, R. J., Schindler, C. W., & Pinkston, J. W. (2016). Conditioned stimuli's role in relapse: Preclinical research on Pavlovian-instrumental-transfer. *Psychopharmacology*, *233*, 1933–1944.
Leach, K., & Gregory, K. J. (2017). Molecular insights into allosteric modulation of Class C G protein-coupled receptors. *Pharmacological Research*, *116*, 105–118.
Lebourgeois, S., Vilpoux, C., Jeanblanc, J., Acher, F., Marie, N., Noble, F., et al. (2018). Pharmacological activation of mGlu4 and mGlu7 receptors, by LSP2-9166, reduces ethanol consumption and relapse in rat. *Neuropharmacology*, *133*, 163–170.
Lee, J. Y., Choe, E. S., Yang, C. H., Choi, K. H., Cheong, J. H., Jang, C. G., et al. (2016). The mGluR5 antagonist MPEP suppresses the expression and reinstatement, but not the acquisition, of the ethanol-conditioned place preference in mice. *Pharmacology, Biochemistry, and Behavior*, *140*, 33–38.
Lee, K. M., Coehlo, M., McGregor, H. A., Waltermire, R. S., & Szumlinski, K. K. (2015). Binge alcohol drinking elicits persistent negative affect in mice. *Behavioural Brain Research*, *291*, 385–398.
Lee, K. M., Coehlo, M. A., Solton, N. R., & Szumlinski, K. K. (2017). Negative affect and excessive alcohol intake incubate during protracted withdrawal from binge-drinking in adolescent, but not adult, mice. *Frontiers in Psychology*, *8*, 1128.
Lee, K. M., Coelho, M. A., Class, M. A., Sern, K. R., Bocz, M. D., & Szumlinski, K. K. (2018). mGlu5 receptor blockade within the nucleus Accumbens Shell reduces behavioral indices of alcohol withdrawal-induced anxiety in mice. *Frontiers in Pharmacology*, *9*, 1306.
Lee, K. M., Coelho, M. A., Class, M. A., & Szumlinski, K. K. (2018). mGlu5-dependent modulation of anxiety during early withdrawal from binge-drinking in adult and adolescent male mice. *Drug and Alcohol Dependence*, *184*, 1–11.
Lee, K. M., Coelho, M. A., McGregor, H. A., Solton, N. R., Cohen, M., & Szumlinski, K. K. (2016). Adolescent mice are resilient to alcohol withdrawal-induced anxiety and changes in indices of glutamate function within the nucleus Accumbens. *Frontiers in Cellular Neuroscience*, *10*, 265.

Lee, K. M., Coelho, M. A., Sern, K. R., Class, M. A., Bocz, M. D., & Szumlinski, K. K. (2017). Anxiolytic effects of buspirone and MTEP in the Porsolt Forced Swim Test. *Chronic Stress (Thousand Oaks)*, *1*, 1–9.

Leurquin-Sterk, G., Ceccarini, J., Crunelle, C. L., de Laat, B., Verbeek, J., Deman, S., et al. (2018). Lower limbic metabotropic glutamate receptor 5 availability in alcohol dependence. *Journal of Nuclear Medicine*, *59*, 682–690.

Leurquin-Sterk, G., Ceccarini, J., Crunelle, C. L., Weerasekera, A., de Laat, B., Himmelreich, U., et al. (2018). Cerebral dopaminergic and glutamatergic transmission relate to different subjective responses of acute alcohol intake: An in vivo multimodal imaging study. *Addiction Biology*, *23*, 931–944.

Levey, D. F., Le-Niculescu, H., Frank, J., Ayalew, M., Jain, N., Kirlin, B., et al. (2014). Genetic risk prediction and neurobiological understanding of alcoholism. *Translational Psychiatry*, *4*, e391.

Li, X., D'Souza, M. S., Nino, A. M., Doherty, J., Cross, A., & Markou, A. (2016). Attenuation of nicotine-taking and nicotine-seeking behavior by the mGlu2 receptor positive allosteric modulators AZD8418 and AZD8529 in rats. *Psychopharmacology*, *233*, 1801–1814.

Li, X., & Markou, A. (2015). Metabotropic glutamate receptor 7 (mGluR7) as a target for the treatment of psychostimulant dependence. *CNS & Neurological Disorders Drug Targets*, *14*, 738–744.

Liechti, M. E., Lhuillier, L., Kaupmann, K., & Markou, A. (2007). Metabotropic glutamate 2/3 receptors in the ventral tegmental area and the nucleus accumbens shell are involved in behaviors relating to nicotine dependence. *The Journal of Neuroscience*, *27*, 9077–9085.

Litman, R. E., Smith, M. A., Doherty, J. J., Cross, A., Raines, S., Gertsik, L., et al. (2016). AZD8529, a positive allosteric modulator at the mGluR2 receptor, does not improve symptoms in schizophrenia: A proof of principle study. *Schizophrenia Research*, *172*, 152–157.

Lominac, K. D., Kapasova, Z., Hannun, R. A., Patterson, C., Middaugh, L. D., & Szumlinski, K. K. (2006). Behavioral and neurochemical interactions between group 1 mGluR antagonists and ethanol: Potential insight into their anti-addictive properties. *Drug and Alcohol Dependence*, *85*, 142–156.

Lopez, M. F., & Becker, H. C. (2014). Operant ethanol self-administration in ethanol dependent mice. *Alcohol*, *48*, 295–299.

Lum, E. N., Campbell, R. R., Rostock, C., & Szumlinski, K. K. (2014). mGluR1 within the nucleus accumbens regulates alcohol intake in mice under limited-access conditions. *Neuropharmacology*, *79*, 679–687.

Maisel, N. C., Blodgett, J. C., Wilbourne, P. L., Humphreys, K., & Finney, J. W. (2013). Meta-analysis of naltrexone and acamprosate for treating alcohol use disorders: When are these medications most helpful? *Addiction*, *108*, 275–293.

Mantsch, J. R., Baker, D. A., Funk, D., Le, A. D., & Shaham, Y. (2016). Stress-induced reinstatement of drug seeking: 20 years of Progress. *Neuropsychopharmacology*, *41*, 335–356.

McBride, W. J., Murphy, J. M., & Ikemoto, S. (1999). Localization of brain reinforcement mechanisms: Intracranial self-administration and intracranial place-conditioning studies. *Behavioural Brain Research*, *101*, 129–152.

McCool, B. A., & Chappell, A. M. (2012). Using monosodium glutamate to initiate ethanol self-administration in inbred mouse strains. *Addiction Biology*, *17*, 121–131.

McGeehan, A. J., & Olive, M. F. (2003). The mGluR5 antagonist MPEP reduces the conditioned rewarding effects of cocaine but not other drugs of abuse. *Synapse*, *47*, 240–242.

McMillen, B. A., Crawford, M. S., Kulers, C. M., & Williams, H. L. (2005). Effects of a metabotropic, mglu5, glutamate receptor antagonist on ethanol consumption by genetic drinking rats. *Alcohol and Alcoholism*, *40*, 494–497.

Meinhardt, M. W., Hansson, A. C., Perreau-Lenz, S., Bauder-Wenz, C., Stahlin, O., Heilig, M., et al. (2013). Rescue of infralimbic mGluR2 deficit restores control over drug-seeking behavior in alcohol dependence. *The Journal of Neuroscience*, *33*, 2794–2806.

Melendez, R. I. (2011). Intermittent (every-other-day) drinking induces rapid escalation of ethanol intake and preference in adolescent and adult C57BL/6J mice. *Alcoholism, Clinical and Experimental Research*, *35*, 652–658.

Metten, P., Schlumbohm, J. P., Huang, L. C., Greenberg, G. D., Hack, W. R., Spence, S. E., et al. (2018). An alcohol withdrawal test battery measuring multiple behavioral symptoms in mice. *Alcohol*, *68*, 19–35.

Meyers, J. L., Salling, M. C., Almli, L. M., Ratanatharathorn, A., Uddin, M., Galea, S., et al. (2015). Frequency of alcohol consumption in humans; the role of metabotropic glutamate receptors and downstream signaling pathways. *Translational Psychiatry*, *5*, e586.

Miller, W. R., & Wilbourne, P. L. (2002). Mesa Grande: A methodological analysis of clinical trials of treatments for alcohol use disorders. *Addiction*, *97*, 265–277.

Mishra, D., Zhang, X., & Chergui, K. (2012). Ethanol disrupts the mechanisms of induction of long-term potentiation in the mouse nucleus accumbens. *Alcoholism, Clinical and Experimental Research*, *36*, 2117–2125.

Muller Herde, A., Mihov, Y., Kramer, S. D., Mu, L., Adamantidis, A., Ametamey, S. M., et al. (2019). Chronic nicotine exposure alters metabotropic glutamate receptor 5: Longitudinal PET study and Behavioural assessment in rats. *Neurotoxicity Research*, *36*, 806–816.

Nickols, H. H., & Conn, P. J. (2014). Development of allosteric modulators of GPCRs for treatment of CNS disorders. *Neurobiology of Disease*, *61*, 55–71.

Nikiforuk, A., Popik, P., Drescher, K. U., van Gaalen, M., Relo, A. L., Mezler, M., et al. (2010). Effects of a positive allosteric modulator of group II metabotropic glutamate receptors, LY487379, on cognitive flexibility and impulsive-like responding in rats. *The Journal of Pharmacology and Experimental Therapeutics*, *335*, 665–673.

Niswender, C. M., & Conn, P. J. (2010). Metabotropic glutamate receptors: Physiology, pharmacology, and disease. *Annual Review of Pharmacology and Toxicology*, *50*, 295–322.

Obara, I., Bell, R. L., Goulding, S. P., Reyes, C. M., Larson, L. A., Ary, A. W., et al. (2009). Differential effects of chronic ethanol consumption and withdrawal on homer/glutamate receptor expression in subregions of the accumbens and amygdala of P rats. *Alcoholism, Clinical and Experimental Research*, *33*, 1924–1934.

O'Brien, N. L., Way, M. J., Kandaswamy, R., Fiorentino, A., Sharp, S. I., Quadri, G., et al. (2014). The functional GRM3 Kozak sequence variant rs148754219 affects the risk of schizophrenia and alcohol dependence as well as bipolar disorder. *Psychiatric Genetics*, *24*, 277–278.

Olive, M. F., McGeehan, A. J., Kinder, J. R., McMahon, T., Hodge, C. W., Janak, P. H., et al. (2005). The mGluR5 antagonist 6-methyl-2-(phenylethynyl)pyridine decreases ethanol consumption via a protein kinase C epsilon-dependent mechanism. *Molecular Pharmacology*, *67*, 349–355.

Parkitna, J. R., Sikora, M., Golda, S., Golembiowska, K., Bystrowska, B., Engblom, D., et al. (2013). Novelty-seeking behaviors and the escalation of alcohol drinking after abstinence in mice are controlled by metabotropic glutamate receptor 5 on neurons expressing dopamine d1 receptors. *Biological Psychiatry*, *73*, 263–270.

Pecknold, J. C., McClure, D. J., Appeltauer, L., Wrzesinski, L., & Allan, T. (1982). Treatment of anxiety using fenobam (a nonbenzodiazepine) in a double-blind standard (diazepam) placebo-controlled study. *Journal of Clinical Psychopharmacology*, *2*, 129–133.

Pelkey, K. A., Yuan, X., Lavezzari, G., Roche, K. W., & McBain, C. J. (2007). mGluR7 undergoes rapid internalization in response to activation by the allosteric agonist AMN082. *Neuropharmacology*, *52*, 108–117.

Porter, R. H., Jaeschke, G., Spooren, W., Ballard, T. M., Buttelmann, B., Kolczewski, S., et al. (2005). Fenobam: A clinically validated nonbenzodiazepine anxiolytic is a potent, selective, and noncompetitive mGlu5 receptor antagonist with inverse agonist activity. *The Journal of Pharmacology and Experimental Therapeutics*, *315*, 711–721.

Renteria, R., Baltz, E. T., & Gremel, C. M. (2018). Chronic alcohol exposure disrupts top-down control over basal ganglia action selection to produce habits. *Nature Communications*, *9*, 211.

Renteria, R., Jeanes, Z. M., & Morrisett, R. A. (2014). Ethanol attenuation of long-term depression in the nucleus accumbens can be overcome by activation of TRPV1 receptors. *Alcoholism, Clinical and Experimental Research*, *38*, 2763–2769.

Sacks, J. J., Gonzales, K. R., Bouchery, E. E., Tomedi, L. E., & Brewer, R. D. (2015). 2010 national and state costs of excessive alcohol consumption. *American Journal of Preventive Medicine*, *49*, e73–e79.

Salih, H., Anghelescu, I., Kezic, I., Sinha, V., Hoeben, E., Van Nueten, L., et al. (2015). Pharmacokinetic and pharmacodynamic characterisation of JNJ-40411813, a positive allosteric modulator of mGluR2, in two randomised, double-blind phase-I studies. *Journal of Psychopharmacology*, *29*, 414–425.

Salling, M. C., Faccidomo, S., & Hodge, C. W. (2008). Nonselective suppression of operant ethanol and sucrose self-administration by the mGluR7 positive allosteric modulator AMN082. *Pharmacology, Biochemistry, and Behavior*, *91*, 14–20.

Samson, H. H., & Czachowski, C. L. (2003). Behavioral measures of alcohol self-administration and intake control: Rodent models. *International Review of Neurobiology*, *54*, 107–143.

Schroeder, J. P., Overstreet, D. H., & Hodge, C. W. (2005). The mGluR5 antagonist MPEP decreases operant ethanol self-administration during maintenance and after repeated alcohol deprivations in alcohol-preferring (P) rats. *Psychopharmacology*, *179*, 262–270.

Schroeder, J. P., Spanos, M., Stevenson, J. R., Besheer, J., Salling, M., & Hodge, C. W. (2008). Cue-induced reinstatement of alcohol-seeking behavior is associated with increased ERK1/2 phosphorylation in specific limbic brain regions: Blockade by the mGluR5 antagonist MPEP. *Neuropharmacology*, *55*, 546–554.

Scofield, M. D., Heinsbroek, J. A., Gipson, C. D., Kupchik, Y. M., Spencer, S., Smith, A. C., et al. (2016). The nucleus Accumbens: Mechanisms of addiction across drug classes reflect the importance of glutamate homeostasis. *Pharmacological Reviews*, *68*, 816–871.

Sharko, A. C., & Hodge, C. W. (2008). Differential modulation of ethanol-induced sedation and hypnosis by metabotropic glutamate receptor antagonists in C57BL/6J mice. *Alcoholism, Clinical and Experimental Research*, *32*, 67–76.

Sidhpura, N., Weiss, F., & Martin-Fardon, R. (2010). Effects of the mGlu2/3 agonist LY379268 and the mGlu5 antagonist MTEP on ethanol seeking and reinforcement are differentially altered in rats with a history of ethanol dependence. *Biological Psychiatry*, *67*, 804–811.

Simonyi, A., Christian, M. R., Sun, A. Y., & Sun, G. Y. (2004). Chronic ethanol-induced subtype- and subregion-specific decrease in the mRNA expression of metabotropic glutamate receptors in rat hippocampus. *Alcoholism, Clinical and Experimental Research*, *28*, 1419–1423.

Sinclair, C. M., Cleva, R. M., Hood, L. E., Olive, M. F., & Gass, J. T. (2012). mGluR5 receptors in the basolateral amygdala and nucleus accumbens regulate cue-induced reinstatement of ethanol-seeking behavior. *Pharmacology, Biochemistry, and Behavior*, *101*, 329–335.

Spanagel, R. (2017). Animal models of addiction. *Dialogues in Clinical Neuroscience*, *19*, 247–258.

Spanagel, R., Noori, H. R., & Heilig, M. (2014). Stress and alcohol interactions: Animal studies and clinical significance. *Trends in Neurosciences*, *37*, 219–227.

Spear, L. P. (2018). Effects of adolescent alcohol consumption on the brain and behaviour. *Nature Reviews. Neuroscience, 19*, 197–214.
Stahle, L. K. R., Jonzon, B., Eriksson, B., & Kagedal, M. (2012). Safety evaluation of the mGluR5 antagonists AZD9272, AZD2066 and AZD2516 in healthy volunteers and patients with neuropathic pain or major deppresive disorder. In *14th world congress on pain, Aug 27–31, Milan, Italy*.
Stennett, B. A., Padovan-Hernandez, Y., & Knackstedt, L. A. (2019). Sequential cocaine-alcohol self-administration produces adaptations in rat nucleus accumbens core glutamate homeostasis that are distinct from those produced by cocaine self-administration alone. *Neuropsychopharmacology, 45*, 441–450.
Stewart, R. B., & Grupp, L. A. (1981). An investigation of the interaction between the reinforcing properties of food and ethanol using the place preference paradigm. *Progress in Neuro-Psychopharmacology, 5*, 609–613.
Su, L. D., Sun, C. L., & Shen, Y. (2010). Ethanol acutely modulates mGluR1-dependent long-term depression in cerebellum. *Alcoholism, Clinical and Experimental Research, 34*, 1140–1145.
Sukoff Rizzo, S. J., Leonard, S. K., Gilbert, A., Dollings, P., Smith, D. L., Zhang, M. Y., et al. (2011). The metabotropic glutamate receptor 7 allosteric modulator AMN082: A monoaminergic agent in disguise? *The Journal of Pharmacology and Experimental Therapeutics, 338*, 345–352.
Szumlinski, K. K., Ary, A. W., Lominac, K. D., Klugmann, M., & Kippin, T. E. (2008). Accumbens Homer2 overexpression facilitates alcohol-induced neuroplasticity in C57BL/6J mice. *Neuropsychopharmacology, 33*, 1365–1378.
Terbeck, S., Akkus, F., Chesterman, L. P., & Hasler, G. (2015). The role of metabotropic glutamate receptor 5 in the pathogenesis of mood disorders and addiction: Combining preclinical evidence with human positron emission tomography (PET) studies. *Frontiers in Neuroscience, 9*, 86.
Thiele, T. E., & Navarro, M. (2014). "Drinking in the dark" (DID) procedures: A model of binge-like ethanol drinking in non-dependent mice. *Alcohol, 48*, 235–241.
Tolliver, G. A., Sadeghi, K. G., & Samson, H. H. (1988). Ethanol preference following the sucrose-fading initiation procedure. *Alcohol, 5*, 9–13.
Valyear, M. D., Villaruel, F. R., & Chaudhri, N. (2017). Alcohol-seeking and relapse: A focus on incentive salience and contextual conditioning. *Behavioural Processes, 141*, 26–32.
Van Skike, C. E., Goodlett, C., & Matthews, D. B. (2019). Acute alcohol and cognition: Remembering what it causes us to forget. *Alcohol, 79*, 105–125.
Varnas, K., Cselenyi, Z., Arakawa, R., Nag, S., Stepanov, V., Moein, M. M., et al. (2019). The pro-psychotic metabotropic glutamate receptor compounds fenobam and AZD9272 share binding sites with monoamine oxidase-B inhibitors in humans. *Neuropharmacology, 162*, 107809.
Vendruscolo, L. F., & Roberts, A. J. (2014). Operant alcohol self-administration in dependent rats: Focus on the vapor model. *Alcohol, 48*, 277–286.
Venniro, M., Caprioli, D., & Shaham, Y. (2016). Animal models of drug relapse and craving: From drug priming-induced reinstatement to incubation of craving after voluntary abstinence. *Progress in Brain Research, 224*, 25–52.
Vranjkovic, O., Winkler, G., & Winder, D. G. (2018). Ketamine administration during a critical period after forced ethanol abstinence inhibits the development of time-dependent affective disturbances. *Neuropsychopharmacology, 43*, 1915–1923.
Wilcox, M. V., Cuzon Carlson, V. C., Sherazee, N., Sprow, G. M., Bock, R., Thiele, T. E., et al. (2014). Repeated binge-like ethanol drinking alters ethanol drinking patterns and depresses striatal GABAergic transmission. *Neuropsychopharmacology, 39*, 579–594.

Wills, T. A., Baucum, A. J., 2nd, Holleran, K. M., Chen, Y., Pasek, J. G., Delpire, E., et al. (2017). Chronic intermittent alcohol disrupts the GluN2B-associated proteome and specifically regulates group I mGlu receptor-dependent long-term depression. *Addiction Biology*, *22*, 275–290.

Windisch, K. A., & Czachowski, C. L. (2018). Effects of group II metabotropic glutamate receptor modulation on ethanol- and sucrose-seeking and consumption in the rat. *Alcohol*, *66*, 77–85.

Wise, R. A. (1973). Voluntary ethanol intake in rats following exposure to ethanol on various schedules. *Psychopharmacologia*, *29*, 203–210.

Wise, R. A., & Bozarth, M. A. (1987). A psychomotor stimulant theory of addiction. *Psychological Review*, *94*, 469–492.

Wood, C. M., Nicolas, C. S., Choi, S. L., Roman, E., Nylander, I., Fernandez-Teruel, A., et al. (2016). Prevalence and influence of cys407* Grm2 mutation in Hannover-derived Wistar rats: mGlu2 receptor loss links to alcohol intake, risk taking and emotional behaviour. *Neuropharmacology*, *115*, 128–138.

World Health Organization. (2014). *Global status report on alcohol and health*. World Health Organization.

Wu, H., Wang, C., Gregory, K. J., Han, G. W., Cho, H. P., Xia, Y., et al. (2014). Structure of a class C GPCR metabotropic glutamate receptor 1 bound to an allosteric modulator. *Science*, *344*, 58–64.

Xia, Y., Ma, D., Hu, J., Tang, C., Wu, Z., Liu, L., et al. (2012). Effect of metabotropic glutamate receptor 3 genotype on N-acetylaspartate levels and neurocognition in non-smoking, active alcoholics. *Behavioral and Brain Functions*, *8*, 42.

Xia, Y., Wu, Z., Ma, D., Tang, C., Liu, L., Xin, F., et al. (2014). Association of single-nucleotide polymorphisms in a metabotropic glutamate receptor GRM3 gene subunit to alcohol-dependent male subjects. *Alcohol and Alcoholism*, *49*, 256–260.

Xu, Y., & Li, Z. (2019). Imaging metabotropic glutamate receptor system: Application of positron emission tomography technology in drug development. *Medicinal Research Reviews*, *39*, 1892–1922.

Yang, H. J., Zhang, H. Y., Bi, G. H., He, Y., Gao, J. T., & Xi, Z. X. (2017). Deletion of type 2 metabotropic glutamate receptor decreases sensitivity to cocaine reward in rats. *Cell Reports*, *20*, 319–332.

Yin, H. H., & Knowlton, B. J. (2006). The role of the basal ganglia in habit formation. *Nature Reviews. Neuroscience*, *7*, 464–476.

Yoneyama, N., Crabbe, J. C., Ford, M. M., Murillo, A., & Finn, D. A. (2008). Voluntary ethanol consumption in 22 inbred mouse strains. *Alcohol*, *42*, 149–160.

Zammataro, M., Chiechio, S., Montana, M. C., Traficante, A., Copani, A., Nicoletti, F., et al. (2011). mGlu2 metabotropic glutamate receptors restrain inflammatory pain and mediate the analgesic activity of dual mGlu2/mGlu3 receptor agonists. *Molecular Pain*, *7*, 6.

Zhao, Y., Dayas, C. V., Aujla, H., Baptista, M. A., Martin-Fardon, R., & Weiss, F. (2006). Activation of group II metabotropic glutamate receptors attenuates both stress and cue-induced ethanol-seeking and modulates c-fos expression in the hippocampus and amygdala. *The Journal of Neuroscience*, *26*, 9967–9974.

Zhou, Z., Karlsson, C., Liang, T., Xiong, W., Kimura, M., Tapocik, J. D., et al. (2013). Loss of metabotropic glutamate receptor 2 escalates alcohol consumption. *Proceedings of the National Academy of Sciences of the United States of America*, *110*, 16963–16968.

CHAPTER NINE

Allosteric modulation of muscarinic receptors in alcohol and substance use disorders

Leigh C. Walker, Andrew J. Lawrence*
Florey Institute of Neuroscience and Mental Health, University of Melbourne, Parkville, VIC, Australia
*Corresponding author: e-mail address: andrew.lawrence@florey.edu.au

Contents

Advances in Pharmacology, Volume 88
ISSN 1054-3589
https://doi.org/10.1016/bs.apha.2020.01.003

Abstract

Alcohol and substance use disorders are chronic relapsing disorders, characterized by a compulsion to take drugs and loss of control in limiting intake. The impact of alcohol and substance abuse on morbidity and mortality is very high worldwide, and treatment options are inadequate at a population level. There is a need for the discovery and development of novel pharmacotherapies to treat alcohol and substance use disorders. The recent development of subtype selective muscarinic acetylcholine receptor (mAChR) allosteric modulators, is rapidly increasing our understanding of this system and revealing great promise for disease treatment. In this chapter, we will present and integrate the current literature regarding the role of mAChRs in drug and alcohol abuse with emerging evidence using novel allosteric modulators targeting specific mAChR subtypes. We will focus on the potential of M_1, M_4 and M_5 mAChRs in the treatment of alcohol, psychostimulant and opioid dependence, using evidence from preclinical studies to predict their utility in treating different stages of the addiction cycle. Overall, preclinical evidence suggests allosteric modulation of mAChRs may provide promise as potential treatment options for alcohol and substance abuse in reducing consumption, facilitating abstinence and preventing relapse.

Abbreviations

Ach acetylcholine
AUD alcohol use disorder
BLA basolateral amygdala
CCK cholecystokinin
CFB cholinergic basal forebrain
CIN cholinergic interneuron
CNS central nervous system
CPP conditioned place preference
D_1 dopamine 1 receptor
D_2 dopamine 2 receptor
DG dentate gyrus
dMSN direct pathway MSN
FDA federal drug association
FR fixed ratio
GPCR G protein-coupled receptors
iMSN indirect pathway MSN
KO knock out
LDTg laterodorsal tegmental nucleus
mAChR muscarinic acetylcholine receptor
MS medial septum
MSN medium spiny neurons
nAChR nicotinic acetylcholine receptors
NAM negative allosteric modulator
nbM nucleus basalis of Meynert
NIDA National Institute on Drug Abuse

PAM	positive allosteric modulator
PFC	prefrontal cortex
PPTg	pedunculopontine tegmental nucleus
PR	progressive ratio
PTSD	post-traumatic stress disorder
PV	parvalbumin
SN	substantia nigra
SUD	substance use disorder

1. Introduction

Alcohol and substance dependence are chronic relapsing diseases characterized by compulsive drug taking despite negative consequences. These disorders are a major socioeconomic burden on society with misuse and related substance use disorders affecting millions of people worldwide. In the United States, 66.7 million people reported binge drinking in the past month and 27.1 million people were current users of illicit drugs or misused prescription drugs (SAMHSA, 2014). Alcohol misuse leads to 88,000 deaths in the United States each year (Stahre, Roeber, Kanny, Brewer, & Zhang, 2014) and opioids lead to over 70,000 overdose deaths. Opioid overdose deaths have more than tripled over the last decade, with rates increasing from 16,849 in 1999 to 70,237 in 2017 (NIDA, 2019). Aside from the individual cost, alcohol misuse and alcohol use disorders (AUD) alone costs the United States approximately $249 billion in lost productivity, health care expenses and other criminal justice costs (CDC, 2016), while other substance use disorders (SUD) costs the American economy an estimated $193 billion (Birnbaum et al., 2011; NDIC, 2011).

Treatment options for drug abuse and dependence are inadequate (Kranzler & Soyka, 2018; Walker & Lawrence, 2018). There are currently 3 FDA approved therapeutics for AUD; Disulfiram, which inhibits acetaldehyde metabolism causing unpleasant symptoms upon alcohol intake, thus acting as a deterrent (Vallari & Pietruszko, 1982); Naltrexone, an opioid receptor antagonist (Niciu & Arias, 2013); and Acamprosate, used to reduce relapse in already abstinent alcoholics (Al Qatari, Khan, Harris, & Littleton, 2001; Spanagel et al., 2014). These medications can be effective in certain populations of individuals with AUD, however, at a population level they suffer from adverse side effects, low rates of compliance and high rate of relapse (Kranzler & Soyka, 2018; Lyon, 2017). For opioid dependence, opioid agonists, including methadone and buprenorphine are approved by the FDA to help with detoxification. While methadone and buprenorphine are generally a safer, less reinforcing substitute for other opiates, they have abuse liability if not administered under supervision (Maxwell & McCance-Katz, 2010). Naltrexone is also FDA approved for the treatment of opioid dependence and may be useful to maintain abstinence in highly motivated individuals, however, adverse side effects are prevalent (Schuckit, 2016). There are no current FDA approved medications for psychostimulant dependence. This, in combination with the limitations of treatments for AUD and opioid dependence highlight the need for development of better pharmacotherapies to treat AUD and SUD.

Because of the role of acetylcholine (ACh) in reward (Cragg, Exley, & Clements, 2005; Williams & Adinoff, 2008), and higher order cognitive processes, including learning and memory (Pepeu & Giovannini, 2004), ACh may play an important role in the processes underpinning drug and alcohol dependence. To date, research has highlighted the potential of muscarinic acetylcholine receptors (mAChRs) in neurocognitive disorders, such as Alzheimer's disease, Parkinson's disease and schizophrenia (Bosboom, Stoffers, & Wolters, 2003; Mesulam, Guillozet, Shaw, & Quinn, 2002; Raedler et al., 2003), with relatively less consideration given to their role in addictive disorders. The recent advancement of subtype selective mAChR allosteric compounds have allowed greater understanding of the specific receptor contributions to different components of substance abuse and dependence including consumption, abstinence and relapse. Moreover, the National Institute on Drug Abuse (NIDA), has recently named the M_5 mAChRs in their top 10 targets for the treatment of opioid use disorder (Rasmussen, White, & Acri, 2019). In this chapter we give a brief overview of animal models of addiction, the expression and role of mAChRs in reward circuitry and discuss the current evidence and potential for allosteric modulation of M_1, M_4 and M_5 mAChRs in the treatment of alcohol and other substance use disorders.

2. Acetylcholine

ACh was first identified in 1914 by Sir Henry Hallett Dale for its actions on heart tissue, and in 1921, Otto Loewi confirmed ACh as a neurotransmitter. This was the first neurotransmitter to be identified, and for their work they received the 1936 Nobel Prize in Physiology or Medicine. While ACh acts as a neurotransmitter at the neuromuscular junction; within the central nervous system (CNS), it primarily acts as a neuromodulator, altering neuronal excitability, neurotransmitter release and coordinating the firing of groups of neurons (Rice & Cragg, 2004; Wonnacott, 1997; Zhang & Sulzer, 2004).

CNS cholinergic neurons arise from multiple discrete sources, they project widely throughout the brain to modulate cognitive, affective, and behavioral functions. The cholinergic basal forebrain (CBF), is classically segregated into four main regions, the nucleus basalis of Meynert (nbM, Ch1), medial septum (MS, Ch2), and vertical and horizontal bands of the diagonal band of Broca (Ch3 and Ch4), which generally innervate the cortex, amygdala, and hippocampal formation (Fig. 1). Additionally, populations of cholinergic neurons reside in the hindbrain pedunculopontine tegmental nucleus (PPTg; Ch5) and the laterodorsal tegmental nucleus (LDTg; Ch6), which generally provide innervation to the midbrain and hindbrain regions (Mesulam, Mufson, Wainer, & Levey, 1983). Another major population of cholinergic interneurons (CINs) reside within the striatum, which provide tonic activity onto local striatal circuitry (Mesulam, Mufson, Levey, & Wainer, 1983; Mesulam, Mufson, Wainer, et al., 1983; Phelps, Houser, & Vaughn, 1985; Wainer et al., 1984). While CINs were thought to be the main source of ACh within the striatum, recently the PPTg and LDTg have also been shown to innervate the striatum in a topographically specific manner, targeting CINs (Assous & Tepper, 2019; Dautan, Hacioğlu Bay, Bolam, Gerdjikov, & Mena-Segovia, 2016; Dautan et al., 2014). Another innervation from the parafascicular nucleus to the striatum has also been shown to preferentially target CINs (Mandelbaum et al., 2019). While CINs only make up approximately 1–2% of all striatal neurons they possess extensive axonal arborizations that allow them to exert a disproportionate influence over striatal signaling (Kreitzer, 2009). In addition to these groups, smaller cholinergic populations are located in the cerebral cortex, olfactory bulb, hypothalamus, medial habenula and paratrigeminal nucleus (Jeong, Woo, Chua, & Jo, 2016; Krosnowski et al., 2012; López et al., 2019; Mufson, Martin, Mash, Wainer, & Mesulam, 1986; von Engelhardt, Eliava, Meyer, Rozov, & Monyer, 2007).

The effects of ACh are mediated through two classes of receptors: metabotropic muscarinic receptors (mAChR) and ionotropic nicotinic receptors (nAChR). mAChRs are slow-acting, G protein-coupled receptors (GPCRs) that mediate their responses by activating a cascade of intracellular pathways. There are five distinct mAChR subtypes (M_1—M_5) that regulate the activity of a diverse array of central and peripheral functions in the

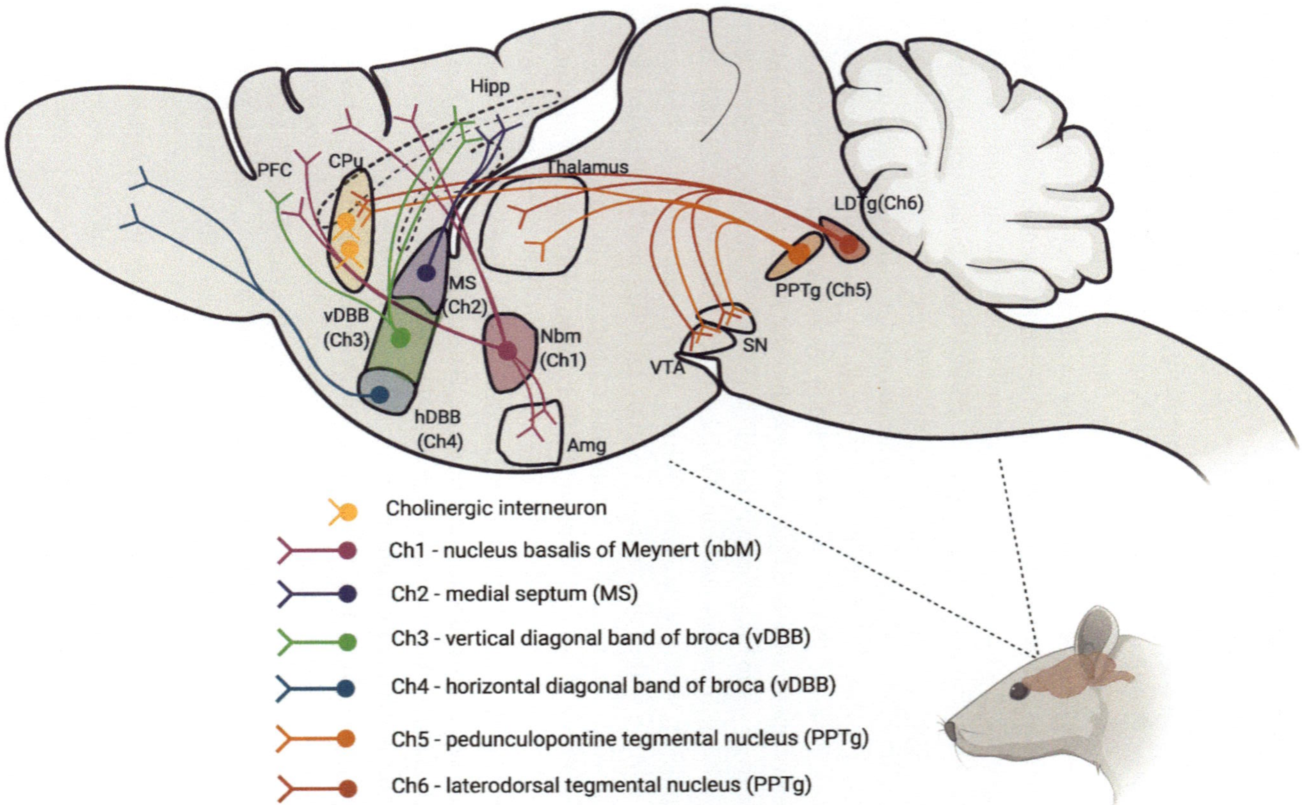

Fig. 1 Illustrated overview of cholinergic pathways in the rodent brain. Cholinergic projections include the nucleus basalis of Meynert (nbM, Ch1), medial septum (MS, Ch2), and vertical and horizontal bands of the diagonal band of Broca (Ch3 and Ch4) projecting to the hippocampus, thalamus, olfactory bulb, and cortical region. Cholinergic pontomesencephalon neurons include the pedunculopontine tegmental nuclei (PPTg, Ch5) and laterodorsal tegmental (LDTg, Ch6) regions projecting to hindbrain, thalamus and striatum. Cholinergic interneurons (CINs) also reside within the dorsal (CPu) and ventral striatum (Acb).

human body but differ in their synaptic and anatomical localization as well as functional coupling to heterotrimeric G proteins. M_1, M_3, and M_5 mAChRs primarily couple through Gq effector proteins, subsequently increasing inositol 1,4,5-phosphate signaling and Ca^{2+} mobilization, while M_2 and M_4 mAChRs couple to Gi/o proteins, inhibiting downstream adenylyl cyclase activation (Offermanns et al., 1994; Peralta, Ashkenazi, Winslow, Ramachandran, & Capon, 1988; Peralta et al., 1988).

Dysregulation of cholinergic systems have been implicated in a variety of neuropsychiatric disorders including schizophrenia, Alzheimer's disease, alcohol and substance use disorders (Langmead & Christopoulos, 2014; Mufson, Counts, Perez, & Ginsberg, 2008; Sarter, Nelson, & Bruno, 2005). While previous genetic models and nonsubtype selective drugs targeting mAChRs have given insight into the role of these receptors in various behaviors and disease models, the lack of selective drugs has hindered progress and clinical development. The recent advancement of mAChR allosteric modulators has permitted greater understanding of discrete subtype roles and the clinical potential of these compounds in the treatment of neuropsychiatric disorders including AUD and SUDs.

3. Animal models of drug addiction

Much of the evidence in understanding the role of mAChRs in AUD and SUDs comes from animal models of addiction. Although no animal model fully emulates the human condition, animal models permit more detailed examination of mechanisms and neural adaptations underpinning aberrant addiction-like behaviors. To elucidate the role of mAChRs in addiction several paradigms including fixed ratio (FR) and progressive ratio (PR) operant self-administration, extinction-reinstatement and conditioned place preference (CPP) paradigms have been employed. In self-administration studies animals are trained to perform a response (commonly lever press or nose poke) in order to obtain a drug reward. This can be delivered orally via a receptacle, for alcohol, or intravenously, for other drugs of abuse (Koob, Bloom, & Kupfer, 1995). The reinforcing properties of the drug can be assessed by altering the number of responses required to obtain the drug. FR schedules, in which a fixed number of responses are required for drug delivery are often used to assess a drug's reinforcing effects. By altering the number of responses required or drug concentration, animals will adjust their rate of responding to compensate (e.g., increase or decrease to titrate dose) (Arnold & Roberts, 1997). On the other hand, to

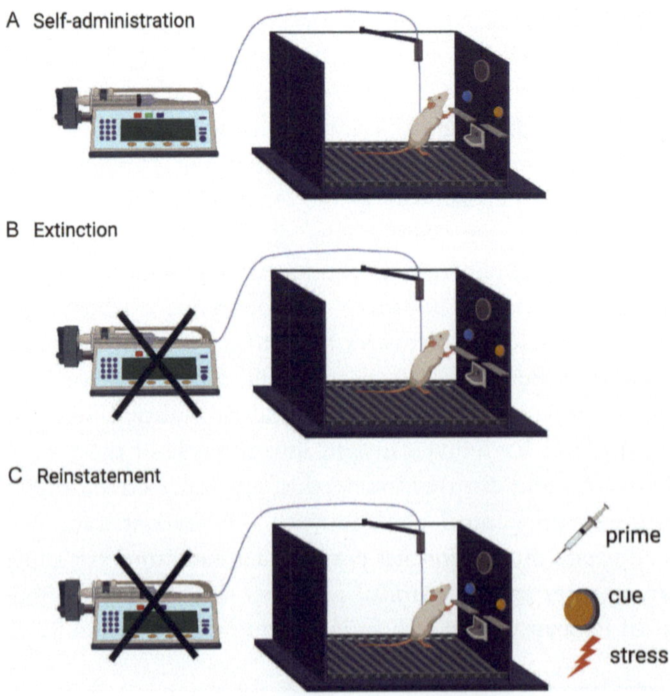

Fig. 2 Schematic of the extinction-reinstatement animal model of drug seeking. The extinction-reinstatement paradigm can be used to examine drug seeking behavior. First animals are trained stably self-administer the drug reward in an operant conditioning chamber. Once stable, the responding is extinguished. During extinction, the drug reinforcer and any drug associated cues are removed, and the animal learns that the action previously associated with drug delivery no longer elicits a reward. Once lever pressing has been extinguished, reinstatement of drug seeking can be measured as the return to lever responding, despite the absence of reward. Reinstatement can be elicited in several ways, including exposure to a drug prime, exposure to a drug associated cue or context or exposure to a stressor.

examine the motivation of an animal to obtain the drug, the difficulty of the required responding can be altered. In a PR schedule response requirements are increased after each delivery of the reinforcer, until the animal will no longer respond, determining a breakpoint (Stafford, LeSage, & Glowa, 1998).

To assess relapse like behavior in the extinction-reinstatement model (Fig. 2), animals are trained first to stably self-administer before responding is extinguished by removing the drug as a reinforcer and any drug associated cues (Shaham, Shalev, Lu, De Wit, & Stewart, 2003). Therefore, the animal learns the operant lever (or nose poke) previously associated with drug delivery no longer elicits a reward, commonly termed extinction. Extinction is not mediated by "erasing" the memory of stimulus-response association, but instead by development of additional memory that is distinct from acquisition (Myers & Davis, 2002). Following extinction, reinstatement of responding previously associated with drug reinforcement, in the absence of drug delivery can be elicited several ways; exposure to a drug prime (Brown, Short, & Lawrence, 2010); re-exposure to a drug associated cue (Jupp, Krstew, Dezsi, & Lawrence, 2011); re-exposure to a drug associated context or environment (Campbell et al., 2019; Crombag, Bossert, Koya, & Shaham, 2008); or exposure to a stressor (Shaham, Erb, & Stewart, 2000; Walker, Kastman, & Lawrence, 2019).

The CPP procedure is commonly used to assess the reinforcing properties of drugs of abuse. In a standard CPP, animals receive a drug in one environment or "context" and a "nondrug" substance (usually the drug's vehicle) in another distinct environment. Following repeat pairings, animals (typically in a drug-free state) are given a choice to move freely between the two environments, and the amount of time spent in the drug-associated context is taken as an index of preference for the drug (Bardo & Bevins, 2000; Koob et al., 1995). To examine craving or relapse-like behavior, CPP can be extinguished by multiple pairings of a nondrug substance with the previously drug associated context and reinstatement of CPP examined through the subsequent administration of the drug.

4. mAChR expression in reward circuitry

Anatomical mapping of GPCRs is often challenging, this is no different for mAChRs, with a lack of subtype specific (validated and/or commercially available) antibodies. The distribution of mAChRs throughout the rodent brain have recently been reviewed in detail (Lebois, Thorn, Edgerton, Popiolek, & Xi, 2018), here we summarize the distribution of each of the mAChR subtypes, focusing on regions important for aberrant behaviors associated with addiction (Fig. 3). All five muscarinic receptors are expressed in the brain and periphery, but receptor abundance varies between regions. M_1, M_2 and M_4 mAChRs are the major subtypes expressed in most brain regions, with M_3 and M_5 exhibiting more discrete patterns of expression (Lebois et al., 2018). Further, cellular localization and action of mAChR receptor subtypes differ, and this brain region specific. For example, M_1, M_3 and M_5 Gq coupled receptors most often expressed postsynaptically to modulate membrane resistance, however, M_5 receptors

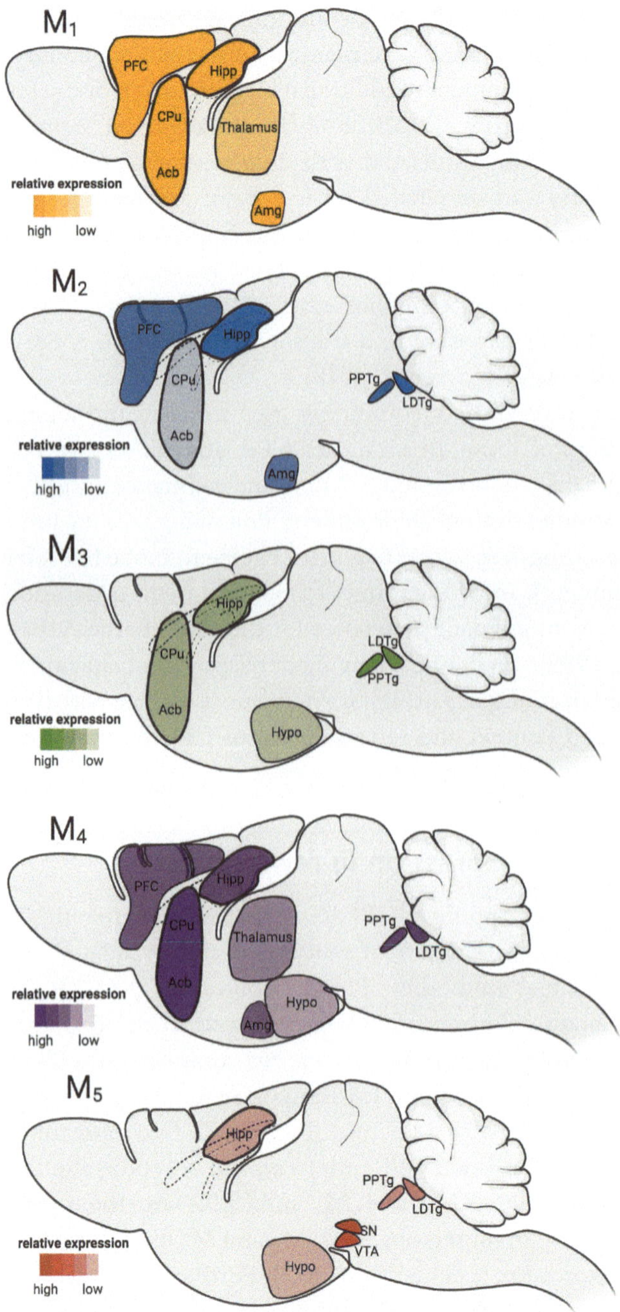

Fig. 3 Illustrated overview of mAChR expression in rodent reward circuitry. Distribution of M_1 (yellow), M_2 (blue), M_3 (green), M_4 (purple), and M_5 (red) muscarinic acetylcholine (ACh) receptors in brain regions implicated in reward. Relative expression of each receptor subtype is indicated by its respective color gradient. M_1 mAChRs are highly

are also expressed presynaptically on dopaminergic terminal from the substantia nigra (SN) to the dorsal striatum (Shin, Adrover, Wess, & Alvarez, 2015). And while Gi/o coupled M_2 and M_4 receptors are often expressed presynaptically, acting to regulate neurotransmitter release, in some regions they also produce inhibitory postsynaptic responses in subsets of neurons. An example of this being the striatum, where M_4 mAChRs are expressed postsynaptically on medium spiny neurons (MSN) (Pancani et al., 2014).

4.1 M_1 mAChRs

The M_1 mAChR is the most abundantly expressed in the CNS including the basal ganglia, hippocampus and amygdala. M_1 mAChR has been identified within the striatum, predominantly on dendrites of both direct (D_1; dMSN) and indirect (D_2; iMSN) pathway medium spiny projection neurons, where they function to increase excitability and facilitate synaptic plasticity (Calabresi, Centonze, Gubellini, Pisani, & Bernardi, 1998; Carr & Surmeier, 2007; Lv et al., 2017; Zhang, Yamada, Gomeza, Basile, & Wess, 2002). Within the hippocampal formation M_1 receptors are densely expressed on pyramidal neurons throughout the CA subfields, subiculum as well as the dentate gyrus (DG) granular layer (Levey, Edmunds, Koliatsos, Wiley, & Heilman, 1995; Rouse, Gilmor, & Levey, 1998; Rouse & Levey, 1996; Volpicelli & Levey, 2004). Here M_1 mAChRs act to increase the intrinsic excitability of parvalbumin (PV) and cholecystokinin (CCK) interneurons, which provide strong feedforward inhibition onto pyramidal neurons (Yi et al., 2014). M_1 receptors are also expressed in the prefrontal cortex (PFC) (Carr & Surmeier, 2007; Navarria et al., 2015) and amygdala, especially the basolateral amygdala (BLA) (Muller, Mascagni, Zaric, & McDonald, 2013).

---

expressed in the cortex, hippocampus, dorsal (CPu) and ventral (Acb) striatum, with low levels detected in the thalamus. M_2 mAChRs are densely expressed in the cortex, hippocampus and hindbrain pedunculopontine tegmental nuclei (PPTg) and laterodorsal tegmental (LDTg) regions, with lower expression observed in the amygdala and CPu and Acb. M_2 mAChRs are also expressed widely throughout the periphery. M_3 mAChRs are expressed diffusely throughout the striatum, hypothalamus, hippocampus and hindbrain LDTg and PPTg. High levels of M_3 mAChRs also exist in the periphery. M_4 mAChRs are highly expressed in striatal regions, moderately expressed across the cortex, thalamus and hippocampus, with low levels also detected within the amygdala, hypothalamus, thalamus and hindbrain LDTg and PPTg. M_5 mAChR expression is most densely expressed within the midbrain ventral tegmental area (VTA) and substantia nigra (SN), with low diffuse expression also detected in the hypothalamus, hippocampus and hindbrain LDTg and PPTg.

4.2 M_2 mAChR

The M_2 mAChR plays a major role in modulating cholinergic tone and broadly modulating circuit function as autoreceptors (Billard, Binch, Crosby, & McQuade, 1995; Douglas, Baghdoyan, & Lydic, 2001; Hersch & Levey, 1995; Levey et al., 1995; Rouse et al., 1998). The M_2 mAChR is expressed at low levels in striatum, specifically M_2 receptors are expressed on CINs where they act directly as autoreceptors, suppressing ACh release (Bernard, Laribi, Levey, & Bloch, 1998; Billard et al., 1995; Rouse, Thomas, & Levey, 1997; Vilaró, Palacios, & Mengod, 1994; Vilaro, Wiederhold, Palacios, & Mengod, 1992) and also to indirectly modulate dopamine release from dopamine terminals (Kuroiwa et al., 2012; Threlfell et al., 2010). While M_2 expression is lower than M_1 expression in the hippocampus, M_2 receptors are thought to be the predominant cholinergic autoreceptors that suppress ACh release and GABA release in the hippocampus (Levey et al., 1995; Rouse et al., 1998; Rouse & Levey, 1996; Volpicelli & Levey, 2004). M_2 mAChR are also expressed on hindbrain PPTg and LDTg cholinergic neurons (Vilaro et al., 1992; Vilaró et al., 1994). These neurons innervate thalamic and midbrain regions, and express M_2 receptors on their terminals (Vilaro et al., 1992; Vilaró et al., 1994) that can act as autoreceptors to inhibit ACh release (Coleman, Lydic, & Baghdoyan, 2004) and also regulate midbrain dopamine levels (Kohlmeier, Ishibashi, Wess, Bickford, & Leonard, 2012; Tzavara et al., 2004). The M_2 mAChR expression has also been detected within the amygdala, largely confined to the glutamatergic and somatostatin positive neurons in the BLA, with some expression also observed in somatostatin containing neurons of the CeA (McDonald & Mascagni, 2011).

4.3 M_3 mAChR

M_3 mAChR is expressed at low levels, diffusely throughout the hippocampus, hypothalamus and striatum (Levey, Edmunds, Heilman, Desmond, & Frey, 1994). Highest labeling density is observed within the pyramidal neurons of the CA1 and CA3 regions on CCK+ neurons, where they control firing frequency (Cea-del Rio et al., 2010). M_3 mAChRs are also expressed on PPTg and LDTg midbrain neurons (Vilaro et al., 1992; Vilaró et al., 1994).

4.4 M_4 mAChR

M_4 mAChRs are widely distributed throughout reward circuitry including the basal ganglia, hippocampus, amygdala, and thalamus. In the striatum M_4

mAChRs are expressed presynaptically on cortico-striatal neurons, where they modulate glutamate release onto both D_1 dMSNs and D_2 iMSNs (Pancani et al., 2014). Further, they are expressed as autoreceptors on the axonal terminals of cholinergic interneurons (Threlfell et al., 2010), and postsynaptically on D_1 dMSNs where they modulate dopamine release through a cannabinoid receptor dependent mechanism (Foster et al., 2016; Ince, Ciliax, & Levey, 1997; Threlfell et al., 2010; Yan, Flores-Hernandez, & Surmeier, 2001). Within the hippocampus M_4 mAChRs are expressed at high levels in the DG and subiculum, with moderate expression within the CA1–CA3 fields (Levey et al., 1995; Rouse et al., 1998; Rouse & Levey, 1996). Some expression has also been observed within the thalamus, amygdala, PFC and hindbrain PPTg and LDTg (Levey, 1993; Levey, Kitt, Simonds, Price, & Brann, 1991; Sugaya, Clamp, Bryan, & McKinney, 1997; Vilaró et al., 1994).

4.5 M_5 mAChRs

M_5 mAChRs have very discrete expression throughout the rodent brain. They are the major subtype expressed within the ventral midbrain including the ventral tegmental area (VTA) and SNc, with more sparse expression across other brain regions (Vilaró, Palacios, & Mengod, 1990). Within the VTA, approximately half of the TH-labeled cells expressed M_5 mRNA, while 80% of TH+ cells colabeled with M_5 in the SNc (Gould et al., 2019). M_5 also shows high coexpression with the D_2 DA receptor, which is another marker of dopamine expressing neurons in the SNc (Weiner, Levey, & Brann, 1990). Contrastingly, less than 15% of cells within the VTA or SNc expressing vGAT coexpressed the M_5 mAChR (Gould et al., 2019). The M_5 receptor is also expressed within the pyramidal cells of the CA1 field, and ventral subiculum, but absent from the CA3 field, the lateral habenula, ventromedial hypothalamus (VMH) and the PPTg and LDTg as visualized by in situ hybridization (Sugaya et al., 1997; Vilaró et al., 1990, 1994).

4.6 Peripheral expression

M_3 is the predominant muscarinic subtype expressed in the periphery being found in the gastrointestinal tract, glands, lung, pancreas, bladder, prostate and testis (Bymaster, McKinzie, Felder, & Wess, 2003; Ito et al., 2009; Matsui et al., 2000). The M_2 mAChR is the second most predominant subtype expressed in the periphery. Specifically, M_2 mAChRs are located in the heart, gastrointestinal tract, bladder and submandibular gland. Many of the adverse pharmacological effects of M_2 and M_3 modulation are attributed to these peripheral actions (Bymaster et al., 2003; Ito et al., 2009; Matsui et al., 2000). The M_1, M_4 and M_5 subtypes are mainly confined to the CNS; however, M_1 is expressed in prostate, where it may influence cell proliferation and growth in prostate cancer (Mannan Baig et al., 2017), while M_4 and M_5 are expressed within the bladder and testis. The limited peripheral expression of M_1, M_4 and M_5 have made them more desirable for CNS clinical development.

5. Effects of drugs of abuse on mAChR expression

Early studies in the 1980s using either involuntary alcohol self-administration or liquid diet, linked alcohol exposure with changes in mAChR expression (Muller, Britton, & Seeman, 1980; Rabin et al., 1980). This was followed by cocaine in the early 1990s (Zeigler, Lipton, Toga, & Ellison, 1991) and more recently, gene array studies have shown oxycodone alters expression of mAChR mRNAs within the brain (Zhang et al., 2014).

While it is clear that drug and alcohol exposure impacts mAChR expression, the exact time course in different brain regions type is not well understood. In male Sprague Dawley rats, expression of mAChRs after 5 days slow release cocaine administration was examined. In the hippocampus mAChR expression was increased 12 h into withdrawal but decreased 2 and 21 days later (Lipton, Olsen, & Ellison, 1995). Further, in the striatum, 12 h and 2 days after withdrawal, mAChR expression was increased, but a decrease was observed after 21 days (Lipton et al., 1995), highlighting the dynamic nature of mAChR expression in relation to drugs of abuse. Further, route of administration and drug dose also seem to influence mAChR expression. While bolus administration of cocaine (20 mg/kg/daily for 5 days) showed no alteration in mAChR expression, administration via a slow release pellet (103 mg total over 5 days), caused dysregulation throughout the striatum, amygdala and hippocampus (Zeigler et al., 1991).

Most early examinations of mAChRs were undertaken using non-subtype selective measures. While these are useful, several drawbacks exist. Binding of ACh to select subtypes results in different signaling cascades and downstream effector proteins. In theory, an upregulation of M_1, M_3 or M_5 receptors may be equivalent to downregulation of M_2 or M_4 receptors, whereby if they occur as consequences of the same behavior, nonselective mAChR assays would not be able to differentiate. The advancement of sequencing and large discovery driven data sets has allowed the identification of subtype specific mAChR mRNA alterations following drug administration. Studies examining oxycodone self-administration suggest *chrm3* and *chrm5* are upregulated in the dorsal striatum, while *chrm2* and *chrm5* are downregulated in the ventral striatum after 14 days voluntary self-administration in male C57BL6/J mice (Mayer-Blackwell et al., 2014; Zhang et al., 2018, 2014). Further, *chrm4* expression in the ventral striatum was negatively correlated with the amount of oxycodone self-administered (Zhang et al., 2018). The caveat with these studies being that they measure mRNA expression, not direct mAChR protein expression or function, which have been shown to diverge in many cases. Overall, while many factors may influence the conflicting results observed with mAChR expression following drug administration, investigation of subtype selective modulation warrants further examination.

6. mAChR allosteric modulators

Classical mAChR ligands used in early preclinical and clinical studies lacked true receptor subtype selectivity, resulting in numerous dose-limiting adverse effects and failure in clinical development (Shekhar et al., 2008). Recently, subtype selective mAChR ligands that bind to allosteric sites, topographically distinct from the orthosteric binding site of ACh, have been developed (Brady et al., 2008; Bubser et al., 2014; Byun et al., 2014). Examples of such compounds are shown in Fig. 4. These compounds have several advantages over orthosteric ligands. First, orthosteric binding sites are more highly conserved across mAChR subtypes, while allosteric modulation has allowed for development of more subtype selective mAChR compounds (Kruse et al., 2013). Further, these compounds only act as positive (PAM) or negative (NAMs) allosteric modulators when the endogenous ligand is present, maintaining more natural spatiotemporal scale (Kruse et al., 2013). Finally, allosteric modulation allows more a more nuanced manipulation of ACh signaling. This may allow for more fine-tuned responses as a consequence of PAM or NAM activity, proving particularly important in diseases, such as AUD and SUDs where tight physiological regulation is vital.

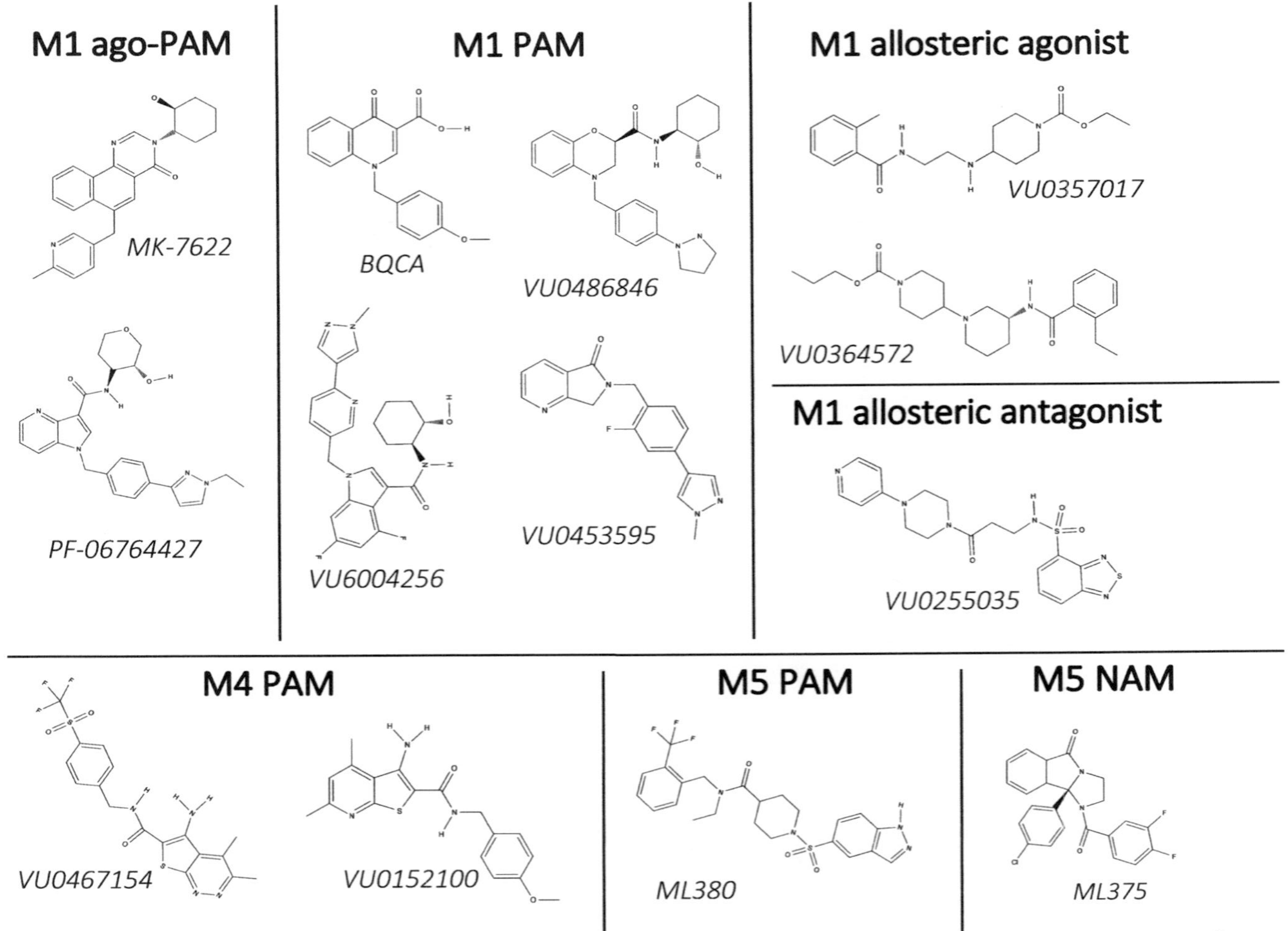

Fig. 4 Allosteric compounds used to understand drug consumption and seeking.

Several highly selective compounds have been developed and have been used in preclinical examination of neuropsychiatric disorders. Currently, the M_4 PAM VU0467154 has the best in vitro potency and pharmacokinetic properties for preclinical examination (Bubser et al., 2014; Byun et al., 2014). VU0467154 does not directly activate the M_4 receptor, instead it potentiates the ACh response by increasing the affinity of ACh for the M_4 receptor (Bubser et al., 2014). Further, this compound has limited side effects in rodent models (Bubser et al., 2014; Byun et al., 2014), and does not lead to tolerance upon repeated dosing (Gould et al., 2018). The M_4 PAM VU6005806 represents another high-quality rodent tool compound for preclinical studies (Engers et al., 2019), however it has yet to be examined in rodent models of addiction. The M_5 NAM, ML375, was identified through a functional high-throughput screen (Gentry et al., 2013). ML375 is the first M_5 selective NAM with favorable selectivity, potency and CNS penetration (Gentry et al., 2013). However, ML375 has a long elimination half-life of $\sim$80 h in rat which can be problematic in rodent paradigms where repeat dosing is required. The newly developed VU6008667, a M_5 NAM with similar potency to ML375 has recently been described (McGowan et al., 2017). VU6008667 has a half-life of $\sim$2.5 h in rat and superior solubility, making it a more desirable in vivo tool, but has yet to be examined in addictive-like behaviors (McGowan et al., 2017).

7. The utility of targeting mAChRs for preventing drug acquisition and maintenance

7.1 Evidence from KO studies and nonselective compounds

Drugs of abuse hijack the mesolimbic dopaminergic reward pathways through a variety of mechanisms, resulting in increased dopamine transmission within the striatum (Di Chiara & Imperato, 1988). The modulation of dopamine release by drugs of abuse has long been studied as a target to treat drug abuse by reducing the rewarding effects associated with alcohol or substance consumption (Nutt, Lingford-Hughes, Erritzoe, & Stokes, 2015). mAChR subtypes have been shown to directly or indirectly modulate the mesolimbic dopamine pathway, suggesting there may be a variety of mechanisms by which mAChRs could modulate one or more of these circuits.

Using mAChR subtype KO mice, researchers have shown M_1 KO mice have enhanced dopamine transmission in the accumbens (Acb) and have a greater response to amphetamine administration (Gerber et al., 2001).

These results suggest M_1 receptors within the striatum modulate dopamine release. M_1 KO mice showed decreased conditioned place preference to cocaine and morphine, although confounding effects on learning and memory could underpin these observations (Carrigan & Dykstra, 2007). M_5 mAChRs are expressed on dopamine terminals from the midbrain, where they potentiate striatal dopamine release (Bendor et al., 2010; Shin et al., 2015; Yamada et al., 2001) and M_5 KO mice exhibit reduced morphine CPP, cocaine self-administration, but not food self-administration (Basile et al., 2002; Fink-Jensen et al., 2003; Thomsen et al., 2005). However, recently Wang and colleagues found M_5 KO mice displayed a morphine CPP in a similar manner to their wildtype counterparts, but other drug associated behaviors such as extinction and reinstatement were impaired (Wang, 2017). In contrast to the reductions observed in M_1 and M_5 KO mice, M_4 KO mice show increased cocaine and alcohol self-administration (de la Cour et al., 2015; Schmidt et al., 2011). While the M_1/M_4 agonist, xanomeline, produced a rightward shift in the cocaine dose-response curve in mice (Thomsen et al., 2010, 2012), and increased the choice for food over cocaine in rats (Thomsen, Fulton, & Caine, 2014). Within the striatum, M_4 receptors are expressed on D_1 direct pathway MSNs, cholinergic interneurons and glutamatergic projections from the prefrontal cortex, where they inhibit dopamine release indirectly (Jeon et al., 2010; Shin et al., 2015). In line with this, M_4 KO mice have impaired cocaine induced dopamine release in the Acb (Schmidt et al., 2011) and hyperactive D_1 MSNs.

The basolateral amygdala (BLA) is another region which expresses mAChRs (primarily M_1 and M_4) and is important for encoding drug associated cues. Administration of the nonselective mAChR antagonist scopolamine into the BLA of mice prior to acquisition of cocaine self-administration disrupted cue-induced reinstatement of cocaine seeking (See, McLaughlin, & Fuchs, 2003). However, when administered after cocaine self-administration was acquired, scopolamine had no effect on cue-induced reinstatement behaviors (See et al., 2003), suggesting a role of BLA mAChRs in acquisition of drug associations, but not when the association has previously been formed.

Together these results suggest the M_4 and M_5 receptors may hold value in the treatment of drug acquisition and maintenance. However, compensatory developmental effects in KO mouse models and nonselective compounds can overshadow behavioral outcomes. Below we discuss some recent findings using novel subtype specific allosteric modulators which have shed more light on specific roles of the M_4 and M_5 mAChRs.

7.2 Recent evidence from allosteric compounds

Evidence from KO mouse models suggest positive allosteric modulation of the M_4 mAChR and negative allosteric modulation of M_5 mAChRs may be useful in preclinical models of drug self-administration. The M_4 PAM, VU0152100, reduced cocaine self-administration and cocaine-induced striatal dopamine increase, without affecting motor performance. These effects were not observed in M_4 KO mice, suggesting a M_4 dependent mechanism (Dencker et al., 2012). Further, selective deletion of M_4 receptors from D_1 receptor neurons, resulted in an intermediate reduction of cocaine self-administration following VU0152100 administration. This indicates that VU0152100 in part, regulates dopamine release via M_4 receptors colocalized on D_1 receptor expressing neurons (Dencker et al., 2012).

The M_5 NAM, ML375, when administered systemically also decreased self-administration of alcohol, cocaine and opiates in a dose related manner (Berizzi et al., 2018; Gould et al., 2019; Gunter et al., 2018). These effects were specific to drug, with no differences in natural reward administration observed (Berizzi et al., 2018; Gould et al., 2019), however, a small reduction in sucrose responding was observed by Gunter and colleagues, in a fixed ratio, but not PR schedule (Gunter et al., 2018). Further, no locomotor deficits were observed (Berizzi et al., 2018; Gould et al., 2019; Gunter et al., 2018), nor any effects on food self-administration (Gould et al., 2019). The dorsal striatum has been implicated as a region important for M_5 mAChR actions in drug self-administration. Intra-cranial microinjections of ML375, directly into the dorsal striatum showed the lateral, but not the medial division, are involved in attenuating alcohol self-administration after long term exposure (Berizzi et al., 2018). This may, in part, be attributed to the role of acetylcholine in mediating habitual behaviors, as rats were trained for an extended period, which has previously been shown to lead to habitual operant responding for alcohol (Corbit, Nie, & Janak, 2012). Interestingly, the M_5 PAM, ML380, did not alter alcohol self-administration when administered in either the medial or lateral division of the dorsal striatum.

Collectively, these findings suggest either enhancement of M_4 receptor signaling, or inhibition of M_5 receptor signaling may have potential for treating drug and alcohol abuse and reducing long-term consumption (Table 1). Indeed, the M_5 mAChR was recently included in NIDA top 10 drugs for development for the treatment of opioid use disorder

Table 1 The role of mAChR allosteric compounds in drug self-administration.

Target	Compound	Ligand type	Drug	Schedule	Outcome	Reference
M_4	VU0152100	PAM	Cocaine	Fixed ratio	Decreased	Dencker et al. (2012)
M_5	ML375	NAM	Alcohol	Fixed ratio	Decreased	Berizzi et al. (2018)
	ML375	NAM	Cocaine	Fixed ratio	Decreased	Gunter et al. (2018)
	ML375	NAM	Cocaine	Progressive ratio	Decreased	Gunter et al. (2018)
	ML375	NAM	Oxycodone	Fixed ratio	Decreased	Gould et al. (2019)
	ML375	NAM	Oxycodone	Progressive ratio	Decreased	Gould et al. (2019)
	ML375	NAM	Remifentanil	Fixed ratio	Decreased	Gould et al. (2019)
	ML375	NAM	Remifentanil	Progressive ratio	Decreased	Gould et al. (2019)
Region specific						
Intra-DLS						
M_5	ML375	NAM	Alcohol	Fixed ratio	Decreased	Berizzi et al. (2018)
	ML380	PAM	Alcohol	Fixed ratio	No effect	Berizzi et al. (2018)
Intra-DMS						
M_5	ML375	NAM	Alcohol	Fixed ratio	No effect	Berizzi et al. (2018)
	ML380	PAM	Alcohol	Fixed ratio	No effect	Berizzi et al. (2018)

(Rasmussen et al., 2019). Current literature suggests the mechanisms underpinning reduced drug taking may be conserved across drug class to some extent, suggesting a common mechanism. However, this requires further elucidation.

8. The utility of targeting mAChRs for extinction facilitation

8.1 Evidence from KO studies and nonselective compounds

Improvement of cognitive functions through cognitive enhancers have been proposed as treatment strategy for addiction. Cognitive enhancers are thought to hold utility in facilitating extinction of conditioned responses to drug associated cues and contexts (Dhonnchadha & Kantak, 2011; Kaplan & Moore, 2011; Perry & Lawrence, 2017; Walker & Lawrence, 2018). mAChRs have long been implicated in memory and cognitive functions, with nonselective antagonists, such as scopolamine, having powerful effects on memory and learning (Davis, Thomas, & Adams, 1971; Robbins et al., 1997). Therefore, mAChRs may provide utility in facilitating drug extinction.

ACh is a critical component of hippocampal memory formation (Grecksch, Ott, & Matthies, 1978; Jaffard, Destrade, Durkin, & Ebel, 1979). Examination of mAChR KO mouse models have implicated all mAChR receptor subtypes in cognition and memory. M_1 KO mice show deficits in a range of cognitive processes including working memory, learning and consolidation, but not behavioral flexibility (Anagnostaras et al., 2003; Bartko et al., 2011; Shinoe, Matsui, Taketo, & Manabe, 2005). M_2 KO mice have deficits in various cognitive domains including working memory, spatial learning, and behavioral flexibility (Bainbridge et al., 2008; Seeger et al., 2004; Tzavara et al., 2003), while M_3 KO mice show deficits in fear conditioning and memory (Poulin et al., 2010). M_4 KO mice show normal spatial reference, working and episodic-like memory, but show deficits in fear conditioning (Bubser et al., 2014; Koshimizu, Leiter, & Miyakawa, 2012; Thomsen et al., 2012). Finally, M_5 KO mice display enhanced CPP extinction (Wang, 2017), however, they have impaired spatial and nonspatial memory, which may be linked to cerebrovascular deficits observed in the M_5 KO mouse line (Araya et al., 2006).

The M_1 and M_4 mAChR are most well studied for their roles in the cognition-enhancing effects of ACh signaling. The reduction of M_1 mAChR has been associated with severity of dementia in subjects with

AD (Potter et al., 2011; Tsang et al., 2006). Further, M_1 antagonists have been shown to impair cognitive function (Zhao et al., 2018), while, agonism of M_1/M_4 receptors can enhance cognitive functioning in rodent models (Galloway, Lebois, Shagarabi, Hernandez, & Manns, 2014); an effect that seems to translate to the clinic as the M_1/M_4 receptor agonist, Xanomeline, improves cognitive function and behavioral symptoms in AD patients and individuals with schizophrenia. Within the striatum M_1 receptor stimulation heightens the excitability of D_1 MSNs, increasing striatal responsiveness to glutamatergic corticostriatal input and facilitates inhibition of behavior (Ding, Guzman, Peterson, Goldberg, & Surmeier, 2010; Goldberg, Ding, & Surmeier, 2012; Shen et al., 2007). Drug addiction is often associated with behavioral inflexibility that is thought to contribute to addictive behaviors by reducing an addicts' ability to control their behavior toward the drug (Furlong & Corbit, 2018; Verdejo-Garcia et al., 2015). Several selective orthosteric agonists and antagonist have also shown M_1 stimulation enhances behavioral flexibility (Brandeis et al., 1995; Ragozzino et al., 2012). M1 receptors in the striatum (McCool, Patel, Talati, & Ragozzino, 2008), prefrontal cortex (Shirey et al., 2009) and hippocampus (Xiong et al., 2019) have been implicated in mediating flexible shifting in rodent models, the latter via phosphorylation of GluA2 subunits. Recently, novel M_1 and M_4 mAChR allosteric compounds have been used to begin dissecting the relative contributions of the M_1 vs the M_4 receptors in these cognitive domains.

8.2 Recent evidence from allosteric compounds

Using subtype selective mAChR allosteric compounds, scientists are beginning to unravel the subtype contributions to cognitive function (Table 2). Xanomeline, has shown great promise in reducing cognitive deficits in an early proof of concept trial in patients with schizophrenia (Shekhar et al., 2008) and patients with AD (Bodick et al., 1997). However, the dose-limiting off-target gastrointestinal side effects, attributed to peripheral M_2 and M_3 activation prevented clinical development (McArthur, Gray, & Schreiber, 2010). The development of selective allosteric modulators/agonists of the M_1, M_4 mAChRs have allowed preclinical examination of specific M_1 and M_4 effects in learning and memory, including drug associated behaviors.

The M_1 allosteric agonists VU0357017 and VU0364572 robustly improved hippocampal-dependent learning in rats in a novel object recognition test, the Morris water maze and contextual fear conditioning

Table 2 The role of mAChR allosteric compounds in memory and extinction.

Target	Compound	Ligand type	Behavior	Outcome	Reference
M_1	VU0357017	Allosteric agonist	Morris water maze	No effect	Digby et al. (2012)
	VU0357017	Allosteric agonist	Contextual fear conditioning	Increased acquisition	Digby et al. (2012)
	VU0357017	Allosteric agonist	Cocaine self-administration—extinction	No effect	Stoll, Hart, Lindsley, and Thomsen (2018)
	VU0364572	Allosteric agonist	Contextual fear conditioning	Increased acquisition	Digby et al. (2012)
	VU0364572	Allosteric agonist	Morris water maze	Increased memory retention	Digby et al. (2012)
	VU0364572	Allosteric agonist	Novel object recognition test	Increased memory[a]	Galloway et al. (2014)
	BQCA	PAM	Novel object recognition test	Increased memory[a]	Galloway et al. (2014)
	VU0453595	PAM	Stress enhanced fear learning	Enhanced extinction	Maksymetz et al. (2019)
	VU0453595	PAM	Novel object recognition test	Increased memory	Moran et al. (2018)
	VU0486846	PAM	Novel object recognition test	Increased memory	Rook et al. (2018)
	VU6004256	PAM	Novel object recognition test	Increased memory	Rook et al. (2017)

Continued

Table 2 The role of mAChR allosteric compounds in memory and extinction.—cont'd

Target	Compound	Ligand type	Behavior	Outcome	Reference
	MK-7622	Ago-PAM	Novel object recognition test	No effect	Moran et al. (2018)
	PF-06764427	Ago-PAM	Novel object recognition test	No effect	Rook et al. (2017)
	VU0255035	Allosteric antagonist	Contextual fear extinction	Impaired extinction	Maksymetz et al. (2019)
	VU0255035	Allosteric antagonist	Auditory fear extinction	No effect	Maksymetz et al. (2019)
M_4	VU0467154	PAM	Pairwise discrimination task	Increased acquisition and memory consolidation	Gould et al. (2018)
	VU0467154	PAM	Conditioned place preference	Enhanced CPP extinction	Dall et al. (2017)
	VU0152100	PAM	Novel object recognition test	Increased memory[a]	Galloway et al. (2014)
	VU0152100	PAM	Cocaine self-administration—extinction	No effect	Stoll et al. (2018)
Combination	VU0152100 +	PAM	Cocaine self-administration—extinction	Enhanced drug extinction	Stoll et al. (2018)
	VU0357017	Allosteric agonist			

[a]Only in rats with baseline impairments.

paradigms (Digby et al., 2012; Galloway et al., 2014; Lebois, Trimper, Hu, Levey, & Manns, 2016). In line with this, the M_1 PAM (BQCA) has also been shown to increase memory performance in a novel object recognition test, similar to VU0364572 (Galloway et al., 2014). Interestingly the effects on object recognition were only observed in rats with low baseline, with some potential detrimental effects observed in rats with higher basal memory function (Galloway et al., 2014). Administration of the M_1 allosteric antagonist VU0255035 also revealed a role for M_1 mAChRs in contextual fear extinction, with mice displaying significantly higher freezing to the context on recall day, compared with vehicle-treated controls (Maksymetz et al., 2019). Interestingly, VU0255035 did not alter auditory-cued fear extinction. Electrophysiological recordings suggest inputs to the PFC from the ventral hippocampus and BLA, but not thalamus or mediodorsal nucleus, may underpin these behaviors (Maksymetz et al., 2019). Examination of ago-PAMs, which exert both endogenous agonist and PAM activity, have shown M1 PAMs that lack agonist activity have less side effects and greater cognitive enhancing activities (Moran et al., 2018; Rook et al., 2017, 2018). While the PAMs VU045395, VU0486848 and VU6004256 increased memory in the novel object recognition task, ago-PAMs MK-7622 and PF-06764427 had no effect in the same task, but showed greater side effect profiles (Moran et al., 2018; Rook et al., 2017, 2018).

Allosteric modulation of the M_4 receptor using the selective PAM VU0467154, dose dependently accelerated rates of learning and acquisition in a pairwise discrimination task when administered daily, for 10 days, prior to the behavioral task (Gould et al., 2018). These effects were absent in M_4 mAChR KO mice and persisted when VU0467154 was administered directly after the pairwise discrimination task, suggesting the cognitive enhancing effects of M_4 mAChR PAMs may be mediated in part through mechanisms of memory consolidation versus encoding or acquisition (Gould et al., 2018). Further, VU0467154 administered 30 min prior to cocaine conditioned place preference (CPP) extinction sessions facilitated extinction at a greater rate (Dall et al., 2017), however the timing of treatment was not examined in this study. Another M_4 PAM, VU0152100 has also been shown to improve the memory performance of rats, but only ones which had poorer performance at baseline (Galloway et al., 2014). When tested in an extinction model of cocaine self-administration in mice, VU0152100 in combination with a selective M_1 agonist VU0357017, increased the rate of extinction by more than 50%. Interestingly, VU0357017 or VU0152100 administered alone did not alter the rate of extinction. However, administration of the M_1/M_4 agonist xanomeline-treated mice extinguished in a similar manner, suggesting a synergistic role for M_1 and M_4 mAChRs in extinction facilitation (Stoll et al., 2018). In contrast to the effects of VU0467154 enhancing memory consolidation (Gould et al., 2018), the timing in which xanomeline was administered did not alter extinction facilitation, suggesting this is not due to consolidation (Stoll et al., 2018). Further examination of M_1 and M_4 allosteric compounds is warranted to understand the potential synergistic effects in facilitation of drug extinction.

9. Reinstatement of drug seeking

9.1 Evidence from KO studies and nonselective compounds

Relapse to drug taking after a period of abstinence is a major hurdle in the treatment of addiction, with up to 90% of addicts relapsing, the majority within the first 3 months of abstinence (Sinha, 2001). In rodents, relapse can be modeled using conditioned place preference and operant extinction-reinstatement models (see animal models section above).

These paradigms have implicated M_1/M_4 mAChRs in cocaine induced reinstatement using the nonselective agonist, xanomeline (Stoll et al., 2018), while M_5 KO mice show a decreased reinstatement to a cocaine CPP (Wang, 2017). Further, opposing effects of M_4 KO have been observed, based on their cellular localization. Mice lacking M_4 mAChRs globally in D_1 receptor neurons displayed greater cocaine seeking and drug-primed reinstatement than their littermate controls in a CPP paradigm (Klawonn et al., 2018). This coincided with greater impulsivity in the 5-choice-serial-reaction-time-task (5CSRTT). In contrast, mice lacking M_4 mAChRs globally on cholinergic (Choline acetyltransferase, ChAT+) neurons showed dysfunction in their ability to acquire both natural reward and cocaine conditioning, suggesting impairments in learning (Klawonn et al., 2018). Together these results suggest subpopulations of M_4 receptors may drive diverging behaviors. While this study examined M_4 mAChR deletions on all cholinergic neurons, loci specific knockdowns would be useful to untangle this dichotomy. D1 MSNs and cholinergic interneurons (CINs) within the striatum may be of particular interest as the cholinergic system within the striatum has been linked to behavioral flexibility (Bell, Lindner, Langdon, Mullins, & Christakou, 2019) and modulation of the central dopaminergic "reward" system (Jeon et al., 2010). M_4 mAChRs on CINs act via negative feedback to regulate cholinergic neuron output, while M_4 mAChRs expressed postsynaptically on D_1 MSNs directly modulate their activity (Jeon et al., 2010) as well as indirectly modulating presynaptic dopamine release (Foster et al., 2016). Therefore, indirectly reducing D_1 MSN signaling via M_4 mAChR activation/enhancement may provide a nuanced mechanism to retune striatal function in relation to aberrant drug seeking behaviors.

9.2 Recent evidence from allosteric compounds

Similar to their effects in reducing drug self-administration, mAChR allosteric modulators are also involved in relapse to drug seeking (Table 3). The M_4 PAM VU0467154 reduced reinstatement of a CPP (Dall et al., 2017), while the M_5 NAM, ML375, reduced cue-induced reinstatement of alcohol (Berizzi et al., 2018) and opiate seeking (Gould et al., 2019). However, where these actions are mediated are unknown. As discussed above, M_5 receptors are expressed on dopaminergic projections from the SN to the ventral and dorsal striatum. M_5 signaling in the dorsolateral striatum modulates alcohol self-administration, but whether this mechanism is conserved in relapse behavior is unknown. M_5 receptors are also expressed on dopaminergic neurons in the VTA (Gould et al., 2019), where the nonselective muscarinic receptor antagonist, scopolamine, reduces cue-induced cocaine seeking (Nunes et al., 2019). Cholinergic innervations from the LDTg and PPTg synapse onto dopaminergic neurons within the VTA. In turn, these neurons primarily innervate the Acb, and local administration of nonselective cholinergic agonists and antagonists within the ventral midbrain reduce dopamine release within the Acb (Lester, Miller, & Blaha, 2010; Shin et al., 2015). The neurocircuitry underpinning M_5 mAChR

Table 3 The role of mAChR allosteric compounds in relapse to drug seeking.

Target	Compound	Ligand type	Drug	Behavior	Outcome	Reference
M_4	VU0467154	PAM	Cocaine	Conditioned place preference	Decreased	Dall et al. (2017)
M_5	ML375	NAM	Alcohol	Cue-induced reinstatement	Decreased	Berizzi et al. (2018)
	ML375	NAM	Oxycodone	Cue reactivity	Decreased	Gould et al. (2019)

modulation of dopamine release and subsequent relapse behaviors require further examination. Further, research has also implicated VTA mAChR signaling in stress and anxiety behaviors associated with drug withdrawal (Nunes et al., 2019; Small, Nunes, Hughley, & Addy, 2016), while the M_1 PAM, VU0453595, enhanced fear extinction in a rodent model of post-traumatic stress disorder (PTSD) (Maksymetz et al., 2019). This suggests mAChRs could also mediate stress-induced relapse to drug seeking, however, further experiments are required to examine this.

10. Conclusion

In summary, mAChRs are promising targets for several aspects of AUD and SUD treatment. M_1 PAMs/allosteric agonists may provide utility in extinction facilitation, but this may require combination with M_4 PAMs which needs further examination. The mechanism of cognitive enhancement via memory formation compared to consolidation or increased behavioral flexibility also requires elucidation. M_4 PAMs show promise in the treatment of drug consumption and maintenance, extinction facilitation and relapse to drug seeking. However, loci specific roles of the M_4 receptor and the mechanism/s in which it modulates drug consumption and seeking are required. VU0467154 is a desirable candidate for clinical development, however, this has been prevented as it was found to be 35 times less potent at human M_4 compared to rodent (Wood et al., 2017). Attempts to develop M_4 PAMs with desirable efficacy and potency at the human M_4 receptor are ongoing (Engers et al., 2019; Temple et al., 2019). However, to date, no candidates for potential clinical development have been identified (Engers et al., 2019; Temple et al., 2019). However, since allosteric modulators bind to less conserved regions on the receptor, there is further challenges in ensuring these selective compounds have the same efficacy across species. Several M_1 PAMs are currently in clinical trial for Alzheimer's disease (Table 4), which may allow for repurposing for the indication of AUD or SUD if proven safe and effective in improving cognition.

M_5 NAMs show great promise for the treatment of drug and alcohol use disorders, however, ML375 has been limited by solubility and long half-life preventing repeat dosing. In fact, the majority of our current understanding of all mAChR allosteric modulators are based on single dose studies. If these compounds are to be useful for clinical development, it is likely they would require chronic administration without inducing tolerance. The M_4 PAM,

Table 4 Muscarinic compounds in clinical development.

Target	Compound	Ligand type	Indication	Phase	Stage	Clinical trial ID
M_1	VU319	PAM	Alzheimer disease	Phase 1	Recruiting	NCT03220295
	MK-7622	PAM	Alzheimer disease	Phase 2	Terminated [a]	NCT01852110
	TAK-071	PAM	Mild cognitive impairment/mild Alzheimer disease	Phase 1	Completed	NCT02769065
	HTL0018318	Agonist	Alzheimer disease	Phase 1b	Completed	NCT03456349
	HTL0018318	Agonist	Dementia with Lewy bodies	Phase 2	Terminated [b]	NCT03592862
M_4	HTL0016878	Agonist	Alzheimer disease	Phase 1	Recruiting	NCT03244228
M_1/M_4	KarXT (xanomeline + trospium chloride)	Nonselective M_1/M_4 agonist + peripherally restricted muscarinic antagonist	Schizophrenia	Phase 2	Active, not recruiting	NCT03697252

[a]Terminated due to efficacy.
[b]Terminated due to safety concerns.

VU0467154, recently demonstrated no alterations in plasma or brain levels of VU0467154, or tolerance after 10 days of repeat dosing (Gould et al., 2018). With the development of the short acting M_5 NAM, VU6008667 (McGowan et al., 2017), repeat dosing and potential effects of M_5 NAMs on tolerance or receptor alterations can be conducted.

Preclinical evidence suggests the abilities of M_4 mAChR PAMs and M_5 mAChR NAMs to reduce drug consumption and seeking extends across drug class, with beneficial effects observed in alcohol, cocaine and opiate use. However, understanding the mechanisms by which M_1, M_4 and M_5 mAChRs exert their anti-addictive effects is of great importance. This may help us to understand whether combination treatments could act synergistically to provide even more benefit compared to targeting a single mAChR subtype. While allosteric modulators generally have the benefit of acting in a more nuanced manner to potentiate ACh signaling on an endogenously temporal-spatial scale, one pitfall of is the reliance on endogenous ACh tone for signaling (Kruse et al., 2013). This leaves allosteric modulators susceptible to changes over disease progression, whereby basal ACh tone may be altered. If ACh tone is decreased, PAMs may not be enough to compensate for the reduced ACh tone and restore ACh signaling and a selective agonist may be more appropriate. However, some allosteric modulators do exert endogenous agonist activity. Ago-PAMs can induce activation in the absence of orthosteric agonist in addition to increasing potency/and efficacy of orthosteric agonists (Foster & Conn, 2017). The difference in mechanism of action can impact both the side-effect profiles and therapeutic potential of these compounds (Alt et al., 2016). For example, the highly potent M1 ago-PAMs MK-7622 and PF-06764427 produce excessive M1 activation, which is thought to induce agonist activity in the PFC and ultimately impair cognitive function (Moran et al., 2018). Understanding these potential changes will be crucial for future development. Further, there is a lack of research conducted in female rodents. Several studies have suggested potential sex differences in cholinergic system (Hall et al., 2017; Kirry, Durigan, Twining, & Gilmartin, 2019). Therefore, the role of mAChRs in females requires exploration and validation.

While single nucleotide polymorphisms (SNPs) in the *CHRM1* and *CHRM2* gene are associated with nicotine addiction (Lou et al., 2006; Mobascher et al., 2010), there are limited studies examining the role of mAChRs in nicotine dependence. nAChRs have been extensively studied, leading to the identification of varenicline (Chantix®/Champix®), a smoking cessation drug that acts predominantly as a partial agonist at

$\alpha 4\beta 2$ nAChRs (Coe et al., 2005; Gonzales et al., 2006; Tonstad et al., 2006). However, adverse side effects limit the effectiveness of varenicline (Thomas, Martin, Knipe, Higgins, & Gunnell, 2015). Understanding the role of mAChRs in nicotine dependence warrants examination. There is evidence of synergistic actions of muscarinic and nicotinic receptor actions on memory and attention in human subjects (Ellis et al., 2006; Green et al., 2005). "Cocktail" treatments combining selective muscarinic and nicotinic compounds may allow for greater efficacy at lower doses with less adverse side effects, which may be useful in the treatment of nicotine and other drug/alcohol dependence. Future examination is required to understand these interactions.

Overall, there converging preclinical evidence to suggest allosteric modulation of mAChRs is a viable target for AUD and SUDs. Recent advances in the development of highly selective mAChR compounds have allowed detailed examination of mAChR subtypes at multiple stages of the addiction cycle. While these studies are overwhelmingly positive, our understanding of mAChR allosteric modulation in AUD and SUD is only just beginning. The potential of mAChR allosteric modulators as a treatment for other neuropsychiatric disorders including Alzheimer's and schizophrenia has aided in the development of mAChR compounds. In fact, several mAChR compounds are currently in clinical trial, or preclinical development, advancing toward a clinically viable treatment option. More research is required to understand the pharmacological properties underpinning the efficacy of allosteric mAChR compounds which will help to drive development of compounds which have the greatest chance of clinical success.

Acknowledgments

This research was supported by an NHMRC Project Grant to A.J.L. (1120576) of which A.J.L. is a Principal Research Fellow (1116930). We acknowledge the Victorian State Government Operational Infrastructure Program.

Conflict of interest statement

The authors have no conflicts of interest to declare.

References

Al Qatari, M., Khan, S., Harris, B., & Littleton, J. (2001). Acamprosate is neuroprotective against glutamate-induced excitotoxicity when enhanced by ethanol withdrawal in neocortical cultures of fetal rat brain. *Alcoholism: Clinical and Experimental Research*, *25*(9), 1276–1283.

Alt, A., Pendri, A., Bertekap, R. L., Li, G., Benitex, Y., Nophsker, M., et al. (2016). Evidence for classical cholinergic toxicity associated with selective activation of M1 muscarinic receptors. *Journal of Pharmacology and Experimental Therapeutics*, *356*(2), 293–304.

Anagnostaras, S. G., Murphy, G. G., Hamilton, S. E., Mitchell, S. L., Rahnama, N. P., Nathanson, N. M., et al. (2003). Selective cognitive dysfunction in acetylcholine M 1 muscarinic receptor mutant mice. *Nature Neuroscience*, *6*(1), 51.

Araya, R., Noguchi, T., Yuhki, M., Kitamura, N., Higuchi, M., Saido, T. C., et al. (2006). Loss of M5 muscarinic acetylcholine receptors leads to cerebrovascular and neuronal abnormalities and cognitive deficits in mice. *Neurobiology of Disease*, *24*(2), 334–344.

Arnold, J. M., & Roberts, D. C. (1997). A critique of fixed and progressive ratio schedules used to examine the neural substrates of drug reinforcement. *Pharmacology Biochemistry and Behavior*, *57*(3), 441–447.

Assous, M., & Tepper, J. M. (2019). Excitatory extrinsic afferents to striatal interneurons and interactions with striatal microcircuitry. *European Journal of Neuroscience*, *49*(5), 593–603.

Bainbridge, N. K., Koselke, L. R., Jeon, J., Bailey, K. R., Wess, J., Crawley, J. N., et al. (2008). Learning and memory impairments in a congenic C57BL/6 strain of mice that lacks the M2 muscarinic acetylcholine receptor subtype. *Behavioural Brain Research*, *190*(1), 50–58.

Bardo, M., & Bevins, R. A. (2000). Conditioned place preference: What does it add to our preclinical understanding of drug reward? *Psychopharmacology*, *153*(1), 31–43.

Bartko, S. J., Romberg, C., White, B., Wess, J., Bussey, T. J., & Saksida, L. M. (2011). Intact attentional processing but abnormal responding in M1 muscarinic receptor-deficient mice using an automated touchscreen method. *Neuropharmacology*, *61*(8), 1366–1378.

Basile, A. S., Fedorova, I., Zapata, A., Liu, X., Shippenberg, T., Duttaroy, A., et al. (2002). Deletion of the M5 muscarinic acetylcholine receptor attenuates morphine reinforcement and withdrawal but not morphine analgesia. *Proceedings of the National Academy of Sciences of the United States of America*, *99*(17), 11452–11457.

Bell, T., Lindner, M., Langdon, A., Mullins, P. G., & Christakou, A. (2019). Regional striatal cholinergic involvement in human behavioural flexibility. *Journal of Neuroscience*, *39*, 5740–5749.

Bendor, J., Lizardi-Ortiz, J. E., Westphalen, R. I., Brandstetter, M., Hemmings, H. C., Sulzer, D., et al. (2010). AGAP1/AP-3-dependent endocytic recycling of M5 muscarinic receptors promotes dopamine release. *The EMBO Journal*, *29*(16), 2813–2826.

Berizzi, A. E., Perry, C. J., Shackleford, D. M., Lindsley, C. W., Jones, C. K., Chen, N. A., et al. (2018). Muscarinic M 5 receptors modulate ethanol seeking in rats. *Neuropsychopharmacology*, *43*(7), 1510.

Bernard, V., Laribi, O., Levey, A. I., & Bloch, B. (1998). Subcellular redistribution of m2 muscarinic acetylcholine receptors in striatal interneurons in vivo after acute cholinergic stimulation. *Journal of Neuroscience*, *18*(23), 10207–10218.

Billard, W., Binch, H., Crosby, G., & McQuade, R. D. (1995). Identification of the primary muscarinic autoreceptor subtype in rat striatum as m2 through a correlation of in vivo microdialysis and in vitro receptor binding data. *Journal of Pharmacology and Experimental Therapeutics*, *273*(1), 273–279.

Birnbaum, H. G., White, A. G., Schiller, M., Waldman, T., Cleveland, J. M., & Roland, C. L. (2011). Societal costs of prescription opioid abuse, dependence, and misuse in the United States. *Pain Medicine*, *12*(4), 657–667.

Bodick, N. C., Offen, W. W., Levey, A. I., Cutler, N. R., Gauthier, S. G., Satlin, A., et al. (1997). Effects of xanomeline, a selective muscarinic receptor agonist, on cognitive function and behavioral symptoms in Alzheimer disease. *Archives of Neurology*, *54*(4), 465–473.

Bosboom, J., Stoffers, D., & Wolters, E. C. (2003). The role of acetylcholine and dopamine in dementia and psychosis in Parkinson's disease. In R. Horowski et al. (Eds.)*Advances in research on neurodegeneration* (pp. 185–195). Springer.

Brady, A. E., Jones, C. K., Bridges, T. M., Kennedy, J. P., Thompson, A. D., Heiman, J. U., et al. (2008). Centrally active allosteric potentiators of the M4 muscarinic acetylcholine receptor reverse amphetamine-induced hyperlocomotor activity in rats. *Journal of Pharmacology and Experimental Therapeutics*, *327*(3), 941–953.

Brandeis, R., Sapir, M., Hafif, N., Abraham, S., Oz, N., Stein, E., et al. (1995). AF150 (S): A new functionally selective M1 agonist improves cognitive performance in rats. *Pharmacology Biochemistry and Behavior*, *51*(4), 667–674.

Brown, R. M., Short, J. L., & Lawrence, A. J. (2010). Identification of brain nuclei implicated in cocaine-primed reinstatement of conditioned place preference: A behaviour dissociable from sensitization. *PLoS One*, *5*(12), e15889.

Bubser, M., Bridges, T. M., Dencker, D., Gould, R. W., Grannan, M., Noetzel, M. J., et al. (2014). Selective activation of M4 muscarinic acetylcholine receptors reverses MK-801-induced behavioral impairments and enhances associative learning in rodents. *ACS Chemical Neuroscience*, *5*(10), 920–942.

Bymaster, F. P., McKinzie, D. L., Felder, C. C., & Wess, J. (2003). Use of M 1–M 5 muscarinic receptor knockout mice as novel tools to delineate the physiological roles of the muscarinic cholinergic system. *Neurochemical Research*, *28*(3–4), 437–442.

Byun, N. E., Grannan, M., Bubser, M., Barry, R. L., Thompson, A., Rosanelli, J., et al. (2014). Antipsychotic drug-like effects of the selective M 4 muscarinic acetylcholine receptor positive allosteric modulator VU0152100. *Neuropsychopharmacology*, *39*(7), 1578.

Calabresi, P., Centonze, D., Gubellini, P., Pisani, A., & Bernardi, G. (1998). Endogenous ACh enhances striatal NMDA-responses via M1-like muscarinic receptors and PKC activation. *European Journal of Neuroscience*, *10*(9), 2887–2895.

Campbell, E. J., Flanagan, J. P., Walker, L. C., Hill, M. K., Marchant, N. J., & Lawrence, A. J. (2019). Anterior insular cortex is critical for the propensity to relapse following punishment-imposed abstinence of alcohol seeking. *Journal of Neuroscience*, *39*(6), 1077–1087.

Carr, D. B., & Surmeier, D. J. (2007). M1 muscarinic receptor modulation of Kir2 channels enhances temporal summation of excitatory synaptic potentials in prefrontal cortex pyramidal neurons. *Journal of Neurophysiology*, *97*(5), 3432–3438.

Carrigan, K. A., & Dykstra, L. A. (2007). Behavioral effects of morphine and cocaine in M1 muscarinic acetylcholine receptor-deficient mice. *Psychopharmacology*, *191*(4), 985–993.

CDC. (2016). *Centers for Disease Control Prevention, excessive drinking is draining the US economy*. CDC.

Cea-del Rio, C. A., Lawrence, J. J., Tricoire, L., Erdelyi, F., Szabo, G., & McBain, C. J. (2010). M3 muscarinic acetylcholine receptor expression confers differential cholinergic modulation to neurochemically distinct hippocampal basket cell subtypes. *Journal of Neuroscience*, *30*(17), 6011–6024.

Coe, J. W., Brooks, P. R., Vetelino, M. G., Wirtz, M. C., Arnold, E. P., Huang, J., et al. (2005). Varenicline: An $\alpha 4\beta 2$ nicotinic receptor partial agonist for smoking cessation. *Journal of Medicinal Chemistry*, *48*(10), 3474–3477.

Coleman, C., Lydic, R., & Baghdoyan, H. (2004). M2 muscarinic receptors in pontine reticular formation of C57BL/6J mouse contribute to rapid eye movement sleep generation. *Neuroscience*, *126*(4), 821–830.

Corbit, L. H., Nie, H., & Janak, P. H. (2012). Habitual alcohol seeking: Time course and the contribution of subregions of the dorsal striatum. *Biological Psychiatry*, *72*(5), 389–395.

Cragg, S. J., Exley, R., & Clements, M. A. (2005). Striatal acetylcholine control of reward-related dopamine signalling. In J. P. Bolam, C. A. Ingham, & P. J. Magill (Eds.), *The basal ganglia VIII* (pp. 99–108). Springer.

Crombag, H. S., Bossert, J. M., Koya, E., & Shaham, Y. (2008). Context-induced relapse to drug seeking: A review. *Philosophical Transactions of the Royal Society, B: Biological Sciences*, *363*(1507), 3233–3243.

Dall, C., Weikop, P., Dencker, D., Molander, A. C., Wörtwein, G., Conn, P. J., et al. (2017). Muscarinic receptor M4 positive allosteric modulators attenuate central effects of cocaine. *Drug and Alcohol Dependence*, *176*, 154–161.

Dautan, D., Hacioğlu Bay, H., Bolam, J. P., Gerdjikov, T. V., & Mena-Segovia, J. (2016). Extrinsic sources of cholinergic innervation of the striatal complex: A whole-brain mapping analysis. *Frontiers in Neuroanatomy*, *10*, 1.

Dautan, D., Huerta-Ocampo, I., Witten, I. B., Deisseroth, K., Bolam, J. P., Gerdjikov, T., et al. (2014). A major external source of cholinergic innervation of the striatum and nucleus accumbens originates in the brainstem. *Journal of Neuroscience*, *34*(13), 4509–4518.

Davis, J. W., Thomas, R. K., Jr., & Adams, H. (1971). Interactions of scopolamine and physostigmine with ECS and one trial learning. *Physiology & Behavior*, *6*(3), 219–222.

de la Cour, C., Sørensen, G., Wortwein, G., Weikop, P., Dencker, D., Fink-Jensen, A., et al. (2015). Enhanced self-administration of alcohol in muscarinic acetylcholine M4 receptor knockout mice. *European Journal of Pharmacology*, *746*, 1–5.

Dencker, D., Weikop, P., Sørensen, G., Woldbye, D. P., Wörtwein, G., Wess, J., et al. (2012). An allosteric enhancer of M 4 muscarinic acetylcholine receptor function inhibits behavioral and neurochemical effects of cocaine. *Psychopharmacology*, *224*(2), 277–287.

Dhonnchadha, B. Á. N., & Kantak, K. M. (2011). Cognitive enhancers for facilitating drug cue extinction: Insights from animal models. *Pharmacology Biochemistry and Behavior*, *99*(2), 229–244.

Di Chiara, G., & Imperato, A. (1988). Drugs abused by humans preferentially increase synaptic dopamine concentrations in the mesolimbic system of freely moving rats. *Proceedings of the National Academy of Sciences of the United States of America*, *85*(14), 5274–5278.

Digby, G. J., Noetzel, M. J., Bubser, M., Utley, T. J., Walker, A. G., Byun, N. E., et al. (2012). Novel allosteric agonists of M1 muscarinic acetylcholine receptors induce brain region-specific responses that correspond with behavioral effects in animal models. *Journal of Neuroscience*, *32*(25), 8532–8544.

Ding, J. B., Guzman, J. N., Peterson, J. D., Goldberg, J. A., & Surmeier, D. J. (2010). Thalamic gating of corticostriatal signaling by cholinergic interneurons. *Neuron*, *67*(2), 294–307.

Douglas, C. L., Baghdoyan, H. A., & Lydic, R. (2001). M2 muscarinic autoreceptors modulate acetylcholine release in prefrontal cortex of C57BL/6J mouse. *Journal of Pharmacology and Experimental Therapeutics*, *299*(3), 960–966.

Ellis, J. R., Ellis, K. A., Bartholomeusz, C. F., Harrison, B. J., Wesnes, K. A., Erskine, F. F., et al. (2006). Muscarinic and nicotinic receptors synergistically modulate working memory and attention in humans. *International Journal of Neuropsychopharmacology*, *9*(2), 175–189.

Engers, D. W., Melancon, B. J., Gregro, A. R., Bertron, J. L., Bollinger, S. R., Felts, A. S., et al. (2019). VU6005806/AZN-00016130, an advanced M4 positive allosteric modulator (PAM) profiled as a potential preclinical development candidate. *Bioorganic & Medicinal Chemistry Letters*, *29*(14), 1714–1718.

Fink-Jensen, A., Fedorova, I., Wörtwein, G., Woldbye, D. P., Rasmussen, T., Thomsen, M., et al. (2003). Role for M5 muscarinic acetylcholine receptors in cocaine addiction. *Journal of Neuroscience Research*, *74*(1), 91–96.

Foster, D. J., & Conn, P. J. (2017). Allosteric modulation of GPCRs: New insights and potential utility for treatment of schizophrenia and other CNS disorders. *Neuron*, *94*(3), 431–446.

Foster, D. J., Wilson, J. M., Remke, D. H., Mahmood, M. S., Uddin, M. J., Wess, J., et al. (2016). Antipsychotic-like effects of M4 positive allosteric modulators are mediated by CB2 receptor-dependent inhibition of dopamine release. *Neuron*, *91*(6), 1244–1252.

Furlong, T. M., & Corbit, L. H. (2018). Drug addiction: Augmented habit learning or failure of goal-directed control? In R. Morris, A. Bornstein, & A. Shenhav (Eds.), *Goal-directed decision making*, (pp. 367–386). Elsevier.

Galloway, C. R., Lebois, E. P., Shagarabi, S. L., Hernandez, N. A., & Manns, J. R. (2014). Effects of selective activation of M1 and M4 muscarinic receptors on object recognition memory performance in rats. *Pharmacology*, *93*(1–2), 57–64.

Gentry, P. R., Kokubo, M., Bridges, T. M., Kett, N. R., Harp, J. M., Cho, H. P., et al. (2013). Discovery of the first M5-selective and CNS penetrant negative allosteric modulator (NAM) of a muscarinic acetylcholine receptor:(S)-9b-(4-Chlorophenyl)-1-(3, 4-difluorobenzoyl)-2, 3-dihydro-1 H-imidazo [2, 1-a] isoindol-5 (9b H)-one (ML375). *Journal of Medicinal Chemistry*, *56*(22), 9351–9355.

Gerber, D. J., Sotnikova, T. D., Gainetdinov, R. R., Huang, S. Y., Caron, M. G., & Tonegawa, S. (2001). Hyperactivity, elevated dopaminergic transmission, and response to amphetamine in M1 muscarinic acetylcholine receptor-deficient mice. *Proceedings of the National Academy of Sciences of the United States of America*, *98*(26), 15312–15317.

Goldberg, J. A., Ding, J. B., & Surmeier, D. J. (2012). Muscarinic modulation of striatal function and circuitry. In A. Fryer, A. Christopoulos, & N. Nathanson (Eds.), *Muscarinic receptors* (pp. 223–241). Springer.

Gonzales, D., Rennard, S. I., Nides, M., Oncken, C., Azoulay, S., Billing, C. B., et al. (2006). Varenicline, an α4β2 nicotinic acetylcholine receptor partial agonist, vs sustained-release bupropion and placebo for smoking cessation: A randomized controlled trial. *JAMA*, *296*(1), 47–55.

Gould, R. W., Grannan, M. D., Gunter, B. W., Ball, J., Bubser, M., Bridges, T. M., et al. (2018). Cognitive enhancement and antipsychotic-like activity following repeated dosing with the selective M4 PAM VU0467154. *Neuropharmacology*, *128*, 492–502.

Gould, R. W., Gunter, B. W., Bubser, M., Matthews, R. T., Teal, L. B., Ragland, M. G., et al. (2019). Acute negative allosteric modulation of M5 muscarinic acetylcholine receptors inhibits oxycodone self-administration and cue-induced reactivity with no effect on antinociception. *ACS Chemical Neuroscience*, *10*(8), 3740–3750.

Grecksch, G., Ott, T., & Matthies, H. (1978). Influence of post-training intrahippocampally applied oxotremorine on the consolidation of a brightness discrimination. *Pharmacology Biochemistry and Behavior*, *8*(3), 215–218.

Green, A., Ellis, K. A., Ellis, J., Bartholomeusz, C. F., Ilic, S., Croft, R. J., et al. (2005). Muscarinic and nicotinic receptor modulation of object and spatial n-back working memory in humans. *Pharmacology Biochemistry and Behavior*, *81*(3), 575–584.

Gunter, B. W., Gould, R. W., Bubser, M., McGowan, K. M., Lindsley, C. W., & Jones, C. K. (2018). Selective inhibition of M5 muscarinic acetylcholine receptors attenuates cocaine self-administration in rats. *Addiction Biology*, *23*(5), 1106–1116.

Hall, B. J., Abreu-Villaça, Y., Cauley, M., Junaid, S., White, H., Kiany, A., et al. (2017). The ventral hippocampal muscarinic cholinergic system plays a key role in sexual dimorphisms of spatial working memory in rats. *Neuropharmacology*, *117*, 106–113.

Hersch, S. M., & Levey, A. I. (1995). Diverse pre-and post-synaptic expression of m1–m4 muscarinic receptor proteins in neurons and afferents in the rat neostriatum. *Life Sciences*, *56*(11 – 12), 931–938.

Ince, E., Ciliax, B. J., & Levey, A. I. (1997). Differential expression of D1 and D2 dopamine and m4 muscarinic acetylcholine receptor proteins in identified striatonigral neurons. *Synapse*, *27*(4), 357–366.

Ito, Y., Oyunzul, L., Seki, M., Fujino, T., Matsui, M., & Yamada, S. (2009). Quantitative analysis of the loss of muscarinic receptors in various peripheral tissues in M1–M5 receptor single knockout mice. *British Journal of Pharmacology*, *156*(7), 1147–1153.

Jaffard, R., Destrade, C., Durkin, T., & Ebel, A. (1979). Memory formation as related to genotypic or experimental variations of hippocampal cholinergic activity in mice. *Physiology & Behavior, 22*(6), 1093–1096.

Jeon, J., Dencker, D., Wörtwein, G., Woldbye, D. P., Cui, Y., Davis, A. A., et al. (2010). A subpopulation of neuronal M4 muscarinic acetylcholine receptors plays a critical role in modulating dopamine-dependent behaviors. *Journal of Neuroscience, 30*(6), 2396–2405.

Jeong, J. H., Woo, Y. J., Chua, S., Jr., & Jo, Y.-H. (2016). Single-cell gene expression analysis of cholinergic neurons in the arcuate nucleus of the hypothalamus. *PLoS One, 11*(9) e0162839.

Jupp, B., Krstew, E., Dezsi, G., & Lawrence, A. (2011). Discrete cue-conditioned alcohol-seeking after protracted abstinence: Pattern of neural activation and involvement of orexin1 receptors. *British Journal of Pharmacology, 162*(4), 880–889.

Kaplan, G. B., & Moore, K. A. (2011). The use of cognitive enhancers in animal models of fear extinction. *Pharmacology Biochemistry and Behavior, 99*(2), 217–228.

Kirry, A. J., Durigan, D. J., Twining, R. C., & Gilmartin, M. R. (2019). Estrous cycle stage gates sex differences in prefrontal muscarinic control of fear memory formation. *Neurobiology of Learning and Memory, 161*, 26–36.

Klawonn, A. M., Wilhelms, D. B., Lindström, S. H., Singh, A. K., Jaarola, M., Wess, J., et al. (2018). Muscarinic M4 receptors on cholinergic and dopamine D1 receptor-expressing neurons have opposing functionality for positive reinforcement and influence impulsivity. *Frontiers in Molecular Neuroscience, 11*, 139.

Kohlmeier, K. A., Ishibashi, M., Wess, J., Bickford, M. E., & Leonard, C. S. (2012). Knockouts reveal overlapping functions of M2 and M4 muscarinic receptors and evidence for a local glutamatergic circuit within the laterodorsal tegmental nucleus. *Journal of Neurophysiology, 108*(10), 2751–2766.

Koob, G. F., Bloom, F., & Kupfer, D. (1995). Animal models of drug addiction. In F. E. Bloom & D. J. Kupfer (Eds.), *Psychopharmacology: The fourth generation in progress* (pp. 759–772). Raven Press.

Koshimizu, H., Leiter, L. M., & Miyakawa, T. (2012). M 4 muscarinic receptor knockout mice display abnormal social behavior and decreased prepulse inhibition. *Molecular Brain, 5*(1), 10.

Kranzler, H. R., & Soyka, M. (2018). Diagnosis and pharmacotherapy of alcohol use disorder: A review. *JAMA, 320*(8), 815–824.

Kreitzer, A. C. (2009). Physiology and pharmacology of striatal neurons. *Annual Review of Neuroscience, 32*, 127–147.

Krosnowski, K., Ashby, S., Sathyanesan, A., Luo, W., Ogura, T., & Lin, W. (2012). Diverse populations of intrinsic cholinergic interneurons in the mouse olfactory bulb. *Neuroscience, 213*, 161–178.

Kruse, A. C., Ring, A. M., Manglik, A., Hu, J., Hu, K., Eitel, K., et al. (2013). Activation and allosteric modulation of a muscarinic acetylcholine receptor. *Nature, 504*(7478), 101.

Kuroiwa, M., Hamada, M., Hieda, E., Shuto, T., Sotogaku, N., Flajolet, M., et al. (2012). Muscarinic receptors acting at pre-and post-synaptic sites differentially regulate dopamine/DARPP-32 signaling in striatonigral and striatopallidal neurons. *Neuropharmacology, 63*(7), 1248–1257.

Langmead, C. J., & Christopoulos, A. (2014). Functional and structural perspectives on allosteric modulation of GPCRs. *Current Opinion in Cell Biology, 27*, 94–101.

Lebois, E., Thorn, C., Edgerton, J., Popiolek, M., & Xi, S. (2018). Muscarinic receptor subtype distribution in the central nervous system and relevance to aging and Alzheimer's disease. *Neuropharmacology, 136*, 362–373.

Lebois, E. P., Trimper, J. B., Hu, C., Levey, A. I., & Manns, J. R. (2016). Effects of selective M1 muscarinic receptor activation on hippocampal spatial representations and neuronal oscillations. *ACS Chemical Neuroscience*, 7(10), 1393–1405.

Lester, D. B., Miller, A. D., & Blaha, C. D. (2010). Muscarinic receptor blockade in the ventral tegmental area attenuates cocaine enhancement of laterodorsal tegmentum stimulation-evoked accumbens dopamine efflux in the mouse. *Synapse*, *64*(3), 216–223.

Levey, A. I. (1993). Immunological localization of m1–m5 muscarinic acetylcholine receptors in peripheral tissues and brain. *Life Sciences*, *52*(5–6), 441–448.

Levey, A., Edmunds, S., Heilman, C., Desmond, T. J., & Frey, K. A. (1994). Localization of muscarinic m3 receptor protein and M3 receptor binding in rat brain. *Neuroscience*, *63*(1), 207–221.

Levey, A., Edmunds, S., Koliatsos, V., Wiley, R., & Heilman, C. (1995). Expression of m1-m4 muscarinic acetylcholine receptor proteins in rat hippocampus and regulation by cholinergic innervation. *Journal of Neuroscience*, *15*(5), 4077–4092.

Levey, A. I., Kitt, C., Simonds, W., Price, D., & Brann, M. (1991). Identification and localization of muscarinic acetylcholine receptor proteins in brain with subtype-specific antibodies. *Journal of Neuroscience*, *11*(10), 3218–3226.

Lipton, J. W., Olsen, R. W., & Ellison, G. D. (1995). Length of continuous cocaine exposure determines the persistence of muscarinic and benzodiazepine receptor alterations. *Brain Research*, *676*(2), 378–385.

López, A. J., Jia, Y., White, A. O., Kwapis, J. L., Espinoza, M., Hwang, P., et al. (2019). Medial habenula cholinergic signaling regulates cocaine-associated relapse-like behavior. *Addiction Biology*, *24*(3), 403–413.

Lou, X.-Y., Ma, J. Z., Payne, T. J., Beuten, J., Crew, K. M., & Li, M. D. (2006). Gene-based analysis suggests association of the nicotinic acetylcholine receptor β1 subunit (CHRNB1) and M1 muscarinic acetylcholine receptor (CHRM1) with vulnerability for nicotine dependence. *Human Genetics*, *120*(3), 381–389.

Lv, X., Dickerson, J. W., Rook, J. M., Lindsley, C. W., Conn, P. J., & Xiang, Z. (2017). M1 muscarinic activation induces long-lasting increase in intrinsic excitability of striatal projection neurons. *Neuropharmacology*, *118*, 209–222.

Lyon, J. (2017). More treatments on deck for alcohol use disorder. *JAMA*, *317*(22), 2267–2269.

Maksymetz, J., Joffe, M. E., Moran, S. P., Stansley, B. J., Li, B., Temple, K., et al. (2019). M1 muscarinic receptors modulate fear-related inputs to the prefrontal cortex: Implications for novel treatments of posttraumatic stress disorder. *Biological Psychiatry*, *85*(12), 989–1000.

Mandelbaum, G., Taranda, J., Haynes, T. M., Hochbaum, D. R., Huang, K. W., Hyun, M., et al. (2019). Distinct cortical-thalamic-striatal circuits through the parafascicular nucleus. *Neuron*, *102*(3), 636–652. e637.

Mannan Baig, A., Khan, N. A., Effendi, V., Rana, Z., Ahmad, H., & Abbas, F. (2017). Differential receptor dependencies: Expression and significance of muscarinic M1 receptors in the biology of prostate cancer. *Anti-Cancer Drugs*, *28*(1), 75–87.

Matsui, M., Motomura, D., Karasawa, H., Fujikawa, T., Jiang, J., Komiya, Y., et al. (2000). Multiple functional defects in peripheral autonomic organs in mice lacking muscarinic acetylcholine receptor gene for the M3 subtype. *Proceedings of the National Academy of Sciences of the United States of America*, *97*(17), 9579–9584.

Maxwell, J. C., & McCance-Katz, E. F. (2010). Indicators of buprenorphine and methadone use and abuse: What do we know? *The American Journal on Addictions*, *19*(1), 73–88.

Mayer-Blackwell, B., Schlussman, S., Butelman, E., Ho, A., Ott, J., Kreek, M., et al. (2014). Self administration of oxycodone by adolescent and adult mice affects striatal neurotransmitter receptor gene expression. *Neuroscience*, *258*, 280–291.

McArthur, R. A., Gray, J., & Schreiber, R. (2010). Cognitive effects of muscarinic M1 functional agonists in non-human primates and clinical trials. *Current Opinion in Investigational Drugs*, *11*(7), 740–760.

McCool, M. F., Patel, S., Talati, R., & Ragozzino, M. E. (2008). Differential involvement of M1-type and M4-type muscarinic cholinergic receptors in the dorsomedial striatum in task switching. *Neurobiology of Learning and Memory*, *89*(2), 114–124.

McDonald, A. J., & Mascagni, F. (2011). Neuronal localization of M2 muscarinic receptor immunoreactivity in the rat amygdala. *Neuroscience*, *196*, 49–65.

McGowan, K. M., Nance, K. D., Cho, H. P., Bridges, T. M., Conn, P. J., Jones, C. K., et al. (2017). Continued optimization of the M5 NAM ML375: Discovery of VU6008667, an M5 NAM with high CNS penetration and a desired short half-life in rat for addiction studies. *Bioorganic & Medicinal Chemistry Letters*, *27*(6), 1356–1359.

Mesulam, M., Guillozet, A., Shaw, P., & Quinn, B. (2002). Widely spread butyrylcholinesterase can hydrolyze acetylcholine in the normal and Alzheimer brain. *Neurobiology of Disease*, *9*(1), 88–93.

Mesulam, M. M., Mufson, E. J., Levey, A. I., & Wainer, B. H. (1983). Cholinergic innervation of cortex by the basal forebrain: Cytochemistry and cortical connections of the septal area, diagonal band nuclei, nucleus basalis (substantia innominata), and hypothalamus in the rhesus monkey. *Journal of Comparative Neurology*, *214*(2), 170–197.

Mesulam, M., Mufson, E., Wainer, B., & Levey, A. (1983). Central cholinergic pathways in the rat: An overview based on an alternative nomenclature (Ch1–Ch6). *Neuroscience*, *10*(4), 1185–1201.

Mobascher, A., Rujescu, D., Mittelstrass, K., Giegling, I., Lamina, C., Nitz, B., et al. (2010). Association of a variant in the muscarinic acetylcholine receptor 2 gene (CHRM2) with nicotine addiction. *American Journal of Medical Genetics Part B: Neuropsychiatric Genetics*, *153*(2), 684–690.

Moran, S. P., Dickerson, J. W., Cho, H. P., Xiang, Z., Maksymetz, J., Remke, D. H., et al. (2018). M1-positive allosteric modulators lacking agonist activity provide the optimal profile for enhancing cognition. *Neuropsychopharmacology*, *43*(8), 1763.

Mufson, E. J., Counts, S. E., Perez, S. E., & Ginsberg, S. D. (2008). Cholinergic system during the progression of Alzheimer's disease: Therapeutic implications. *Expert Review of Neurotherapeutics*, *8*(11), 1703–1718.

Mufson, E., Martin, T., Mash, D. C., Wainer, B., & Mesulam, M.-M. (1986). Cholinergic projections from the parabigeminal nucleus (Ch8) to the superior colliculus in the mouse: A combined analysis of horseradish peroxidase transport and choline acetyltransferase immunohistochemistry. *Brain Research*, *370*(1), 144–148.

Muller, P., Britton, R. S., & Seeman, P. (1980). The effects of long-term ethanol on brain receptors for dopamine, acetylcholine, serotonin and noradrenaline. *European Journal of Pharmacology*, *65*(1), 31–37.

Muller, J. F., Mascagni, F., Zaric, V., & McDonald, A. J. (2013). Muscarinic cholinergic receptor M1 in the rat basolateral amygdala: Ultrastructural localization and synaptic relationships to cholinergic axons. *Journal of Comparative Neurology*, *521*(8), 1743–1759.

Myers, K. M., & Davis, M. (2002). Behavioral and neural analysis of extinction. *Neuron*, *36*(4), 567–584.

Navarria, A., Wohleb, E. S., Voleti, B., Ota, K. T., Dutheil, S., Lepack, A. E., et al. (2015). Rapid antidepressant actions of scopolamine: Role of medial prefrontal cortex and M1-subtype muscarinic acetylcholine receptors. *Neurobiology of Disease*, *82*, 254–261.

NDIC. (2011). *National Drug Intelligence Center, The economic impact of illicit drug use on American society*. Washington, DC: United States Department of Justice.

Niciu, M. J., & Arias, A. J. (2013). Targeted opioid receptor antagonists in the treatment of alcohol use disorders. *CNS Drugs*, *27*(10), 777–787.

NIDA. (2019). *National Institute on drug abuse, Overdose death rates*. (Updated Jan 2019) Retrieved from https://www.drugabuse.gov/related-topics/trends-statistics/overdose-death-rates.

Nunes, E. J., Bitner, L., Hughley, S. M., Small, K. M., Walton, S. N., Rupprecht, L. E., et al. (2019). Cholinergic receptor blockade in the VTA attenuates cue-induced cocaine-seeking and reverses the anxiogenic effects of forced abstinence. *Neuroscience*, *413*, 252–263.

Nutt, D. J., Lingford-Hughes, A., Erritzoe, D., & Stokes, P. R. (2015). The dopamine theory of addiction: 40 years of highs and lows. *Nature Reviews. Neuroscience*, *16*(5), 305–312.

Offermanns, S., Wieland, T., Homann, D., Sandmann, J., Bombien, E., Spicher, K., et al. (1994). Transfected muscarinic acetylcholine receptors selectively couple to Gi-type G proteins and Gq/11. *Molecular Pharmacology*, *45*(5), 890–898.

Pancani, T., Bolarinwa, C., Smith, Y., Lindsley, C. W., Conn, P. J., & Xiang, Z. (2014). M4 mAChR-mediated modulation of glutamatergic transmission at corticostriatal synapses. *ACS Chemical Neuroscience*, *5*(4), 318–324.

Pepeu, G., & Giovannini, M. G. (2004). Changes in acetylcholine extracellular levels during cognitive processes. *Learning & Memory*, *11*(1), 21–27.

Peralta, E. G., Ashkenazi, A., Winslow, J. W., Ramachandran, J., & Capon, D. J. (1988). Differential regulation of PI hydrolysis and adenylyl cyclase by muscarinic receptor subtypes. *Nature*, *334*(6181), 434.

Peralta, E., Winslow, J., Ashkenazi, A., Smith, D., Ramachandran, J., & Capon, D. (1988). Structural basis of muscarinic acetylcholine receptor subtype diversity. *Trends in Pharmacological Sciences*, *6*(Suppl. 6–11).

Perry, C., & Lawrence, A. (2017). Addiction, cognitive decline and therapy: Seeking ways to escape a vicious cycle. *Genes, Brain and Behavior*, *16*(1), 205–218.

Phelps, P. E., Houser, C. R., & Vaughn, J. E. (1985). Immunocytochemical localization of choline acetyltransferase within the rat neostriatum: A correlated light and electron microscopic study of cholinergic neurons and synapses. *Journal of Comparative Neurology*, *238*(3), 286–307.

Potter, P. E., Rauschkolb, P. K., Pandya, Y., Sue, L. I., Sabbagh, M. N., Walker, D. G., et al. (2011). Pre-and post-synaptic cortical cholinergic deficits are proportional to amyloid plaque presence and density at preclinical stages of Alzheimer's disease. *Acta Neuropathologica*, *122*(1), 49–60.

Poulin, B., Butcher, A., McWilliams, P., Bourgognon, J.-M., Pawlak, R., Kong, K. C., et al. (2010). The M3-muscarinic receptor regulates learning and memory in a receptor phosphorylation/arrestin-dependent manner. *Proceedings of the National Academy of Sciences of the United States of America*, *107*(20), 9440–9445.

Rabin, R., Wolfe, B., Dibner, M., Zahniser, N., Melchior, C., & Molinoff, P. (1980). Effects of ethanol administration and withdrawal on neurotransmitter receptor systems in C57 mice. *Journal of Pharmacology and Experimental Therapeutics*, *213*(3), 491–496.

Raedler, T. J., Knable, M. B., Jones, D. W., Urbina, R. A., Gorey, J. G., Lee, K. S., et al. (2003). In vivo determination of muscarinic acetylcholine receptor availability in schizophrenia. *American Journal of Psychiatry*, *160*(1), 118–127.

Ragozzino, M. E., Artis, S., Singh, A., Twose, T. M., Beck, J. E., & Messer, W. S. (2012). The selective M1 muscarinic cholinergic agonist CDD-0102A enhances working memory and cognitive flexibility. *Journal of Pharmacology and Experimental Therapeutics*, *340*(3), 588–594.

Rasmussen, K., White, D. A., & Acri, J. B. (2019). NIDA's medication development priorities in response to the opioid crisis: Ten most wanted. *Neuropsychopharmacology*, *44*(4), 657.

Rice, M. E., & Cragg, S. J. (2004). Nicotine amplifies reward-related dopamine signals in striatum. *Nature Neuroscience*, 7(6), 583.

Robbins, T., Semple, J., Kumar, R., Truman, M., Shorter, J., Ferraro, A., et al. (1997). Effects of scopolamine on delayed-matching-to-sample and paired associates tests of visual memory and learning in human subjects: Comparison with diazepam and implications for dementia. *Psychopharmacology*, *134*(1), 95–106.

Rook, J. M., Abe, M., Cho, H. P., Nance, K. D., Luscombe, V. B., Adams, J. J., et al. (2017). Diverse effects on M1 signaling and adverse effect liability within a series of M1 ago-PAMs. *ACS Chemical Neuroscience*, *8*(4), 866–883.

Rook, J. M., Bertron, J. L., Cho, H. P., Garcia-Barrantes, P. M., Moran, S. P., Maksymetz, J. T., et al. (2018). A novel M1 PAM VU0486846 exerts efficacy in cognition models without displaying agonist activity or cholinergic toxicity. *ACS Chemical Neuroscience*, *9*(9), 2274–2285.

Rouse, S., Gilmor, M., & Levey, A. (1998). Differential presynaptic and postsynaptic expression of m1–m4 muscarinic acetylcholine receptors at the perforant pathway/granule cell synapse. *Neuroscience*, *86*(1), 221–232.

Rouse, S. T., & Levey, A. L. (1996). Expression of m1-m4 muscarinic acetylcholine receptor immunoreactivity in septohippocampal neurons and other identified hippocampal afferents. *Journal of Comparative Neurology*, *375*(3), 406–416.

Rouse, S. T., Thomas, T. M., & Levey, A. I. (1997). Muscarinic acetylcholine receptor subtype, m2: Diverse functional implications of differential synaptic localization. *Life Sciences*, *60*(13–14), 1031–1038.

SAMHSA. (2014). *Substance Abuse and Mental Health Services Administration, National Survey on Drug Use and Health*. SAMHSA.

Sarter, M., Nelson, C. L., & Bruno, J. P. (2005). Cortical cholinergic transmission and cortical information processing in schizophrenia. *Schizophrenia Bulletin*, *31*(1), 117–138.

Schmidt, L. S., Thomsen, M., Weikop, P., Dencker, D., Wess, J., Woldbye, D. P., et al. (2011). Increased cocaine self-administration in M 4 muscarinic acetylcholine receptor knockout mice. *Psychopharmacology*, *216*(3), 367–378.

Schuckit, M. A. (2016). Treatment of opioid-use disorders. *New England Journal of Medicine*, *375*(4), 357–368.

See, R., McLaughlin, J., & Fuchs, R. (2003). Muscarinic receptor antagonism in the basolateral amygdala blocks acquisition of cocaine-stimulus association in a model of relapse to cocaine-seeking behavior in rats. *Neuroscience*, *117*(2), 477–483.

Seeger, T., Fedorova, I., Zheng, F., Miyakawa, T., Koustova, E., Gomeza, J., et al. (2004). M2 muscarinic acetylcholine receptor knock-out mice show deficits in behavioral flexibility, working memory, and hippocampal plasticity. *Journal of Neuroscience*, *24*(45), 10117–10127.

Shaham, Y., Erb, S., & Stewart, J. (2000). Stress-induced relapse to heroin and cocaine seeking in rats: A review. *Brain Research Reviews*, *33*(1), 13–33.

Shaham, Y., Shalev, U., Lu, L., De Wit, H., & Stewart, J. (2003). The reinstatement model of drug relapse: History, methodology and major findings. *Psychopharmacology*, *168*(1–2), 3–20.

Shekhar, A., Potter, W. Z., Lightfoot, J., Lienemann, D., Pharm, J., Dubé, S., et al. (2008). Selective muscarinic receptor agonist xanomeline as a novel treatment approach for schizophrenia. *American Journal of Psychiatry*, *165*(8), 1033–1039.

Shen, W., Tian, X., Day, M., Ulrich, S., Tkatch, T., Nathanson, N. M., et al. (2007). Cholinergic modulation of Kir2 channels selectively elevates dendritic excitability in striatopallidal neurons. *Nature Neuroscience*, *10*(11), 1458.

Shin, J. H., Adrover, M. F., Wess, J., & Alvarez, V. A. (2015). Muscarinic regulation of dopamine and glutamate transmission in the nucleus accumbens. *Proceedings of the National Academy of Sciences of the United States of America*, *112*(26), 8124–8129.

Shinoe, T., Matsui, M., Taketo, M. M., & Manabe, T. (2005). Modulation of synaptic plasticity by physiological activation of M1 muscarinic acetylcholine receptors in the mouse hippocampus. *Journal of Neuroscience*, *25*(48), 11194–11200.

Shirey, J. K., Brady, A. E., Jones, P. J., Davis, A. A., Bridges, T. M., Kennedy, J. P., et al. (2009). A selective allosteric potentiator of the M1 muscarinic acetylcholine receptor increases activity of medial prefrontal cortical neurons and restores impairments in reversal learning. *Journal of Neuroscience*, *29*(45), 14271–14286.
Sinha, R. (2001). How does stress increase risk of drug abuse and relapse? *Psychopharmacology*, *158*(4), 343–359.
Small, K. M., Nunes, E., Hughley, S., & Addy, N. A. (2016). Ventral tegmental area muscarinic receptors modulate depression and anxiety-related behaviors in rats. *Neuroscience Letters*, *616*, 80–85.
Spanagel, R., Vengeliene, V., Jandeleit, B., Fischer, W.-N., Grindstaff, K., Zhang, X., et al. (2014). Acamprosate produces its anti-relapse effects via calcium. *Neuropsychopharmacology*, *39*(4), 783.
Stafford, D., LeSage, M. G., & Glowa, J. R. (1998). Progressive-ratio schedules of drug delivery in the analysis of drug self-administration: A review. *Psychopharmacology*, *139*(3), 169–184.
Stahre, M., Roeber, J., Kanny, D., Brewer, R. D., & Zhang, X. (2014). Peer reviewed: Contribution of excessive alcohol consumption to deaths and years of potential life lost in the United States. *Preventing Chronic Disease*, *11*, E109.
Stoll, K., Hart, R., Lindsley, C. W., & Thomsen, M. (2018). Effects of muscarinic M 1 and M 4 acetylcholine receptor stimulation on extinction and reinstatement of cocaine seeking in male mice, independent of extinction learning. *Psychopharmacology*, *235*(3), 815–827.
Sugaya, K., Clamp, C., Bryan, D., & McKinney, M. (1997). mRNA for the m4 muscarinic receptor subtype is expressed in adult rat brain cholinergic neurons. *Molecular Brain Research*, *50*(1–2), 305–313.
Temple, K. J., Engers, J. L., Long, M. F., Gregro, A. R., Watson, K. J., Chang, S., et al. (2019). Discovery of a novel 3, 4-dimethylcinnoline carboxamide M4 positive allosteric modulator (PAM) chemotype via scaffold hopping. *Bioorganic & Medicinal Chemistry Letters*, *29*(21), 126678.
Thomas, K. H., Martin, R. M., Knipe, D. W., Higgins, J. P., & Gunnell, D. (2015). Risk of neuropsychiatric adverse events associated with varenicline: Systematic review and meta-analysis. *BMJ*, *350*, h1109.
Thomsen, M., Conn, P. J., Lindsley, C., Wess, J., Boon, J. Y., Fulton, B. S., et al. (2010). Attenuation of cocaine's reinforcing and discriminative stimulus effects via muscarinic M1 acetylcholine receptor stimulation. *Journal of Pharmacology and Experimental Therapeutics*, *332*(3), 959–969.
Thomsen, M., Fulton, B. S., & Caine, S. B. (2014). Acute and chronic effects of the M 1/M 4-preferring muscarinic agonist xanomeline on cocaine vs. food choice in rats. *Psychopharmacology*, *231*(3), 469–479.
Thomsen, M., Lindsley, C. W., Conn, P. J., Wessell, J. E., Fulton, B. S., Wess, J., et al. (2012). Contribution of both M 1 and M 4 receptors to muscarinic agonist-mediated attenuation of the cocaine discriminative stimulus in mice. *Psychopharmacology*, *220*(4), 673–685.
Thomsen, M., Woldbye, D. P., Wörtwein, G., Fink-Jensen, A., Wess, J., & Caine, S. B. (2005). Reduced cocaine self-administration in muscarinic M5 acetylcholine receptor-deficient mice. *Journal of Neuroscience*, *25*(36), 8141–8149.
Threlfell, S., Clements, M. A., Khodai, T., Pienaar, I. S., Exley, R., Wess, J., et al. (2010). Striatal muscarinic receptors promote activity dependence of dopamine transmission via distinct receptor subtypes on cholinergic interneurons in ventral versus dorsal striatum. *Journal of Neuroscience*, *30*(9), 3398–3408.
Tonstad, S., Tønnesen, P., Hajek, P., Williams, K. E., Billing, C. B., Reeves, K. R., et al. (2006). Effect of maintenance therapy with varenicline on smoking cessation: A randomized controlled trial. *JAMA*, *296*(1), 64–71.

Tsang, S. W., Lai, M. K., Kirvell, S., Francis, P. T., Esiri, M. M., Hope, T., et al. (2006). Impaired coupling of muscarinic M1 receptors to G-proteins in the neocortex is associated with severity of dementia in Alzheimer's disease. *Neurobiology of Aging*, *27*(9), 1216–1223.

Tzavara, E. T., Bymaster, F. P., Davis, R. J., Wade, M. R., Perry, K. W., Wess, J., et al. (2004). M4 muscarinic receptors regulate the dynamics of cholinergic and dopaminergic neurotransmission: Relevance to the pathophysiology and treatment of related CNS pathologies. *The FASEB Journal*, *18*(12), 1410–1412.

Tzavara, E., Bymaster, F., Felder, C., Wade, M., Gomeza, J., Wess, J., et al. (2003). Dysregulated hippocampal acetylcholine neurotransmission and impaired cognition in M2, M4 and M2/M4 muscarinic receptor knockout mice. *Molecular Psychiatry*, *8*(7), 673.

Vallari, R. C., & Pietruszko, R. (1982). Human aldehyde dehydrogenase: Mechanism of inhibition of disulfiram. *Science*, *216*(4546), 637–639.

Verdejo-Garcia, A., Clark, L., Verdejo-Roman, J., Albein-Urios, N., Martinez-Gonzalez, J. M., Gutierrez, B., et al. (2015). Neural substrates of cognitive flexibility in cocaine and gambling addictions. *The British Journal of Psychiatry*, *207*(2), 158–164.

Vilaró, M. T., Palacios, J., & Mengod, G. (1990). Localization of m5 muscarinic receptor mRNA in rat brain examined by in situ hybridization histochemistry. *Neuroscience Letters*, *114*(2), 154–159.

Vilaró, M. T., Palacios, J., & Mengod, G. (1994). Multiplicity of muscarinic autoreceptor subtypes? Comparison of the distribution of cholinergic cells and cells containing mRNA for five subtypes of muscarinic receptors in the rat brain. *Molecular Brain Research*, *21*(1–2), 30–46.

Vilaro, M., Wiederhold, K.-H., Palacios, J., & Mengod, G. (1992). Muscarinic M2 receptor mRNA expression and receptor binding in cholinergic and non-cholinergic cells in the rat brain: A correlative study using in situ hybridization histochemistry and receptor autoradiography. *Neuroscience*, *47*(2), 367–393.

Volpicelli, L. A., & Levey, A. I. (2004). Muscarinic acetylcholine receptor subtypes in cerebral cortex and hippocampus. *Progress in Brain Research*, *145*, 59–66.

von Engelhardt, J., Eliava, M., Meyer, A. H., Rozov, A., & Monyer, H. (2007). Functional characterization of intrinsic cholinergic interneurons in the cortex. *Journal of Neuroscience*, *27*(21), 5633–5642.

Wainer, B., Bolam, J., Freund, T., Henderson, Z., Totterdell, S., & Smith, A. (1984). Cholinergic synapses in the rat brain: A correlated light and electron microscopic immunohistochemical study employing a monoclonal antibody against choline acetyltransferase. *Brain Research*, *308*(1), 69–76.

Walker, L. C., Kastman, H. E., & Lawrence, A. J. (2019). Pattern of neural activation following yohimbine-induced reinstatement of alcohol seeking in rats. *European Journal of Neuroscience*. in press (PMID 31066114).

Walker, L. C., & Lawrence, A. J. (2018). Investigational drug therapies in phase I and phase II clinical trials for alcohol use disorders. *Expert Opinion on Investigational Drugs*, *27*(8), 677–690.

Wang, H. G. (2017). M5 muscarinic receptor gene deletion accelerates extinction, but inhibits reinstatement of morphine-conditioned reward in mice. *Journal of Addiction and Preventive Medicine*, *2*(01), 110.

Weiner, D. M., Levey, A. I., & Brann, M. R. (1990). Expression of muscarinic acetylcholine and dopamine receptor mRNAs in rat basal ganglia. *Proceedings of the National Academy of Sciences of the United States of America*, *87*(18), 7050–7054.

Williams, M. J., & Adinoff, B. (2008). The role of acetylcholine in cocaine addiction. *Neuropsychopharmacology*, *33*(8), 1779.

Wonnacott, S. (1997). Presynaptic nicotinic ACh receptors. *Trends in Neurosciences*, *20*(2), 92–98.

Wood, M. R., Noetzel, M. J., Poslusney, M. S., Melancon, B. J., Tarr, J. C., Lamsal, A., et al. (2017). Challenges in the development of an M4 PAM in vivo tool compound: The discovery of VU0467154 and unexpected DMPK profiles of close analogs. *Bioorganic & Medicinal Chemistry Letters*, *27*(2), 171–175.

Xiong, C.-H., Liu, M.-G., Zhao, L.-X., Chen, M.-W., Tang, L., Yan, Y.-H., et al. (2019). M1 muscarinic receptors facilitate hippocampus-dependent cognitive flexibility via modulating GluA2 subunit of AMPA receptors. *Neuropharmacology*, *146*, 242–251.

Yamada, M., Lamping, K. G., Duttaroy, A., Zhang, W., Cui, Y., Bymaster, F. P., et al. (2001). Cholinergic dilation of cerebral blood vessels is abolished in M5 muscarinic acetylcholine receptor knockout mice. *Proceedings of the National Academy of Sciences of the United States of America*, *98*(24), 14096–14101.

Yan, Z., Flores-Hernandez, J., & Surmeier, D. (2001). Coordinated expression of muscarinic receptor messenger RNAs in striatal medium spiny neurons. *Neuroscience*, *103*(4), 1017–1024.

Yi, F., Ball, J., Stoll, K. E., Satpute, V. C., Mitchell, S. M., Pauli, J. L., et al. (2014). Direct excitation of parvalbumin-positive interneurons by M1 muscarinic acetylcholine receptors: Roles in cellular excitability, inhibitory transmission and cognition. *The Journal of Physiology*, *592*(16), 3463–3494.

Zeigler, S., Lipton, J., Toga, A., & Ellison, G. (1991). Continuous cocaine administration produces persisting changes in brain neurochemistry and behavior. *Brain Research*, *552*(1), 27–35.

Zhang, Y., Liang, Y., Randesi, M., Yuferov, V., Zhao, C., & Kreek, M. J. (2018). Chronic oxycodone self-administration altered reward-related genes in the ventral and dorsal striatum of C57BL/6J mice: An RNA-seq analysis. *Neuroscience*, *393*, 333–349.

Zhang, Y., Mayer-Blackwell, B., Schlussman, S. D., Randesi, M., Butelman, E. R., Ho, A., et al. (2014). Extended access oxycodone self-administration and neurotransmitter receptor gene expression in the dorsal striatum of adult C57BL/6 J mice. *Psychopharmacology*, *231*(7), 1277–1287.

Zhang, H., & Sulzer, D. (2004). Frequency-dependent modulation of dopamine release by nicotine. *Nature Neuroscience*, 7(6), 581.

Zhang, W., Yamada, M., Gomeza, J., Basile, A. S., & Wess, J. (2002). Multiple muscarinic acetylcholine receptor subtypes modulate striatal dopamine release, as studied with M1–M5 muscarinic receptor knock-out mice. *Journal of Neuroscience*, *22*(15), 6347–6352.

Zhao, L.-X., Ge, Y.-H., Xiong, C.-H., Tang, L., Yan, Y.-H., Law, P.-Y., et al. (2018). M1 muscarinic receptor facilitates cognitive function by interplay with AMPA receptor GluA1 subunit. *The FASEB Journal*, *32*(8), 4247–4257.

CHAPTER TEN

M1 muscarinic acetylcholine receptors: A therapeutic strategy for symptomatic and disease-modifying effects in Alzheimer's disease?

Miriam Scarpa, Sarah Hesse, Sophie J. Bradley*
The Centre for Translational Pharmacology, Institute of Molecular, Cell and Systems Biology, College of Medical, Veterinary and Life Sciences, University of Glasgow, Glasgow, United Kingdom
*Corresponding author: e-mail address: sophie.bradley@glasgow.ac.uk

Contents

Abstract

The M1 muscarinic acetylcholine receptor (mAChR) plays a crucial role in learning and memory processes and has long been identified as a promising therapeutic target for the improvement of cognitive decline in Alzheimer's disease (AD). As such, clinical trials with xanomeline, a mAChR orthosteric agonist, showed an improvement in cognitive and behavioral symptoms associated with AD. Despite this, the clinical utility of xanomeline was hampered by a lack of M1 receptor selectivity and adverse cholinergic responses attributed to activation of peripheral M2 and M3 mAChRs. More recently, efforts have focused on developing more selective M1 compounds via targeting the less-conserved allosteric binding pockets. As such, positive allosteric modulators (PAMs) have emerged as an exciting strategy to achieve exquisite selectivity for the M1 mAChR in order to deliver improvements in cognitive function in AD. Furthermore, over recent years it

Advances in Pharmacology, Volume 88
ISSN 1054-3589
https://doi.org/10.1016/bs.apha.2019.12.003

has become increasingly apparent that M1 therapeutics may also offer disease-modifying effects in AD, due to the modulation of pathogenic amyloid processing. This article will review the progress made in the development of M1 selective ligands for the treatment of cognitive decline in AD, and will discuss the current evidence that selective targeting of the M1 mAChR could also have the potential to modify AD progression.

Non-standard abbreviations

ACh acetylcholine
AChE acetylcholine esterase
AD Alzheimer's disease
AHL amphetamine-induced hyper-locomotion
Aβ amyloid-β peptide
AICD amyloid precursor protein intranuclear domain
APP amyloid-beta protein precursor
APPsα secreted amyloid protein precursor alpha
BACE1 beta-secretase 1
BF basal forebrain
CVS cardiovascular system
CNS central nervous system
CAT choline acetyltransferase
DB diagonal band
DMTs disease-modifying treatments
GI gastrointestinal
GPCR G protein-coupled receptor
mAChR muscarinic acetylcholine receptor
MS medial septum
NAMs negative allosteric modulators
NFTs neurofibrillary tangles
NALs neutral allosteric ligands
NOR novel object recognition
NB nucleus basalis
PAMs positive allosteric modulators
PSP progressive supranuclear palsy
PKC protein kinase C
SI substantia innominate
TGN *trans*-golgi network

1. Introduction

Alzheimer's disease (AD) is the most common form of dementia and is associated with neuronal atrophy and profound behavioral and cognitive disturbances (Whitehouse et al., 1982). Neuropathologically, AD is characterized by the presence of amyloid plaques, consisting largely of amyloid-β peptide (Aβ), and neurofibrillary tangles (NFTs), formed by hyperphosphorylated tau (Selkoe, 1991b). Several neurotransmitter systems are dysregulated in AD, including cholinergic, glutamatergic, serotonergic, adrenergic and peptidergic pathways (Thathiah & De Strooper, 2011). Early studies in post-mortem AD brain tissue, revealed a significant reduction in the activity of enzymes in presynaptic cholinergic neurons in the cortex and hippocampus (Davies & Maloney, 1976) and the loss of presynaptic cholinergic markers correlates with accumulation of Aβ plaques, NFTs and clinical severity of dementia (Ladner & Lee, 1998). The basal forebrain (BF) provides a major source of cholinergic neurons to the neocortex, hippocampus and amygdala and plays a key role in learning, memory and attentional processes (for detailed review, see Ballinger, Ananth, Talmage, & Role, 2016). The BF is composed of structures that include the medial septal (MS) nuclei, the diagonal band (DB) nuclei, the nucleus basalis (NB) and the substantia innominate (SI). Significant loss of cholinergic neurons within the BF of AD patients, particularly in the NB where >75% reductions in neurons has been demonstrated (Whitehouse et al., 1982), leads to widespread cholinergic denervation and cognitive impairment, giving rise to the cholinergic hypothesis of AD (Coyle, Price, & DeLong, 1983; Greenamyre et al., 1985). Aside from the NMDA antagonist, memantine, which modulates glutamatergic transmission, the current frontline treatment options for AD, based solely on the cholinergic hypothesis, are acetylcholinesterase (AChE) inhibitors, such as donepezil, rivastigmine and galantamine. These inhibitors act to up-regulate cholinergic transmission by inhibiting the breakdown of acetylcholine (ACh) and can temporarily ameliorate some of the symptoms of AD. However, AChE inhibitors have a limited therapeutic potential, they are only efficacious for mild to moderate AD (Neugroschl & Wang, 2011) and long-term treatment with donepezil offers no disease-modifying effects (Courtney et al., 2004). In addition, their non-specific nature represents a major drawback, causing gastrointestinal (GI) and cardiovascular side effects induced by potentiation of peripheral cholinergic signaling, including exocrine secretions, bradycardia and GI distress (Courtney et al., 2004; Inglis, 2002). These dose-limiting side effects result in modest overall efficacy of AChE inhibitors. Furthermore, by global elevation of ACh concentrations, AChE inhibitors have the potential to indirectly activate functionally opposing acetylcholine receptors, which could also account for their limited efficacy in the CNS. Taken together, this highlights the need for receptor subtype- and tissue-specific agonists. Therefore, there remains a significant unmet clinical need to develop novel therapies for AD with improved adverse effect profiles that can treat symptoms associated with AD and also positively modify the underlying pathophysiology.

Given that G protein-coupled receptors (GPCRs) are involved in almost all physiological processes, it is perhaps unsurprising that several subtypes have been implicated in the pathogenesis of AD. GPCRs have the potential to influence a variety of dysfunctional signaling pathways in AD, and over recent years a number of GPCR targets have been evaluated, with 10 GPCR-targeted drugs currently in clinical trials for AD (Hauser, Attwood, Rask-Andersen, Schiöth, & Gloriam, 2017). Of these GPCRs, preclinical and clinical data suggest that muscarinic acetylcholine receptors (mAChRs) may represent a novel therapeutic strategy for symptomatic treatment in AD. Clinical trials with the muscarinic agonist, xanomeline, showed modest improvements in cognitive function in AD patients (Bodick, Offen, Shannon, et al., 1997), and these beneficial effects are thought to be mediated through activation of M1 and/or M4 mAChRs (Thorn et al., 2019). Recent studies have shown that both M1- and M4 mAChR-*selective* ligands may both be beneficial in the treatment of memory deficits, albeit via different mechanisms of action in the CNS (Lebois, Trimper, Hu, Levey, & Manns, 2016; Popiolek et al., 2019; Thorn et al., 2019). Based on the cholinergic hypothesis of AD, however, mAChRs may be anticipated to provide only symptomatic relief of cognitive decline in AD. However, a large body of data now exists to provide evidence that targeting the M1 mAChR can influence amyloid processing and offer disease-modifying effects in neurodegenerative diseases. This article will discuss the progress made thus far in the development of M1 mAChR clinical candidates, with a particular emphasis on allosteric ligands as a strategy to achieve greater subtype selectivity. Furthermore, we will review the evidence that M1 mAChRs may offer a therapeutic target for both symptomatic and disease-modifying effects.

2. Muscarinic acetylcholine receptors (mAChRs)

The mAChR family comprises five distinct subtypes (M1–M5), which are encoded by distinct CHRM genes (Hulme, Birdsall, & Buckley, 1990) and are members of class A (rhodopsin-like) GPCRs (Fredriksson, Lagerström, Lundin, & Schiöth, 2003). Crystal structures of all five mAChR subtypes have now been determined, confirming a common structural architecture across this family of receptors, with a highly-conserved transmembrane core which forms the binding site for the endogenous ligand acetylcholine (Haga et al., 2012; Kruse et al., 2012; Thal et al., 2016; Vuckovic et al., 2019). Crystallization of the entire muscarinic receptor family has revealed important structural differences across the different receptor subtypes, particularly within the extracellular loop regions, providing crucial information that could allow for the rational design of subtype selective muscarinic ligands. Members of this GPCR family also differ in their G protein-selectivity, with M1, M3, and M5 mAChRs preferentially coupling to the pertussis toxin-insensitive $G_{q/11}$ family of G proteins, while the M2 and M4 subtypes preferentially couple to the G_i family, which are pertussis toxin-sensitive (Caulfield & Birdsall, 1998; Felder, 1995; Nathanson, 1987; Wess, 1993).

Muscarinic receptors are widely distributed throughout the body (Levey, 1993; Levey, Kitt, Simonds, Price, & Brann, 1991) and play fundamental roles in many physiological systems (e.g., CNS, cardiovascular system (CVS), GI tract, lungs). The muscarinic cholinergic system plays a crucial role in learning and memory processes (Hasselmo, 1999, 2006; Hasselmo & Bower, 1993; Hasselmo & Sarter, 2011; Sarter & Bruno, 1997) and extensive evidence suggests that cholinergic signaling through muscarinic receptors is impaired in AD (Levey, 1996). For example, it was shown in the late 1970s that cognitive impairment in AD patients correlated with a decrease in choline acetyltransferase (CAT) activity (Perry et al., 1978). Furthermore, in human post-mortem AD tissue, there is a substantial reduction in BF neurons, thereby indicating a reduction in the cholinergic innervation of the neocortex and hippocampus (Whitehouse, Price, Clark, Coyle, & DeLong, 1981; Whitehouse et al., 1982). More specifically, as previously discussed in patients with familial or sporadic forms of AD, a significant loss of cholinergic neuronal cells in the NB has been reported (Whitehouse et al., 1982). While cholinergic neuron density was found to be unchanged in mild cognitive impairment (MCI) and early AD (Gilmor et al., 1999), pretangles and NFTs were observed in the NB as early as MCI and throughout AD progression (Mesulam, Shaw, Mash, & Weintraub, 2004; Rasool, Svendsen, & Selkoe, 1986; Svensson, Alafuzoff, & Nordberg, 1992), highlighting the vulnerability of the NB to neurofibrillary insult in AD. As the NB provides the major cholinergic input to the cortex and amygdala and corresponded changes in cognition with pathology were found, the NB provides an early target for cholinergic therapies (Mesulam, 2004; Mesulam, Mufson, Levey, & Wainer, 1983). The major cholinergic innervation to the hippocampus is derived from the cholinergic neurons of the MS and the DB (reviewed in Dutar, Bassant, Senut, & Lamour, 1995; Melander et al., 1985; Mesulam et al., 1983). Previous studies suggested that these cholinergic neurons are comparably unaffected in AD (Mufson, Bothwell, & Kordower, 1989; Mufson, Cochran, Benzing, & Kordower, 1993). Interestingly a recent study suggested that cholinergic neurons in the BF can control inflammation and innate immune responses in mice suggesting that a disruption of this mechanism in AD could exacerbate pathology (Lehner et al., 2019). M1 mAChRs are abundant in the forebrain, including the cerebral cortex and hippocampus (Levey, 1993; Volpicelli & Levey, 2004), where they are the predominant muscarinic receptor subtype (Bradley et al., 2017) and play a crucial role in learning and memory processes, which are impaired in AD (Fisher, 2008b; Ladner & Lee, 1998). In particular, M1 mAChRs have been demonstrated to regulate specific memory processes such as spatial working memory, episodic memory and acquisition, retention and consolidation (Anagnostaras et al., 2003; Brandeis et al., 1995; Lebois et al., 2016; Nathan et al., 2013). Blockade of muscarinic receptor neurotransmission by administration of non-selective mAChR antagonists, such as scopolamine, produces substantial cognitive deficits in animals and humans (Bartus, Dean, Beer, & Lippa, 1982; Flicker, Serby, & Ferris, 1990; Rusted & Warburton, 1988) and genetic deletion of M1 mAChR in mice leads to deficits in working memory and memory consolidation (Anagnostaras et al., 2003). Although there remains some debate regarding the efficiency of $G_{q/11}$ G protein-coupling to the M1 mAChR in aged and AD brains (Bradley et al., 2017; McQuail et al., 2013; Tsang et al., 2006), importantly the M1 mAChR expression is preserved in AD, since it is localized in post-synaptic neurons (Levey, 1996; Svensson et al., 1992). Therefore, drugs directly activating M1 mAChRs, rather than indirectly via inhibition of endogenous ACh breakdown, would likely retain efficacy as the disease progresses. These observations have been driving research efforts and drug discovery programs toward selective activation of the M1 mAChR for treatment of AD (Fisher, 2008a).

3. M1 mAChR drug development

3.1 Targeting the M1 receptor with orthosteric agonists

Over the past four decades, many pharmaceutical companies have invested in the development of drugs to selectively target M1 mAChRs aimed at symptomatic improvement in AD and schizophrenia. However, despite the overwhelming preclinical evidence to suggest that M1 muscarinic agonists show significant potential as cognition-enhancing drugs, translating these findings to successful clinical outcomes has so far proven challenging. Early attempts were led by Eli Lilly, who demonstrated positive effects of xanomeline, a muscarinic receptor agonist (Fig. 1), in Phase 2 clinical trials (Bodick, Offen, Levey, et al., 1997). The observed positive effects

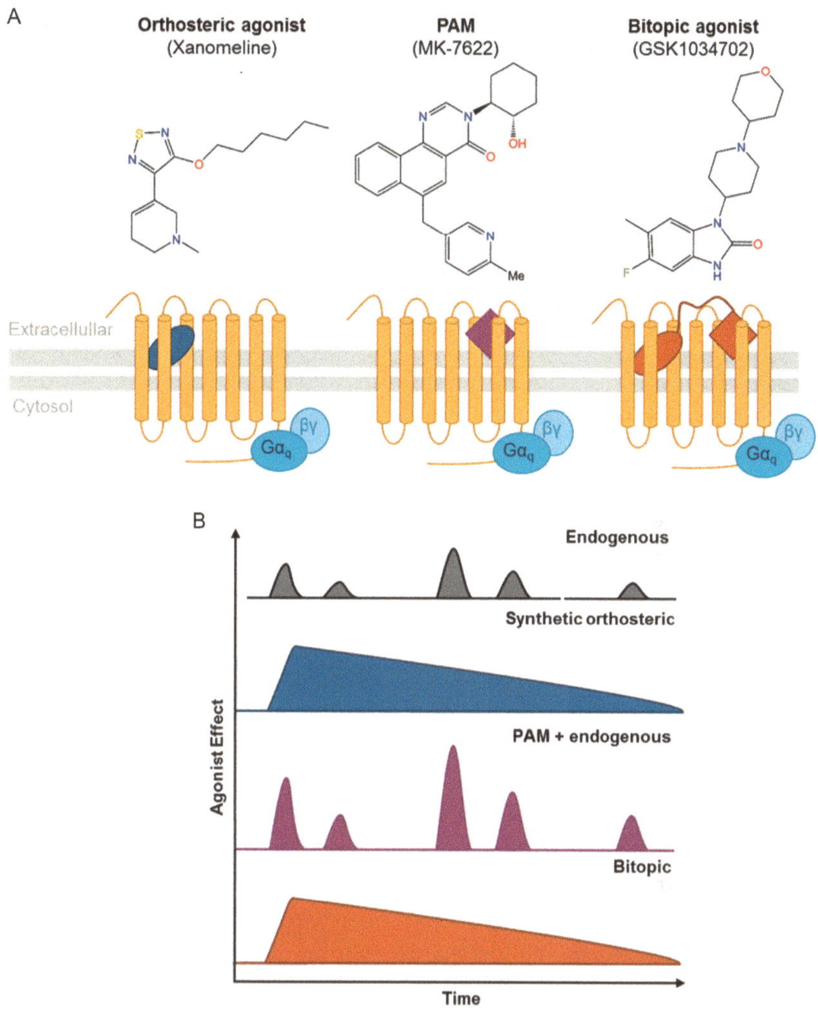

Fig. 1 Different classes of ligands targeting mAChRs. (A) Orthosteric ligands (e.g., xanomeline) target the binding site of the endogenous ligand, acetylcholine, whereas PAMs (e.g., MK-7622) bind to topographically distinct sites. A bitopic ligand (e.g., GSK1034702) binds concomitantly with orthosteric and allosteric sites. Xanomeline, MK-7622 and GSK1034702 are all examples of M1 mAChR ligands, with different mechanisms of action that have been tested in clinical trials. (B) Pure M1 PAMs, lacking intrinsic activity, have the potential to enhance the effects of acetylcholine, while maintaining the spatiotemporal characteristics of endogenous cholinergic signaling. Orthosteric and bitopic ligands will directly activate the receptor until the drug is metabolized from the body.

of xanomeline in improvement of cognitive function and behavioral disturbances in AD patients was the first example of a large-scale clinical trial whereby directly targeting muscarinic receptors could offer an alternative to AChE inhibitors in AD. Efficacy of xanomeline on cognitive function was measured using the Alzheimer's Disease Assessment Scale (ADAS-Cog) and revealed a significant improvement in orientation, constructional praxis, spoken language ability and word-finding difficulty in spontaneous speech. Furthermore, effects of xanomeline on the behavioral symptoms of AD, measured using the Alzheimer's Disease Symptomatology Scale (ADSS), showed most significant improvements in vocal outbursts, suspiciousness, delusions, agitation and hallucinations. These positive outcomes prompted Eli Lilly to conduct a smaller trial of xanomeline in patients with schizophrenia (Shekhar et al., 2008). In this trial, xanomeline efficacy in schizophrenia patients were measured using the Positive and Negative Syndrome Scale (PANSS), the Brief Psychiatric Rating Scale (BPRS) and a battery of cognitive tests. Subjects treated with xanomeline showed improvements in total PANSS and BPRS scores and in cognitive measures, particularly with regards to short-term memory and verbal learning. While these independent clinical trials used different tests to measure study outcomes of two mechanistically distinct diseases, AD and schizophrenia, they similarly demonstrated that xanomeline could have beneficial effects on cognitive function. However, despite these positive effects and the progression of xanomeline to phase 3 clinical trials for AD, the side-effect profile proved to be unsatisfactory, due to the relative lack of M1 selectivity and the action of xanomeline at peripheral M2 and M3 mAChRs, leading to dose-limiting adverse cholinergic side effects such as sweating, salivation and GI disturbances (Melancon, Tarr, Panarese, Wood, & Lindsley, 2013).

Similar to other GPCR families, the conservation of the orthosteric binding pocket of mAChRs (M1–M5), the site of binding for the endogenous ligand acetylcholine, makes the design of highly subtype selective orthosteric ligands extremely challenging (Kruse et al., 2013; Venkatakrishnan et al., 2013). Alternative efforts to improve the subtype selectivity of muscarinic ligands, and therefore minimize peripheral side effects, have focused on targeting the less-conserved binding pockets, and have led to the development of bitopic and allosteric approaches (see below).

Despite this, attempts to develop orthosteric agonists of M1 mAChRs but limit overstimulation or peripheral side effects are currently ongoing. For example, Karuna Therapeutics are optimistic that xanomeline will afford significant clinical benefit in AD and schizophrenia if the side-effect profile can be sufficiently limited (Felder, 2019). Karuna are pursuing clinical trials with KarXT, a co-formulation of xanomeline with trospium chloride—a peripherally restricted muscarinic antagonist to limit activation of peripheral M2 and M3 muscarinic receptors, and have demonstrated improved tolerability in two Phase 1 clinical trials. Recently, Karuna announced the successful outcome of KarXT in Phase 2 trials, with statistically significant improvements in total PANSS score in schizophrenic patients and good overall tolerability.

Furthermore, Sosei-Heptares, in partnership with Allergan, continue to pursue M1 orthosteric agonists for AD. A Phase 1b clinical trial with HTL0009936, demonstrated robust pro-cognitive changes in brain activity even at low doses and this selective compound was well tolerated and devoid of cholinergic side effects associated with previous muscarinic orthosteric agonists. Furthermore, HTL0018318, a selective M1 agonist, has been tested as a potential symptomatic treatment in Phase 1b and Phase 2 clinical trials for AD and other dementias, such as dementia with Lewy bodies. Although reported to be well tolerated in humans after 28 days treatment, Sosei announced the voluntary suspension of their clinical development activities with HTL0018318 due to an unexpected single animal toxicology study in non-human primates.

3.2 Bitopic ligands: A novel approach for selective targeting of M1 mAChR

Following the failure of xanomeline in clinical trials, a number of pharmaceutical companies invested in the development of more muscarinic ligands, giving rise to the emergence of bitopic ligands as an approach to selectively target M1 mAChRs (Fronik, Gaiser, & Sejer Pedersen, 2017; Kruse et al., 2014). Bitopic ligands are compounds with the ability of concomitantly interact with orthosteric and allosteric sites on a single receptor. They are usually single molecular entities characterized by an orthosteric binding and an allosteric binding group chemically attached by a linker (Lane, Sexton, & Christopoulos, 2013).

McN-A-342 was the first M1 mAChR—selective bitopic ligand to be discovered in 1961 (Roszkowski, 1961), initially identified as a selective agonist of the receptor. Later in the 1980s, this compound was described as an allosteric ligand due to its high affinity (Birdsall, Burgen, Hulme, Stockton, & Zigmond, 1983), and subsequently proven to be a bitopic ligand (Valant et al., 2008). The bitopic mode of action was unraveled after progressive truncation of the compound and extensive pharmacological assays, which led to the identification of orthosteric and allosteric fragments (Valant et al., 2008).

As for McN-A-342, the bitopic mode of action has often remained unappreciated for many ligands that were originally described as solely orthosteric or allosteric, and only emerged in later studies. This happens as bitopic ligands display mixed modes of orthosteric or allosteric pharmacology depending on the conditions under which molecular pharmacological assays, such as dissociation kinetic experiments, are performed. In fact, when identifying allosterism, a pre- or co-incubation with orthosteric agonist might hinder the ability of a ligand to bind to the orthosteric site, or when testing for orthosteric binding, the allosteric mode becomes difficult to identify due to the generally low affinity of allosteric binding (Kruse et al., 2014). The discovery of McN-A-342 as a bitopic ligand paved the way to the identification or re-classification of compounds displaying similar pharmacology (Digby et al., 2012; Lebois et al., 2010, 2011; Watt et al., 2011).

GlaxoSmithKline developed GSK1034702 (Fig. 1) as their M1 mAChR clinical candidate, and advanced this compound into clinical trials in 2008 (Nathan et al., 2013). This compound was also initially described as a M1 mAChR-selective allosteric agonist, and reversed scopolamine-induced cognitive deficits in rats (Budzik et al., 2010). GSK1034702 was tested in clinical trials and shown to improve episodic memory in humans with nicotine abstinence-induced cognitive impairments. This compound was reported to be well tolerated but caused adverse GI responses in a proportion of patients (Nathan et al., 2013). GSK1034702 is structurally related to the M1 mAChR bitopic ligand, TBPB, whose mechanism of action was defined by fragmentation studies (Keov et al., 2014, 2013), which implied that GSK1034702 might exhibit a similar mechanism of action. Studies to extensively characterize the pharmacology of GSK1034702 indeed revealed a bitopic mode of action, interacting with the orthosteric binding pocket and concomitantly with an allosteric site (Bradley et al., 2018).

Targeting the M1 mAChR by means of bitopic ligands may offer many advantages as they combine the pharmacology of both orthosteric and allosteric ligands therefore conferring increased selectivity over the first-generation of muscarinic ligands, such as xanomeline. However, as found with GSK1034702, these compounds can still be associated with cholinergic side effects, since they are still able to interact with the highly conserved orthosteric binding pocket, and thereby activate other members of the muscarinic receptor family to drive adverse responses. In addition, bitopic ligand binding to the orthosteric site of muscarinic receptors may lead to engagement of functionally opposing signaling cascades due to the competitive antagonism of ACh, and this property could underlie reduced efficacy of bitopic ligands.

3.3 Development of M1 positive allosteric modulators (PAMs) for AD

An alternative approach to achieve exquisite levels of receptor subtype selectivity is through the development of allosteric ligands. Ligands of this type are able to bind to sites that are topographically distinct from the orthosteric site (from the Ancient Greek allos (ἄλλος) means "other"), and are less conserved across members of the same GPCR subfamily (Fig. 2). The phenomenon of allosterism was firstly observed when enzymes and ion channels displayed cooperative structural changes which were stabilized by preferred ligands (Changeux & Edelstein, 2005).

GPCR allosteric ligand pharmacology is now understood to be as diverse as ligands targeting the orthosteric site, and can range from allosteric agonists, allosteric modulators, neutral allosteric ligands (NALs), ago-PAMs, and each of the types can additionally induce biased signaling. Allosteric agonists directly mediate receptor activation by interacting with a binding domain that is distinct from the orthosteric site. Allosteric modulators can be positive allosteric modulators (PAMs) and negative allosteric modulators (NAMs) (Christopoulos et al., 2014), which respectively potentiate or attenuate the effect of the orthosteric ligand by inducing a molecular rearrangement of the receptor that results in the modulation of its intrinsic affinity for orthosteric ligands and/or orthosteric ligand efficacy. Allosteric modulators can only have effects when an orthosteric ligand is bound to the receptor. NALs bind to allosteric sites but display no cooperativity with orthosteric ligands. Ago-PAMs are able to enhance the potency of the orthosteric ligand similarly to pure PAMs, but in addition they can exert agonism in their own right (Langmead et al., 2006).

The allosteric mechanism of GPCRs is considerably complicated to define, due to the wide range of distinct active states that a GPCR can adopt depending on interactions with both bound ligand(s) and intracellular effectors, e.g., G proteins (Stallaert, Christopoulos, & Bouvier, 2011). Allosteric modulators—with the exception of ago-PAMs, which have intrinsic agonist activity, and can activate the receptor in the absence of the endogenous ligands (Langmead et al., 2006)—require an orthosteric ligand to be bound to the receptor for modulatory action (Bridges & Lindsley, 2008). This implies that receptor modulation would occur in

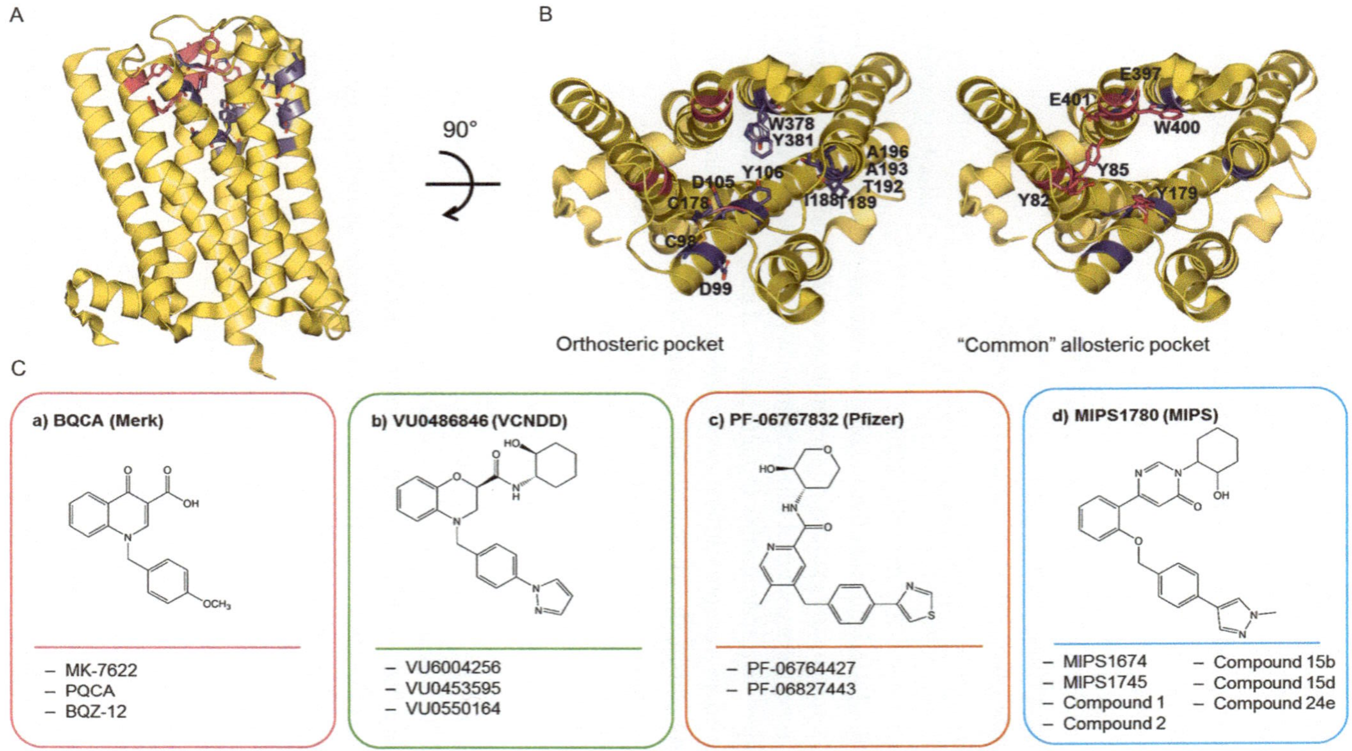

Fig. 2 Structure of the M1 mAChR depicting the orthosteric and allosteric binding pockets. Crystallization of the M1 mAChR revealed a high degree of sequence conservation in the orthosteric binding pocket across M1-M4 mAChRs (Thal et al., 2016). The "common" allosteric binding pocket is comprised of residues within a large extracellular vestibule of the receptors. The M1 mAChR crystal structure is viewed from the (A) membrane or (B) the extracellular side. Images reproduced using the PyMOL Molecular Graphics System, Version 2.0 Schrödinger, LLC. (C) Allosteric drug development for the M1 mAChR has generated an array of PAMs that are based on four distinct chemical scaffolds: BQCA (Ma et al., 2009), VU0486846 (Rook et al., 2018), PF-06767832 (Davoren et al., 2016) and MIPS1780 (Mistry et al., 2016).

a spatial-temporal physiological manner, and its effect can be saturated (Fig. 1). Allosteric modulators with modest cooperativity will exert a limited intrinsic effect, suggesting they may be potentially safer if administered in larger doses, compared to orthosteric compounds (Gregory, Sexton, & Christopoulos, 2007). PAMs represent an encouraging approach for AD treatment for their specificity as well as for their nature as potentiators that would allow to maintain the physiological temporal and spatial cholinergic signaling (Foster, Choi, Conn, & Rook, 2014).

An exemplar ligand is the highly selective, and first prototypical M1 mAChR PAM, benzyl quinolone carboxylic acid (BQCA) (Fig. 2) (Ma et al., 2009). BQCA was developed by Merck and found to possess robust pro-cognitive activity in a scopolamine-induced deficit mouse model, suggesting that this allosteric compound could afford similar cognition-enhancing effects to orthosteric muscarinic ligands. When tested in an amyloid mouse model (Shirey et al., 2009) and prion-infected mice exhibiting terminal neurodegenerative disease (Bradley et al., 2017), BQCA was shown to recover cognitive deficits. Further, a structurally related PAM, PQCA, was subsequently shown to boost cognitive performance in mice, rats and non-human primates (Lange, Cannon, Drott, Kuduk, & Uslaner, 2015; Uslaner et al., 2013). When tested in comparison to donepezil and xanomeline, PQCA was shown to significantly reduce scopolamine-induced memory deficits in monkeys, but was, importantly, devoid of cholinergic side effects that were observed with xanomeline and donepezil, highlighting the potential of M1 PAMs to improve cognitive outcomes in AD without the adverse responses previously noted with orthosteric ligands (Vardigan et al., 2015). Merck also tested PCQA in an aged Tg2576 mouse model overexpressing mutant human amyloid β-protein precursor (APP) and found that this M1 PAM could ameliorate deficits in recognition memory in this mouse model (Puri, Wang, Vardigan, Kuduk, & Uslaner, 2015). Based on the same chemical scaffold, Merck developed MK-7622 (Fig. 1) as their clinical candidate, and effectively showed that MK-7622 was a selective and potent M1 PAM, displaying robust intrinsic activity in the absence of ACh, and effective at reverting scopolamine-induced deficits in non-human primates and in humans (Uslaner et al., 2018). Furthermore, MK-7622 produced electrophysiological effects in both species, as measured by quantitative EEG (Uslaner et al., 2018). However, Merck's clinical trial with MK-7622 was halted for futility in 2016, with a 45 mg adjunctive therapy alongside an AChE inhibitor lacking any improvement in cognitive score or function (Voss et al., 2018). Furthermore, MK-7622 was found to induce cholinergic side effects in around one-fifth of the participants in this study. The failure of this clinical trial could suggest that despite significant preclinical data, a selective M1 PAM can a) still lead to on-target, M1 mAChR-driven, cholinergic adverse effects and b) lack any pro-cognitive activity in AD. Indeed, both Pfizer (Davoren et al., 2016) and Bristol-Myers Squibb (Alt et al., 2016) have published data in agreement with this notion, demonstrating that highly selective M1 ligands can drive cholinergic toxicity and behavioral convulsions.

It should be noted that there now exists a diverse range of structurally distinct M1 PAM chemotypes, arising from Merck, Pfizer, Vanderbilt Centre for Neuroscience Drug Discovery (VCNDD) and Monash Institute for Pharmaceutical Sciences (MIPS) that possess distinct pharmacological properties (Fig. 2). However, it is not well defined as to what type of pharmacological properties are necessary for an M1 PAM to have efficacy in cognition enhancement in AD, while lacking toxic side effects. For example, M1 PAMs that are closely related in structure, PF-06764427 and VU6004256, displaying similar intrinsic agonist activity and in vitro pharmacological profiles while achieving equivalent brain exposures relative to their potency at M1 mAChRs, can have significantly distinct effects in vivo. PF-06764427 induces robust decreases in spontaneous locomotor activity, reverses amphetamine-induced hyper-locomotion (AHL), lacks a significant effect on performance in a novel object recognition (NOR) task and induced cholinergic toxicity and convulsions (Rook et al., 2017). Seizure activity could be observed following administration of 30 mg/kg PF-06764427—a dose that achieved free brain concentrations that were fourfold and 1.9-fold higher than the M1 PAM and M1 allosteric agonist potency, respectively. In contrast, a slightly weaker ago-PAM, VU6004256, had a lesser effect on spontaneous locomotor activity and did not reverse AHL, but produced a profound enhancement of object recognition in the novel object recognition task. Surprisingly, this compound was completely devoid of any adverse effects, despite free brain concentrations reaching fourfold and 1.4-fold higher than the potency of this compound as an M1 PAM and M1 allosteric agonist, respectively (Rook et al., 2017). Although this study did not provide a mechanistic basis for the differences in in vivo effects of these structurally related compounds, it highlights the importance of defining the subtle pharmacological properties in M1 compounds that drive adverse toxic effects in order to develop M1 ligands to deliver maximal therapeutic efficacy in cognitive enhancement.

In more recent studies, Moran, Dickerson, et al. (2018) tested M1 PAMs with high intrinsic activity, MK-7622 and PF-06764427, alongside M1 PAMs that are devoid of intrinsic activity, VU0453595 and VU0550164, for their ability to enhance cognition and drive adverse effects. MK-7622 and PF-06764427 induced severe seizures, whereas VU0453595 did not. Furthermore, MK-7622 did not display efficacy in a NOR test, whereas VU0453595 showed a robust enhancement in object recognition (Moran, Dickerson, et al., 2018). This suggests that M1 PAMs with high levels of intrinsic activity have the potential to overstimulate the M1 mAChR, and induce non-physiological tonic receptor stimulation, leading to disruptions in cognitive function and drive adverse toxic responses (Moran, Dickerson, et al., 2018). Despite this, both Merck and Pfizer continue to challenge the strategy of selective M1 therapeutics, and Pfizer have recently released data to show that an M1 PAM with minimal agonist activity, PF-06827443, can induce cholinergic adverse effects and convulsions (Davoren et al., 2017). However, in subsequent studies, when tested in a range of recombinant and native tissue preparations, PF-06827443, was proven to be a robust ago-PAM (Moran, Cho, et al., 2018), which could account for its associated toxicity. Based on this significant body of preclinical evidence, VCNDD are now moving toward the development of M1 PAMs devoid of intrinsic agonist activity which lack adverse responses while maintaining robust efficacy in cognitive enhancement (Engers et al., 2018; Rook et al., 2018).

The mechanistic basis for M1 ligands driving on-target adverse effects and differences in in vivo efficacies could also be explained by signaling bias. Marlo et al. (2009) showed that two selective M1 PAMs, displaying similar effects in vitro with regards to potentiating the affinity of ACh, could produce distinct effects on phosphoinositide hydrolysis and coupling to phospholipase D (Marlo et al., 2009). Furthermore, the comparison of PF-06764427 and VU6004256 described above (Rook et al., 2017) revealed distinct effects on receptor internalization, with the latter failing to induce measurable internalization. In recent studies using a series of genetically-altered mice expressing M1 receptor mutants have demonstrated that ligands displaying a bias toward phosphorylation-dependent signaling are less likely to induce cholinergic adverse effects and seizures (Bradley et al., 2019, manuscript accepted). Here, the authors found that pilocarpine, a well-characterized muscarinic partial agonist that drives robust seizures despite acting as a partial agonist of muscarinic receptors, showed bias toward G protein-dependent versus phosphorylation-dependent signaling in vitro, whereas the bitopic ligand GSK1034702 displayed no bias across these pathways. When administered in vivo to rats at equivalent occupancy levels, pilocarpine stimulated sixfold increases in phosphoinositide turnover over basal in the cortex, compared to a ~2.5-fold increase stimulated by GSK1034702. This led the authors to conclude that an M1 agonist showing bias toward G protein-dependent signaling, in this case phosphoinositide responses, may result in a greater propensity to induce adverse central and peripheral effects (Bradley et al., 2019; manuscript accepted). Interestingly, Pfizer's M1 PAMs, PF-06767832 and PF-06827443, compounds that drive peripheral cholinergic effects and convulsions, were found to stimulate robust increases in striatal inositol monophosphate levels in vivo (Davoren et al., 2016, 2017). This suggests a possible correlation between the level of G protein-dependent signaling and the propensity for M1 PAMs to induce seizures.

3.4 Orthosteric, bitopic or allosteric: What type of M1 ligand is needed?

Over time, AD is accompanied by progressive neuronal loss, particularly of presynaptic cholinergic neurons (Schliebs & Arendt, 2011). Cognitive deficits and clinical dementia scorings are correlated to reductions in a number of cholinergic markers such as CAT, the enzyme responsible for ACh synthesis, indicating progressive depletion of the neurotransmitter (Davies & Maloney, 1976; Perry, Perry, Blessed, & Tomlinson, 1977). The mechanism of action of current frontline treatments, such as donepezil, is to prevent the breakdown of ACh and boost cholinergic transmission. However, AChE inhibitors have only been approved for mild-to-moderate AD patients (Anand, Gill, & Mahdi, 2014), and they lose efficacy as neurodegeneration progresses, likely due in part to the fact that ACh release from cholinergic neurons is significantly diminished with disease progression. Therefore, there is an unmet need for pharmaceutical therapeutics for mild-moderate and advanced AD, in particular when there are currently hurdles with early diagnosis (Jack et al., 2012).

The rich diversity of M1 mAChR ligands may offer a promising prospective for patient stratification according to disease stages. For example, at preclinical stages of disease, where neuronal injury is not too severe (Jack et al., 2012), administration of a pure M1-PAM that lacks intrinsic activity, would likely restore diminished M1 receptor signaling by increasing the affinity and/or efficacy of the endogenous ligand ACh, maintaining the spatiotemporal signaling characteristics of the endogenous ligand (Fig. 1B) and reducing the likelihood of overstimulation of the receptor leading to adverse responses (Moran, Dickerson, et al., 2018). However, pure PAMs could potentially cause M1-mediated adverse effects without inducing direct receptor overstimulation. For instance, this type of ligand could stabilize the receptor in such conformation that could decrease or prevent receptor internalization (Thomas, Langmead, Wood, & Challiss, 2009). Furthermore, pure PAMs may have the potential to cause seizures by inducing highly synchronous neuronal activity in the CA3-CA1 hippocampal regions, that progressively synchronizes larger populations of neurons at higher doses (Lebois et al., 2016).

Given that pure PAMs are probe-dependent, they may lose their therapeutic efficacy as disease progresses, when levels of endogenous ACh are low due to depletion of cholinergic neurons (Davies & Maloney, 1976; Perry et al., 1977). Ago-PAMs could be an alternative approach to pure PAMs at this stage, as they would be able to activate the receptor in the absence of the endogenous ligand while still conferring exquisite receptor subtype selectivity. It is postulated that ago-PAMs may be more likely to induce side effects associated with receptor overstimulation (Moran, Dickerson, et al., 2018; Rook et al., 2017, 2018). It should be noted, however, that on-target, M1 mAChR-mediated adverse responses, are often tested in wild-type animals. Therefore, M1-selective ligands that lead to severe adverse responses due to receptor overstimulation, may not induce such responses in diseased animals where ACh levels are diminished. It is crucial, therefore, to choose appropriate animal models displaying cholinergic dysfunction akin to AD patients.

Perhaps M1-selective orthosteric or bitopic agonists may have improved therapeutic value in later stages of neurodegeneration, when ACh release is mostly depleted. In fact, this type of ligand would still be able to bind with high affinity and modulate M1 mAChR activity independently of endogenous ACh levels.

In order to fully realize the therapeutic utility of an M1 PAM versus an M1 agonist at different stages of AD severity, it will be critical to elucidate the impact of these distinct pharmacological ligands on hippocampal circuit activity. Previous electrophysiology studies performed on the hippocampus of awake rats demonstrated that systemic administration of an M1 agonist or an M1 PAM similarly promoted synchrony of intrahippocampal neuronal networks, while inducing different patterns of spiking activity (Lebois et al., 2016). These distinct mechanisms of action could lead to differential therapeutic benefits depending on the disease stage. For example, these studies showed that M1 PAMs may be beneficial to improve the intrahippocampal neuronal spiking when the firing of the hippocampal CA3 region is impaired in age-related memory deficits (Wilson, Ikonen, Gallagher, Eichenbaum, & Tanila, 2005), whereas M1 agonists may be preferred when there is significant loss of cholinergic neurons in AD, as the activity would not depend on endogenous ACh release (Lebois et al., 2016).

4. Disease modification potential of M1 mAChRs

As previously mentioned, all currently approved therapeutics for AD have symptomatic rather than disease-modifying properties. The evident need for a new drug that modifies the underlying causes of AD is also reflected in the properties of the compounds currently in the drug development pipeline: in 2018, 112 drugs were registered on clinicaltrials.gov to be in the pipeline for AD, with 63% of these being targeted at disease modification and 22% at symptomatic enhancement of cognition (Cummings, Lee, Ritter, & Zhong, 2018). In 2019, agents aiming to modify disease progression accounted for 73% of the 137 drugs in trials (Cummings, Lee, Ritter, Sabbagh, & Zhong, 2019) in line with the current lack of disease-modifying treatments (DMTs).

Many traditional disease-modifying approaches have focussed on disrupting the production of pathological amyloid, based on the amyloid hypothesis of AD, whereby accumulation and aggregation of Aβ is thought to be central to the etiology of disease (Hardy & Allsop, 1991; Hardy & Higgins, 1992; Selkoe, 1991a). This theory has guided development of potential therapeutics, aimed at prevention or clearance of Aβ (Fig. 3). However, a number of clinical trials with a series of β-secretase 1 (BACE1) inhibitors, γ-secretase inhibitors and Aβ-targeted antibodies have largely been terminated due to lack of efficacy, and in some cases a worsening of cognitive function (Doody et al., 2013; Egan et al., 2019; Green et al., 2009; Honig et al., 2018; Hsiao, Rombouts, & Gijsen, 2019).

Given that both extracellular Aβ plaques and intra-neuronal NFTs containing hyperphosphorylated tau are found in AD (Goedert, Wischik, Crowther, Walker, & Klug, 1988; Grundke-Iqbal, Iqbal, Quinlan, et al., 1986; Grundke-Iqbal, Iqbal, Tung, et al., 1986; Ittner & Götz, 2011; Masters et al., 1985), and that NFT load was found to correlate better with cognitive decline, gliosis and synaptic loss compared to Aβ plaques (Arriagada, Growdon, Hedley-Whyte, & Hyman, 1992; Braak & Braak, 1996; Ingelsson et al., 2004; Thal et al., 2000), potential therapeutic approaches targeting tau pathology have been proposed. These include inhibition of tau hyperphosphorylation or aggregation, or promoting the clearance of tau and rescue neuronal plasticity (Iqbal, Liu, & Gong, 2016).

Interestingly, the only tau-based therapeutic currently in Phase 3 clinical trials is TRx0237 (LMTX) (Cummings et al., 2019), a second-generation tau protein aggregation inhibitor trialed by TauRx Therapeutics and

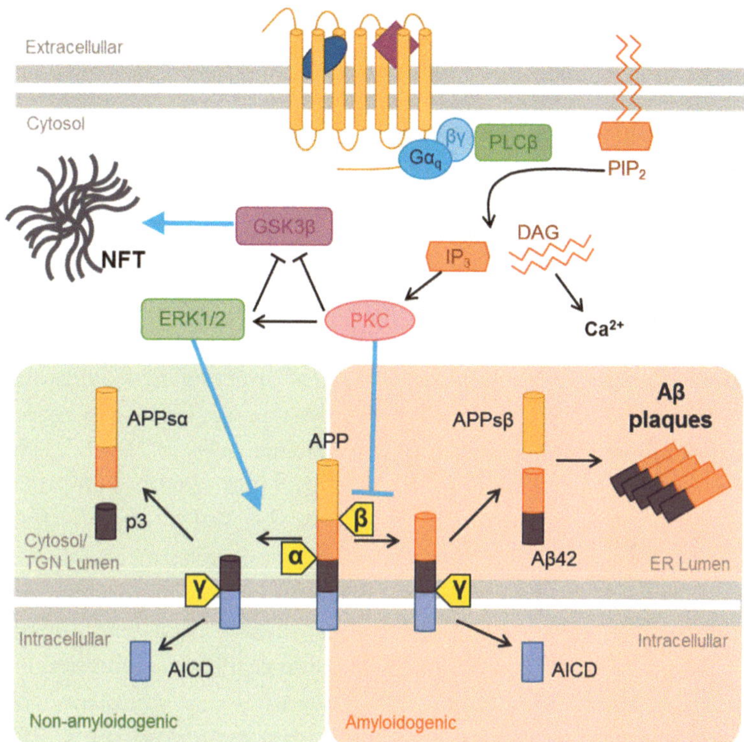

Fig. 3 M1 mAChR regulation of amyloidogenic processing in AD. Proteolytic processing of amyloid precursor protein (APP) occurs broadly via two distinct pathways. In the amyloidogenic pathway, cleavage of APP by β-secretase at the cell surface and in early endosomes (Kinoshita et al., 2003), and the subsequent cleavage by γ-secretase, yield an amyloid precursor protein intracellular domain (AICD), and soluble APPβ and Aβ protein which are secreted and lead to the formation of amyloid β (Aβ) plaques. In the non-amyloidogenic pathway, initial cleavage of APP occurs by α-secretases such as ADAM10 and ADAM17 localized in the Trans-Golgi Network (TGN) or at the plasma membrane (Lammich et al., 1999). These cleave APP within the Aβ peptide region, and therefore, prevent Aβ formation and secretion. M1 mAChRs can enhance non-amyloidogenic APP in vitro via PKC- and ERK1/2-dependent mechanisms, leading to activation of α-secretase and inhibition of β-secretase. Furthermore, M1 mAChR have been shown to regulate formation of NFTs via inhibition of GSK3β to reduce levels of hyperphosphorylated tau.

designed to have improved bioavailability and tolerability properties compared to its precursor form. Two previous Phase 3 trials have suggested that a mono-therapeutic dose of 4 mg twice a day could potentially cause disease-modifying effects with reduced brain atrophy rates in patients with mild AD but this will have to be tested further (Gauthier et al., 2016; Wilcock et al., 2018). Another anti-tau antibody, ABBV-8E12, developed by AbbVie is currently in Phase 2 clinical trials for the tauopathy progressive supranuclear palsy (PSP) (ClinicalTrials.gov ID: NCT02985879) as well as for AD (ClinicalTrials.gov ID: NCT02880956). It has been argued that pure tauopathies such as PSP present better populations for the initial development of tau-based therapeutics in neurodegeneration due to absence of co-pathologies such as amyloid plaques in AD (Boxer et al., 2013, 2014). There have been some reports of the clinical trials in PSP having been halted but this has not been officially confirmed. In light of the failure of all Aβ-targeted therapeutic approaches so far, and the relative infancy of tau approaches, the field is starting to consider other potential targets for disease modification, such as targeting neuroinflammation and neurotransmitter systems, and these now account for a large proportion of compounds in the drug development pipeline (34% of DMT in Phase 3 vs 47% of DMT in Phase 2) (Cummings et al., 2019; Ferrero, Solas, Francis, & Ramirez, 2017; Fu, Wang, & Ip, 2019; Godyń, Jończyk, Panek, & Malawska, 2016; Heneka et al., 2015). Of relevance to the current review is the fact that a large body of evidence now suggests that targeting the M1 receptor may have the potential to offer disease-modifying properties.

Initial indications that M1 mAChRs could regulate the amyloid burden came in the early 1990s, when it was reported that stimulation of M1 mAChRs altered the processing of APP via a protein kinase C (PKC)-dependent mechanism in vitro (Fig. 3) (Buxbaum et al., 1992; Nitsch, Slack, Wurtman, & Growdon, 1992). Clinical studies since demonstrated that activation of M1 mAChR in AD patients reduces the levels of total Aβ in the cerebrospinal fluid (Hock et al., 2000; Nitsch, Deng, Tennis, Schoenfeld, & Growdon, 2000), suggesting that targeting the M1 mAChR may offer therapeutic benefit by reducing Aβ levels. Furthermore, activation of the M1 mAChR in an AD mouse model, 3xTg-AD, has been shown to not only improve cognitive dysfunction, but also to lessen the Aβ and tau pathologies in these mice (Caccamo et al., 2006). The mechanism by which targeting M1 mAChR can reduce amyloid pathology was shown to involve an increase in the α-secretase ADAM17/TACE in vitro, directing processing of APP toward non-amyloidogenic pathways, via independent mechanisms involving both PKC activation and ERK1/2 phosphorylation (Fig. 3) (Buxbaum et al., 1998; Caccamo et al., 2006; Haring et al., 1998). However, acute receptor stimulation or loss of M1 receptors in a transgenic APP mouse model (see below) did not alter expression levels of the α-secretase candidates ADAM10 or ADAM17 in vivo (Davis, Fritz, Wess,

Lah, & Levey, 2010). While these studies established that activation of M1 mAChRs could lead to alterations in amyloid processing and disease-modifying effects, the agonists used in these reports were relatively non-selective, and given that both M1- and M3 mAChRs couple to $G_{q/11}$ pathways and increase secretion of soluble APP (Nitsch et al., 1992), it was unclear that these effects were mediated solely via M1 activation. However, in cultured neurons, carbachol stimulation increased secretion of the APP fragment generated by α-secretase cleavage, termed secreted APP-alpha (APPsα), whereas in neurons derived from M1-deficient mice, this effect was significantly reduced (Davis et al., 2010), indicating that the M1 mAChR is critical for mediating the effects of carbachol on amyloidogenic processing. Furthermore, by crossing the M1 knockout mice with three distinct AD mouse models, APPswe/Ind, 3xTg-AD and Tg-SwDI, it has been demonstrated that loss of the M1 subtype exacerbates neurotoxicity and AD-like pathology (Davis et al., 2010; Medeiros et al., 2011). In APPswe/Ind mice, loss of M1 receptors caused an increase in amyloidogenic processing resulting in greater Aβ plaque accumulation, and a significant reduction in APPsα secretion (Davis et al., 2010). Subsequent studies to analyze the effects of M1 receptor ablation on the tau pathology in 3xTg-AD mice showed that depletion of M1 receptors caused a significant increase in hyperphosphorylated tau via an increase in GSK3β levels (Fig. 3), confirming that loss of M1 receptors causes exacerbation of both amyloid- and tau pathologies in AD mice (Medeiros et al., 2011).

Ablation of M1 receptors has previously been shown to induce cognitive impairments in mice (Anagnostaras et al., 2003), and 3xTg-AD mice also display cognitive deficits (Billings, Oddo, Green, McGaugh, & LaFerla, 2005), when 3xTg-AD mice and M1 knockout mice are crossed, cognitive impairment is significantly worsened (Medeiros et al., 2011). Furthermore, neuroinflammation in AD mouse models is significantly worsened by the loss of M1 receptors, indicated by an increase in both astrocytes and microglia and an upregulation of inflammatory cytokines (Medeiros et al., 2011).

Taken together, these studies establish the M1 receptor as a critical mediator of AD-like pathological features, including amyloid and tau pathology, cognitive impairment and neuroinflammation. Whether newer generations of muscarinic agonist with increased selectivity and/or different pharmacological properties could offer similar (or enhanced) beneficial effects on APP processing in vivo was until recently undetermined.

In 2008, Jones et al. (2008) reported that TBPB increased the secretion of soluble APP and reduced the Aβ burden in vitro (Jones et al., 2008). This has since been tested in vivo with the M1 selective bitopic ligand VU0364572 (Digby et al., 2012) preventing the onset of memory impairments, and reducing the levels of toxic Aβ species and amyloid pathology in the hippocampus and cortex of 5XFAD mice (Lebois et al., 2017). Furthermore, recently, a novel selective allosteric M1 muscarinic and sigma-1 receptor agonist, AF710B, was found to reduce cognitive deficits and amyloid pathology in 3xTg-AD mice (Hall et al., 2018).

Although M1 mAChR PAMs have been shown to have efficacy in alleviating cognitive deficits in AD mouse models (Lange et al., 2015; Ma et al., 2009; Puri et al., 2015; Vardigan et al., 2015), until recently the notion that ligands acting solely via an allosteric site at the M1 receptor could offer both pro-cognitive *and* disease-modifying effects had not been tested. However, recent work has demonstrated that this could be the case. In murine prion disease many of the key features of AD, including extensive gliosis and progressive hippocampal cholinergic neuronal loss, are also present (Bourgognon et al., 2018; Bradley et al., 2017). At early stages of prion disease (9–10 weeks post-inoculation (w.p.i.)) mice show no physical signs of disease, but biochemical and histopathological evidence of disease, as well as behavioral changes such as a decline in burrowing behavior and a deficit in learning and memory, can be observed. As the disease progresses to late stage (12 w.p.i.), mice develop terminal clinical symptoms. Therefore, unlike commonly used mouse models of AD, murine prion disease is a progressive and terminal neurodegenerative disease where the effectiveness of novel M1 mAChR ligands both on memory loss (early stage) and on survival (late stage) can be tested. Using this model, Bradley et al. (2017) recently demonstrated that a highly selective M1 allosteric modulator, BQCA, can significantly extend the lifespan of terminally-sick prion-diseased mice, thereby establishing that M1-selective PAMs also have the potential to achieve clinical efficacy by improving cognitive dysfunction in addition to disease-modifying effects.

5. Conclusion

The M1 mAChR has long been considered an attractive target for the treatment of cognitive impairment in AD. The development of the first-generation, non-selective muscarinic agonists, led to the progression of xanomeline into clinical trials for AD, with positive outcomes on cognitive function and behavioral symptoms. Although this drug displayed dose-limiting side effects that halted its further advancement as an AD treatment, xanomeline paved the way for development of a large array of more selective M1 muscarinic ligands with diverse pharmacological properties, including orthosteric, bitopic and allosteric ligands. Although undisputed as a target for improving cognitive function in AD, whether the M1 receptor is truly a viable target in AD has recently been challenged due to cholinergic toxicity and seizurogenic properties of some highly selective M1 agonists. It is now understood that the overstimulation of cholinergic systems and receptor subtypes underlies these central- and peripheral adverse responses and more recent efforts have focussed on development of ligands that (i) achieve increased subtype selectivity and (ii) limit overstimulation of the M1 mAChR, which can lead to disrupted learning and memory processes and adverse effects. Pure allosteric M1 modulators lacking intrinsic activity may represent an exciting approach to achieve these endpoints—a strategy that is yet to be tested in the clinic. Furthermore, selective orthosteric partial agonists may offer an alternative to restoring M1-mediated transmission while minimizing overstimulation. The field is somewhat divided as to which of these therapeutic strategies may be optimal. It is worthwhile to note that M1 ligands with different mechanisms of action may be efficacious at different disease stages, depending on the severity of the cholinergic dysfunction in AD.

Therefore, it is crucial that preclinical testing of M1 mAChR agonists/modulators is conducted in both healthy and diseased contexts—particularly those which show key features of human neurodegenerative disease, such as progressive neuronal loss and degradation of cholinergic transmission. Clearly there is significant need to define the precise pharmacological properties that are required in an M1 mAChR ligand to deliver therapeutically beneficial effects while avoiding the toxic side effects, and the explosion of structural information may provide critical insight to guide the design of next-generation M1 receptor ligands. Given that all muscarinic receptor clinical trials for AD to date have been prematurely terminated due to adverse effects or futility, whether the M1 mAChR may offer some disease-modification properties is still to be determined. However, a significant body of evidence now suggests that the M1 mAChR has the potential to regulate the processing of pathological amyloid and tau, to alleviate major hallmarks of disease in AD mouse models, and extend lifespan of terminally-sick neurodegenerative mice. Over the next decade, it will be exciting to see the outcome of current and future clinical trials targeting the M1 receptor in AD, both in terms of symptomatic treatment of cognitive decline and progression of disease.

Conflict of interest

The authors have no conflicts of interest to declare.

References

Alt, A., Pendri, A., Bertekap, R. L., Jr., Li, G., Benitex, Y., Nophsker, M., et al. (2016). Evidence for classical cholinergic toxicity associated with selective activation of M1 muscarinic receptors. *The Journal of Pharmacology and Experimental Therapeutics*, *356*(2), 293–304. https://doi.org/10.1124/jpet.115.226910.

Anagnostaras, S. G., Murphy, G. G., Hamilton, S. E., Mitchell, S. L., Rahnama, N. P., Nathanson, N. M., et al. (2003). Selective cognitive dysfunction in acetylcholine M1 muscarinic receptor mutant mice. *Nature Neuroscience*, *6*(1), 51–58. https://doi.org/10.1038/nn992.

Anand, R., Gill, K. D., & Mahdi, A. A. (2014). Therapeutics of Alzheimer's disease: Past, present and future. *Neuropharmacology*, *76*(Pt. A), 27–50. https://doi.org/10.1016/j.neuropharm.2013.07.004.

Arriagada, P. V., Growdon, J. H., Hedley-Whyte, E. T., & Hyman, B. T. (1992). Neurofibrillary tangles but not senile plaques parallel duration and severity of Alzheimer's disease. *Neurology*, *42*(3), 631.

Ballinger, E. C., Ananth, M., Talmage, D. A., & Role, L. W. (2016). Basal forebrain cholinergic circuits and signaling in cognition and cognitive decline. *Neuron*, *91*(6), 1199–1218. https://doi.org/10.1016/j.neuron.2016.09.006.

Bartus, R. T., Dean, R. L., Beer, B., & Lippa, A. S. (1982). The cholinergic hypothesis of geriatric memory dysfunction. *Science*, *217*(4558), 408. Retrieved from http://science.sciencemag.org/content/217/4558/408.abstract.

Billings, L. M., Oddo, S., Green, K. N., McGaugh, J. L., & LaFerla, F. M. (2005). Intraneuronal Abeta causes the onset of early Alzheimer's disease-related cognitive deficits in transgenic mice. *Neuron*, *45*(5), 675–688. https://doi.org/10.1016/j.neuron.2005.01.040.

Birdsall, N. J., Burgen, A. S., Hulme, E. C., Stockton, J. M., & Zigmond, M. J. (1983). The effect of McN-A-343 on muscarinic receptors in the cerebral cortex and heart. *British Journal of Pharmacology*, *78*(2), 257–259. https://doi.org/10.1111/j.1476-5381.1983.tb09388.x.

Bodick, N. C., Offen, W. W., Levey, A. I., et al. (1997). Effects of xanomeline, a selective muscarinic receptor agonist, on cognitive function and behavioral symptoms in Alzheimer disease. *Archives of Neurology*, *54*(4), 465–473.

Bodick, N. C., Offen, W. W., Shannon, H. E., Satterwhite, J., Lucas, R., van Lier, R., et al. (1997). The selective muscarinic agonist xanomeline improves both the cognitive deficits and behavioral symptoms of Alzheimer disease. *Alzheimer Disease and Associated Disorders*, *11*(Suppl. 4), S16–S22. Retrieved from https://www.ncbi.nlm.nih.gov/pubmed/9339268.

Bourgognon, J.-M., Spiers, J. G., Scheiblich, H., Antonov, A., Bradley, S. J., Tobin, A. B., et al. (2018). Alterations in neuronal metabolism contribute to the pathogenesis of prion disease. *Cell Death and Differentiation*, *25*(8), 1408.

Boxer, A. L., Gold, M., Huey, E., Hu, W. T., Rosen, H., Kramer, J., et al. (2013). The advantages of frontotemporal degeneration drug development (part 2 of frontotemporal degeneration: The next therapeutic frontier). *Alzheimer's & Dementia*, *9*(2), 189–198. https://doi.org/10.1016/j.jalz.2012.03.003.

Boxer, A. L., Lang, A. E., Grossman, M., Knopman, D. S., Miller, B. L., Schneider, L. S., et al. (2014). Davunetide in patients with progressive supranuclear palsy: A randomised, double-blind, placebo-controlled phase 2/3 trial. *The Lancet Neurology*, *13*(7), 676–685. https://doi.org/10.1016/S1474-4422(14)70088-2.

Braak, H., & Braak, E. (1996). Evolution of the neuropathology of Alzheimer's disease. *Acta Neurologica Scandinavica*, *94*(S165), 3–12.

Bradley, S. J., Bourgognon, J. M., Sanger, H. E., Verity, N., Mogg, A. J., White, D. J., et al. (2017). M1 muscarinic allosteric modulators slow prion neurodegeneration and restore memory loss. *The Journal of Clinical Investigation*, *127*(2), 487–499. https://doi.org/10.1172/JCI87526.

Bradley, S. J., Molloy, C., Bundgaard, C., Mogg, A. J., Thompson, K. J., Dwomoh, L., et al. (2018). Bitopic binding mode of an M1 muscarinic acetylcholine receptor agonist associated with adverse clinical trial outcomes. *Molecular Pharmacology*, *93*(6), 645. Retrieved from http://molpharm.aspetjournals.org/content/93/6/645.abstract.

Brandeis, R., Sapir, M., Hafif, N., Abraham, S., Oz, N., Stein, E., et al. (1995). AF150(S): A new functionally selective M1 agonist improves cognitive performance in rats. *Pharmacology Biochemistry and Behavior*, *51*(4), 667–674. https://doi.org/10.1016/0091-3057(94)00435-L.

Bridges, T. M., & Lindsley, C. W. (2008). G-protein-coupled receptors: From classical modes of modulation to allosteric mechanisms. *ACS Chemical Biology*, *3*(9), 530–541. https://doi.org/10.1021/cb800116f.

Budzik, B., Garzya, V., Shi, D., Walker, G., Woolley-Roberts, M., Pardoe, J., et al. (2010). Novel N-substituted benzimidazolones as potent, selective, CNS-penetrant, and orally active M1 mAChR agonists. *ACS Medicinal Chemistry Letters*, *1*(6), 244–248. https://doi.org/10.1021/ml100105x.

Buxbaum, J. D., Liu, K. N., Luo, Y., Slack, J. L., Stocking, K. L., Peschon, J. J., et al. (1998). Evidence that tumor necrosis factor alpha converting enzyme is involved in regulated alpha-secretase cleavage of the Alzheimer amyloid protein precursor. *The Journal of Biological Chemistry*, *273*(43), 27765–27767. Retrieved from https://www.ncbi.nlm.nih.gov/pubmed/9774383.

Buxbaum, J. D., Oishi, M., Chen, H. I., Pinkas-Kramarski, R., Jaffe, E. A., Gandy, S. E., et al. (1992). Cholinergic agonists and interleukin 1 regulate processing and secretion of the Alzheimer beta/A4 amyloid protein precursor. *Proceedings of the National Academy of Sciences of the United States of America*, *89*(21), 10075–10078. https://doi.org/10.1073/pnas.89.21.10075.

Caccamo, A., Oddo, S., Billings, L. M., Green, K. N., Martinez-Coria, H., Fisher, A., et al. (2006). M1 receptors play a central role in modulating AD-like pathology in transgenic mice. *Neuron*, *49*(5), 671–682. https://doi.org/10.1016/j.neuron.2006.01.020.

Caulfield, M. P., & Birdsall, N. J. M. (1998). International union of pharmacology. XVII. Classification of muscarinic acetylcholine receptors. *Pharmacological Reviews*, *50*(2), 279. Retrieved from http://pharmrev.aspetjournals.org/content/50/2/279.abstract.

Changeux, J.-P., & Edelstein, S. J. (2005). Allosteric mechanisms of signal transduction. *Science*, *308*(5727), 1424. https://doi.org/10.1126/science.1108595.

Christopoulos, A., Changeux, J.-P., Catterall, W. A., Fabbro, D., Burris, T. P., Cidlowski, J. A., et al. (2014). International union of basic and clinical pharmacology. XC. Multisite pharmacology: Recommendations for the nomenclature of receptor allosterism and allosteric ligands. *Pharmacological Reviews*, *66*, 918–947.

Courtney, C., Farrell, D., Gray, R., Hills, R., Lynch, L., Sellwood, E., et al. (2004). Long-term donepezil treatment in 565 patients with Alzheimer's disease (AD2000): Randomised double-blind trial. *Lancet*, *363*(9427), 2105–2115. https://doi.org/10.1016/S0140-6736(04)16499-4.

Coyle, J. T., Price, D. L., & DeLong, M. R. (1983). Alzheimer's disease: A disorder of cortical cholinergic innervation. *Science*, *219*(4589), 1184–1190. Retrieved from https://www.ncbi.nlm.nih.gov/pubmed/6338589.

Cummings, J., Lee, G., Ritter, A., Sabbagh, M., & Zhong, K. (2019). Alzheimer's disease drug development pipeline: 2019. *Alzheimer's & Dementia: Translational Research & Clinical Interventions*, *5*, 272–293. https://doi.org/10.1016/j.trci.2019.05.008.

Cummings, J., Lee, G., Ritter, A., & Zhong, K. (2018). Alzheimer's disease drug development pipeline: 2018. *Alzheimer's & Dementia: Translational Research & Clinical Interventions*, *4*, 195–214. https://doi.org/10.1016/j.trci.2018.03.009.

Davies, P., & Maloney, A. J. (1976). Selective loss of central cholinergic neurons in Alzheimer's disease. *Lancet*, *2*(8000), 1403. https://doi.org/10.1016/s0140-6736(76)91936-x.

Davis, A. A., Fritz, J. J., Wess, J., Lah, J. J., & Levey, A. I. (2010). Deletion of M1 muscarinic acetylcholine receptors increases amyloid pathology in vitro and in vivo. *The Journal of Neuroscience*, *30*(12), 4190–4196. https://doi.org/10.1523/JNEUROSCI.6393-09.2010.

Davoren, J. E., Garnsey, M., Pettersen, B., Brodney, M. A., Edgerton, J. R., Fortin, J. P., et al. (2017). Design and synthesis of gamma- and delta-lactam M1 positive allosteric modulators (PAMs): Convulsion and cholinergic toxicity of an M1-selective PAM with weak agonist activity. *Journal of Medicinal Chemistry*, *60*(15), 6649–6663. https://doi.org/10.1021/acs.jmedchem.7b00597.

Davoren, J. E., Lee, C. W., Garnsey, M., Brodney, M. A., Cordes, J., Dlugolenski, K., et al. (2016). Discovery of the potent and selective M1 PAM-agonist N-[(3R,4S)-3-hydroxytetrahydro-2H-pyran-4-yl]-5-methyl-4-[4-(1,3-thiazol-4-yl)benzyl]pyridine-2-carboxamide (PF-06767832): Evaluation of efficacy and cholinergic side effects. *Journal of Medicinal Chemistry*, *59*(13), 6313–6328. https://doi.org/10.1021/acs.jmedchem.6b00544.

Digby, G. J., Noetzel, M. J., Bubser, M., Utley, T. J., Walker, A. G., Byun, N. E., et al. (2012). Novel allosteric agonists of M1 muscarinic acetylcholine receptors induce brain region-specific responses that correspond with behavioral effects in animal models. *The Journal of Neuroscience*, *32*(25), 8532–8544. https://doi.org/10.1523/JNEUROSCI.0337-12.2012.

Doody, R. S., Raman, R., Farlow, M., Iwatsubo, T., Vellas, B., Joffe, S., et al. (2013). A phase 3 trial of semagacestat for treatment of Alzheimer's disease. *New England Journal of Medicine*, *369*(4), 341–350. https://doi.org/10.1056/NEJMoa1210951.

Dutar, P., Bassant, M. H., Senut, M. C., & Lamour, Y. (1995). The septohippocampal pathway: Structure and function of a central cholinergic system. *Physiological Reviews*, *75*(2), 393–427. https://doi.org/10.1152/physrev.1995.75.2.393.

Egan, M. F., Kost, J., Voss, T., Mukai, Y., Aisen, P. S., Cummings, J. L., et al. (2019). Randomized trial of verubecestat for prodromal Alzheimer's disease. *New England Journal of Medicine*, *380*(15), 1408–1420. https://doi.org/10.1056/NEJMoa1812840.

Engers, J. L., Childress, E. S., Long, M. F., Capstick, R. A., Luscombe, V. B., Cho, H. P., et al. (2018). VU6007477, a novel M1 PAM based on a pyrrolo[2,3-b]pyridine carboxamide core devoid of cholinergic adverse events. *ACS Medicinal Chemistry Letters*, *9*(9), 917–922. https://doi.org/10.1021/acsmedchemlett.8b00261.

Felder, C. C. (1995). Muscarinic acetylcholine receptors: Signal transduction through multiple effectors. *The FASEB Journal*, *9*(8), 619–625.

Felder, C. C. (2019). GPCR drug discovery-moving beyond the orthosteric to the allosteric domain. *Advances in Pharmacology*, *86*, 1–20. https://doi.org/10.1016/bs.apha.2019.04.002.

Ferrero, H., Solas, M., Francis, P. T., & Ramirez, M. J. (2017). Serotonin 5-HT 6 receptor antagonists in Alzheimer's disease: Therapeutic rationale and current development status. *CNS Drugs*, *31*(1), 19–32.

Fisher, A. (2008a). Cholinergic treatments with emphasis on M1 muscarinic agonists as potential disease-modifying agents for Alzheimer's disease. *Neurotherapeutics*, *5*(3), 433–442. https://doi.org/10.1016/j.nurt.2008.05.002.

Fisher, A. (2008b). M1 muscarinic agonists target major hallmarks of Alzheimer's disease—The pivotal role of brain M1 receptors. *5*, 237–240.

Flicker, C., Serby, M., & Ferris, S. H. (1990). Scopolamine effects on memory, language, visuospatial praxis and psychomotor speed. *Psychopharmacology, 100*(2), 243–250. https://doi.org/10.1007/BF02244414.

Foster, D. J., Choi, D. L., Conn, P. J., & Rook, J. M. (2014). Activation of M1 and M4 muscarinic receptors as potential treatments for Alzheimer's disease and schizophrenia. *Neuropsychiatric Disease and Treatment, 10*, 183–191. https://doi.org/10.2147/ndt.s55104.

Fredriksson, R., Lagerström, M. C., Lundin, L.-G., & Schiöth, H. B. (2003). The G-protein-coupled receptors in the human genome form five main families. phylogenetic analysis, paralogon groups, and fingerprints. *Molecular Pharmacology, 63*(6), 1256. Retrieved from http://molpharm.aspetjournals.org/content/63/6/1256.abstract.

Fronik, P., Gaiser, B. I., & Sejer Pedersen, D. (2017). Bitopic ligands and metastable binding sites: Opportunities for G protein-coupled receptor (GPCR) medicinal chemistry. *Journal of Medicinal Chemistry, 60*(10), 4126–4134. https://doi.org/10.1021/acs.jmedchem.6b01601.

Fu, W.-Y., Wang, X., & Ip, N. Y. (2019). Targeting neuroinflammation as a therapeutic strategy for Alzheimer's disease: Mechanisms, drug candidates, and new opportunities. *ACS Chemical Neuroscience, 10*(2), 872–879. https://doi.org/10.1021/acschemneuro.8b00402.

Gauthier, S., Feldman, H. H., Schneider, L. S., Wilcock, G. K., Frisoni, G. B., Hardlund, J. H., et al. (2016). Efficacy and safety of tau-aggregation inhibitor therapy in patients with mild or moderate Alzheimer's disease: A randomised, controlled, double-blind, parallel-arm, phase 3 trial. *The Lancet, 388*(10062), 2873–2884.

Gilmor, M. L., Erickson, J. D., Varoqui, H., Hersh, L. B., Bennett, D. A., Cochran, E. J., et al. (1999). Preservation of nucleus basalis neurons containing choline acetyltransferase and the vesicular acetylcholine transporter in the elderly with mild cognitive impairment and early Alzheimer's disease. *Journal of Comparative Neurology, 411*(4), 693–704. https://doi.org/10.1002/(SICI)1096-9861(19990906)411:4<693::AID-CNE13>3.0.CO;2-D.

Godyń, J., Jończyk, J., Panek, D., & Malawska, B. (2016). Therapeutic strategies for Alzheimer's disease in clinical trials. *Pharmacological Reports, 68*(1), 127–138. https://doi.org/10.1016/j.pharep.2015.07.006.

Goedert, M., Wischik, C. M., Crowther, R. A., Walker, J. E., & Klug, A. (1988). Cloning and sequencing of the cDNA encoding a core protein of the paired helical filament of Alzheimer disease: Identification as the microtubule-associated protein tau. *Proceedings of the National Academy of Sciences of the United States of America, 85*(11), 4051–4055. https://doi.org/10.1073/pnas.85.11.4051.

Green, R. C., Schneider, L. S., Amato, D. A., Beelen, A. P., Wilcock, G., Swabb, E. A., et al. (2009). Effect of tarenflurbil on cognitive decline and activities of daily living in patients with mild Alzheimer disease: A randomized controlled trial. *JAMA, 302*(23), 2557–2564. https://doi.org/10.1001/jama.2009.1866.

Greenamyre, J. T., Penney, J. B., Young, A. B., D'Amato, C. J., Hicks, S. P., & Shoulson, I. (1985). Alterations in L-glutamate binding in Alzheimer's and Huntington's diseases. *Science, 227*(4693), 1496–1499. Retrieved from https://www.ncbi.nlm.nih.gov/pubmed/2858129.

Gregory, K. J., Sexton, P. M., & Christopoulos, A. (2007). Allosteric modulation of muscarinic acetylcholine receptors. *Current Neuropharmacology, 5*(3), 157–167. https://doi.org/10.2174/157015907781695946.

Grundke-Iqbal, I., Iqbal, K., Quinlan, M., Tung, Y.-C., Zaidi, M. S., & Wisniewski, H. M. (1986). Microtubule-associated protein tau. A component of Alzheimer paired helical filaments. *Journal of Biological Chemistry, 261*(13), 6084–6089.

Grundke-Iqbal, I., Iqbal, K., Tung, Y.-C., Quinlan, M., Wisniewski, H. M., & Binder, L. I. (1986). Abnormal phosphorylation of the microtubule-associated protein tau (tau) in Alzheimer cytoskeletal pathology. *Proceedings of the National Academy of Sciences of the United States of America, 83*(13), 4913–4917.

Haga, K., Kruse, A. C., Asada, H., Yurugi-Kobayashi, T., Shiroishi, M., Zhang, C., et al. (2012). Structure of the human M2 muscarinic acetylcholine receptor bound to an antagonist. *Nature*, *482*(7386), 547–551. https://doi.org/10.1038/nature10753.

Hall, H., Iulita, M. F., Gubert, P., Flores Aguilar, L., Ducatenzeiler, A., Fisher, A., et al. (2018). AF710B, an M1/sigma-1 receptor agonist with long-lasting disease-modifying properties in a transgenic rat model of Alzheimer's disease. *Alzheimers Dement*, *14*(6), 811–823. https://doi.org/10.1016/j.jalz.2017.11.009.

Hardy, J., & Allsop, D. (1991). Amyloid deposition as the central event in the aetiology of Alzheimer's disease. *Trends in Pharmacological Sciences*, *12*(10), 383–388. Retrieved from https://www.ncbi.nlm.nih.gov/pubmed/1763432.

Hardy, J. A., & Higgins, G. A. (1992). Alzheimer's disease: The amyloid cascade hypothesis. *Science*, *256*(5054), 184–185. Retrieved from https://www.ncbi.nlm.nih.gov/pubmed/1566067.

Haring, R., Fisher, A., Marciano, D., Pittel, Z., Kloog, Y., Zuckerman, A., et al. (1998). Mitogen-activated protein kinase-dependent and protein kinase C-dependent pathways link the m1 muscarinic receptor to beta-amyloid precursor protein secretion. *Journal of Neurochemistry*, *71*(5), 2094–2103. Retrieved from https://www.ncbi.nlm.nih.gov/pubmed/9798935.

Hasselmo, M. E. (1999). Neuromodulation: Acetylcholine and memory consolidation. *Trends in Cognitive Sciences*, *3*(9), 351–359. Retrieved from https://www.ncbi.nlm.nih.gov/pubmed/10461198.

Hasselmo, M. E. (2006). The role of acetylcholine in learning and memory. *Current Opinion in Neurobiology*, *16*(6), 710–715. https://doi.org/10.1016/j.conb.2006.09.002.

Hasselmo, M. E., & Bower, J. M. (1993). Acetylcholine and memory. *Trends in Neurosciences*, *16*(6), 218–222. Retrieved from https://www.ncbi.nlm.nih.gov/pubmed/7688162.

Hasselmo, M. E., & Sarter, M. (2011). Modes and models of forebrain cholinergic neuromodulation of cognition. *Neuropsychopharmacology*, *36*(1), 52–73. https://doi.org/10.1038/npp.2010.104.

Hauser, A. S., Attwood, M. M., Rask-Andersen, M., Schiöth, H. B., & Gloriam, D. E. (2017). Trends in GPCR drug discovery: New agents, targets and indications. *Nature Reviews Drug Discovery*, *16*, 829. https://doi.org/10.1038/nrd.2017.178.

Heneka, M. T., Carson, M. J., Khoury, J. E., Landreth, G. E., Brosseron, F., Feinstein, D. L., et al. (2015). Neuroinflammation in Alzheimer's disease. *The Lancet Neurology*, *14*(4), 388–405. https://doi.org/10.1016/S1474-4422(15)70016-5.

Hock, C., Maddalena, A., Heuser, I., Naber, D., Oertel, W., von der Kammer, H., et al. (2000). Treatment with the selective muscarinic agonist talsaclidine decreases cerebrospinal fluid levels of total amyloid beta-peptide in patients with Alzheimer's disease. *Annals of the New York Academy of Sciences*, *920*, 285–291. Retrieved from https://www.ncbi.nlm.nih.gov/pubmed/11193166.

Honig, L. S., Vellas, B., Woodward, M., Boada, M., Bullock, R., Borrie, M., et al. (2018). Trial of solanezumab for mild dementia due to Alzheimer's disease. *New England Journal of Medicine*, *378*(4), 321–330. https://doi.org/10.1056/NEJMoa1705971.

Hsiao, C.-C., Rombouts, F., & Gijsen, H. J. M. (2019). New evolutions in the BACE1 inhibitor field from 2014 to 2018. *Bioorganic & Medicinal Chemistry Letters*, *29*(6), 761–777. https://doi.org/10.1016/j.bmcl.2018.12.049.

Hulme, E. C., Birdsall, N. J. M., & Buckley, N. J. (1990). Muscarinic receptor subtypes. *Annual Review of Pharmacology and Toxicology*, *30*(1), 633–673. https://doi.org/10.1146/annurev.pa.30.040190.003221.

Ingelsson, M., Fukumoto, H., Newell, K., Growdon, J., Hedley-Whyte, E., Frosch, M., et al. (2004). Early Aβ accumulation and progressive synaptic loss, gliosis, and tangle formation in AD brain. *Neurology*, *62*(6), 925–931.

Inglis, F. (2002). The tolerability and safety of cholinesterase inhibitors in the treatment of dementia. *International Journal of Clinical Practice. Supplement*, *127*, 45–63.
Iqbal, K., Liu, F., & Gong, C.-X. (2016). Tau and neurodegenerative disease: The story so far. *Nature Reviews. Neurology*, *12*(1), 15.
Ittner, L. M., & Götz, J. (2011). Amyloid-beta and tau—A toxic pas de deux in Alzheimer's disease. *Nature Reviews. Neuroscience*, *12*(2), 65–72. https://doi.org/10.1038/nrn2967.
Jack, C. R., Jr., Knopman, D. S., Weigand, S. D., Wiste, H. J., Vemuri, P., Lowe, V., et al. (2012). An operational approach to National Institute on Aging-Alzheimer's Association criteria for preclinical Alzheimer disease. *Annals of Neurology*, *71*(6), 765–775. https://doi.org/10.1002/ana.22628.
Jones, C. K., Brady, A. E., Davis, A. A., Xiang, Z., Bubser, M., Tantawy, M. N., et al. (2008). Novel selective allosteric activator of the M1 muscarinic acetylcholine receptor regulates amyloid processing and produces antipsychotic-like activity in rats. *The Journal of Neuroscience*, *28*(41), 10422–10433. https://doi.org/10.1523/JNEUROSCI.1850-08.2008.
Keov, P., López, L., Devine, S. M., Valant, C., Lane, J. R., Scammells, P. J., et al. (2014). Molecular mechanisms of bitopic ligand engagement with the M1 muscarinic acetylcholine receptor. *The Journal of Biological Chemistry*, *289*(34), 23817–23837. https://doi.org/10.1074/jbc.M114.582874.
Keov, P., Valant, C., Devine, S. M., Lane, J. R., Scammells, P. J., Sexton, P. M., et al. (2013). Reverse engineering of the selective agonist TBPB unveils both orthosteric and allosteric modes of action at the M(1) muscarinic acetylcholine receptor. *Molecular Pharmacology*, *84*(3), 425–437. https://doi.org/10.1124/mol.113.087320.
Kinoshita, A., Fukumoto, H., Shah, T., Whelan, C. M., Irizarry, M. C., & Hyman, B. T. (2003). Demonstration by FRET of BACE interaction with the amyloid precursor protein at the cell surface and in early endosomes. *Journal of Cell Science*, *116*(Pt. 16), 3339–3346. https://doi.org/10.1242/jcs.00643.
Kruse, A. C., Hu, J., Pan, A. C., Arlow, D. H., Rosenbaum, D. M., Rosemond, E., et al. (2012). Structure and dynamics of the M3 muscarinic acetylcholine receptor. *Nature*, *482*(7386), 552–556. https://doi.org/10.1038/nature10867.
Kruse, A. C., Kobilka, B. K., Gautam, D., Sexton, P. M., Christopoulos, A., & Wess, J. (2014). Muscarinic acetylcholine receptors: Novel opportunities for drug development. *Nature Reviews Drug Discovery*, *13*, 549. Retrieved from https://doi.org/10.1038/nrd4295.
Kruse, A. C., Ring, A. M., Manglik, A., Hu, J., Hu, K., Eitel, K., et al. (2013). Activation and allosteric modulation of a muscarinic acetylcholine receptor. *Nature*, *504*(7478), 101–106. https://doi.org/10.1038/nature12735.
Ladner, C. J., & Lee, J. M. (1998). Pharmacological drug treatment of Alzheimer disease: The cholinergic hypothesis revisited. *Journal of Neuropathology & Experimental Neurology*, *57*(8), 719–731. https://doi.org/10.1097/00005072-199808000-00001.
Lammich, S., Kojro, E., Postina, R., Gilbert, S., Pfeiffer, R., Jasionowski, M., et al. (1999). Constitutive and regulated alpha-secretase cleavage of Alzheimer's amyloid precursor protein by a disintegrin metalloprotease. *Proceedings of the National Academy of Sciences of the United States of America*, *96*(7), 3922–3927. https://doi.org/10.1073/pnas.96.7.3922.
Lane, J. R., Sexton, P. M., & Christopoulos, A. (2013). Bridging the gap: Bitopic ligands of G-protein-coupled receptors. *Trends in Pharmacological Sciences*, *34*(1), 59–66. https://doi.org/10.1016/j.tips.2012.10.003.
Lange, H. S., Cannon, C. E., Drott, J. T., Kuduk, S. D., & Uslaner, J. M. (2015). The M1 muscarinic positive allosteric modulator PQCA improves performance on translatable tests of memory and attention in rhesus monkeys. *The Journal of Pharmacology and Experimental Therapeutics*, *355*(3), 442–450. https://doi.org/10.1124/jpet.115.226712.

Langmead, C. J., Fry, V. A. H., Forbes, I. T., Branch, C. L., Christopoulos, A., Wood, M. D., et al. (2006). Probing the molecular mechanism of interaction between 4-*n*-butyl-1-[4-(2-methylphenyl)-4-oxo-1-butyl]-piperidine (AC-42) and the muscarinic M $_1$ receptor: Direct pharmacological evidence that AC-42 is an allosteric agonist. *Molecular Pharmacology*, *69*(1), 236. https://doi.org/10.1124/mol.105.017814.

Lebois, E. P., Bridges, T. M., Lewis, L. M., Dawson, E. S., Kane, A. S., Xiang, Z., et al. (2010). Discovery and characterization of novel subtype-selective allosteric agonists for the investigation of M(1) receptor function in the central nervous system. *ACS Chemical Neuroscience*, *1*(2), 104–121. https://doi.org/10.1021/cn900003h.

Lebois, E. P., Digby, G. J., Sheffler, D. J., Melancon, B. J., Tarr, J. C., Cho, H. P., et al. (2011). Development of a highly selective, orally bioavailable and CNS penetrant M1 agonist derived from the MLPCN probe ML071. *Bioorganic & Medicinal Chemistry Letters*, *21*(21), 6451–6455. https://doi.org/10.1016/j.bmcl.2011.08.084.

Lebois, E. P., Schroeder, J. P., Esparza, T. J., Bridges, T. M., Lindsley, C. W., Conn, P. J., et al. (2017). Disease-modifying effects of M1 muscarinic acetylcholine receptor activation in an Alzheimer's disease mouse model. *ACS Chemical Neuroscience*, *8*(6), 1177–1187. https://doi.org/10.1021/acschemneuro.6b00278.

Lebois, E. P., Trimper, J. B., Hu, C., Levey, A. I., & Manns, J. R. (2016). Effects of selective M1 muscarinic receptor activation on hippocampal spatial representations and neuronal oscillations. *ACS Chemical Neuroscience*, 7(10), 1393–1405. https://doi.org/10.1021/acschemneuro.6b00160.

Lehner, K. R., Silverman, H., Adorissio, M., Roy, A., Al-Onaizi, M., Levine, Y., et al. (2019). Forebrain cholinergic signaling regulates innate immune responses and inflammation. *Frontiers in Immunology*, *10*, 585.

Levey, A. I. (1993). Immunological localization of m1–m5 muscarinic acetylcholine receptors in peripheral tissues and brain. *Life Sciences*, *52*(5–6), 441–448. Retrieved from https://www.ncbi.nlm.nih.gov/pubmed/8441326.

Levey, A. I. (1996). Muscarinic acetylcholine receptor expression in memory circuits: Implications for treatment of Alzheimer disease. *Proceedings of the National Academy of Sciences of the United States of America*, *93*(24), 13541. https://doi.org/10.1073/pnas.93.24.13541.

Levey, A. I., Kitt, C. A., Simonds, W. F., Price, D. L., & Brann, M. R. (1991). Identification and localization of muscarinic acetylcholine receptor proteins in brain with subtype-specific antibodies. *The Journal of Neuroscience*, *11*(10), 3218–3226. Retrieved from https://www.ncbi.nlm.nih.gov/pubmed/1941081.

Ma, L., Seager, M. A., Wittmann, M., Jacobson, M., Bickel, D., Burno, M., et al. (2009). Selective activation of the M1 muscarinic acetylcholine receptor achieved by allosteric potentiation. *Proceedings of the National Academy of Sciences of the United States of America*, *106*(37), 15950–15955. https://doi.org/10.1073/pnas.0900903106.

Marlo, J. E., Niswender, C. M., Days, E. L., Bridges, T. M., Xiang, Y., Rodriguez, A. L., et al. (2009). Discovery and characterization of novel allosteric potentiators of M1 muscarinic receptors reveals multiple modes of activity. *Molecular Pharmacology*, *75*(3), 577. https://doi.org/10.1124/mol.108.052886.

Masters, C. L., Simms, G., Weinman, N. A., Multhaup, G., McDonald, B. L., & Beyreuther, K. (1985). Amyloid plaque core protein in Alzheimer disease and Down syndrome. *Proceedings of the National Academy of Sciences of the United States of America*, *82*(12), 4245–4249. https://doi.org/10.1073/pnas.82.12.4245.

McQuail, J. A., Davis, K. N., Miller, F., Hampson, R. E., Deadwyler, S. A., Howlett, A. C., et al. (2013). Hippocampal $G\alpha q/_{11}$ but not $G\alpha o$-coupled receptors are altered in aging. *Neuropharmacology*, *70*, 63–73. https://doi.org/10.1016/j.neuropharm.2013.01.009.

Medeiros, R., Kitazawa, M., Caccamo, A., Baglietto-Vargas, D., Estrada-Hernandez, T., Cribbs, D. H., et al. (2011). Loss of muscarinic M1 receptor exacerbates Alzheimer's disease-like pathology and cognitive decline. *The American Journal of Pathology, 179*(2), 980–991. https://doi.org/10.1016/j.ajpath.2011.04.041.

Melancon, B. J., Tarr, J. C., Panarese, J. D., Wood, M. R., & Lindsley, C. W. (2013). Allosteric modulation of the M1 muscarinic acetylcholine receptor: Improving cognition and a potential treatment for schizophrenia and Alzheimer's disease. *Drug Discovery Today, 18*(23–24), 1185–1199. https://doi.org/10.1016/j.drudis.2013.09.005.

Melander, T., Staines, W. A., Hökfelt, T., Rökaeus, Å., Eckenstein, F., Salvaterra, P. M., et al. (1985). Galanin-like immunoreactivity in cholinergic neurons of the septum-basal forebrain complex projecting to the hippocampus of the rat. *Brain Research, 360*(1), 130–138. https://doi.org/10.1016/0006-8993(85)91228-4.

Mesulam, M. M. (2004). The cholinergic innervation of the human cerebral cortex. In L. Descarries, K. Krnjevic, & M. Steriade (Eds.), *Vol. 145, Progress in brain research* (pp. 67–78). Elsevier.

Mesulam, M. M., Mufson, E. J., Levey, A. I., & Wainer, B. H. (1983). Cholinergic innervation of cortex by the basal forebrain: Cytochemistry and cortical connections of the septal area, diagonal band nuclei, nucleus basalis (substantia innominata), and hypothalamus in the rhesus monkey. *Journal of Comparative Neurology, 214*(2), 170–197.

Mesulam, M., Shaw, P., Mash, D., & Weintraub, S. (2004). Cholinergic nucleus basalis tauopathy emerges early in the aging-MCI-AD continuum. *Annals of Neurology, 55*(6), 815–828. https://doi.org/10.1002/ana.20100.

Mistry, S. N., Jörg, M., Lim, H., Vinh, N. B., Sexton, P. M., Capuano, B., et al. (2016). 4-Phenylpyridin-2-one derivatives: A novel class of positive allosteric modulator of the M1 muscarinic acetylcholine receptor. *Journal of Medicinal Chemistry, 59*(1), 388–409. https://doi.org/10.1021/acs.jmedchem.5b01562.

Moran, S. P., Cho, H. P., Maksymetz, J., Remke, D. H., Hanson, R. M., Niswender, C. M., et al. (2018). PF-06827443 displays robust allosteric agonist and positive allosteric modulator activity in high receptor reserve and native systems. *ACS Chemical Neuroscience, 9*(9), 2218–2224. https://doi.org/10.1021/acschemneuro.8b00106.

Moran, S. P., Dickerson, J. W., Cho, H. P., Xiang, Z., Maksymetz, J., Remke, D. H., et al. (2018). M1-positive allosteric modulators lacking agonist activity provide the optimal profile for enhancing cognition. *Neuropsychopharmacology, 43*(8), 1763–1771. https://doi.org/10.1038/s41386-018-0033-9.

Mufson, E. J., Bothwell, M., & Kordower, J. H. (1989). Loss of nerve growth factor receptor-containing neurons in Alzheimer's disease: A quantitative analysis across subregions of the basal forebrain. *Experimental Neurology, 105*(3), 221–232.

Mufson, E. J., Cochran, E., Benzing, W., & Kordower, J. H. (1993). Galaninergic innervation of the cholinergic vertical limb of the diagonal band (Ch2) and bed nucleus of the Stria terminalis in aging, Alzheimer's disease and down's syndrome (Part 1 of 2). *Dementia and Geriatric Cognitive Disorders, 4*(5), 237–243.

Nathan, P. J., Watson, J., Lund, J., Davies, C. H., Peters, G., Dodds, C. M., et al. (2013). The potent M1 receptor allosteric agonist GSK1034702 improves episodic memory in humans in the nicotine abstinence model of cognitive dysfunction. *International Journal of Neuropsychopharmacology, 16*(4), 721–731. https://doi.org/10.1017/S1461145712000752.

Nathanson, N. M. (1987). Molecular properties of the muscarinic acetylcholine receptor. *Annual Review of Neuroscience, 10*(1), 195–236. https://doi.org/10.1146/annurev.ne.10.030187.001211.

Neugroschl, J., & Wang, S. (2011). Alzheimer's disease: Diagnosis and treatment across the spectrum of disease severity. *Mount Sinai Journal of Medicine: A Journal of Translational and Personalized Medicine*, *78*(4), 596–612. https://doi.org/10.1002/msj.20279.

Nitsch, R. M., Deng, M., Tennis, M., Schoenfeld, D., & Growdon, J. H. (2000). The selective muscarinic M1 agonist AF102B decreases levels of total Abeta in cerebrospinal fluid of patients with Alzheimer's disease. *Annals of Neurology*, *48*(6), 913–918. Retrieved from https://www.ncbi.nlm.nih.gov/pubmed/11117548.

Nitsch, R. M., Slack, B. E., Wurtman, R. J., & Growdon, J. H. (1992). Release of Alzheimer amyloid precursor derivatives stimulated by activation of muscarinic acetylcholine receptors. *Science*, *258*(5080), 304–307. Retrieved from https://www.ncbi.nlm.nih.gov/pubmed/1411529.

Perry, E. K., Perry, R. H., Blessed, G., & Tomlinson, B. E. (1977). Necropsy evidence of central cholinergic deficits in senile dementia. *Lancet*, *1*(8004), 189. https://doi.org/10.1016/s0140-6736(77)91780-9.

Perry, E. K., Tomlinson, B. E., Blessed, G., Bergmann, K., Gibson, P. H., & Perry, R. H. (1978). Correlation of cholinergic abnormalities with senile plaques and mental test scores in senile dementia. *British Medical Journal*, *2*(6150), 1457–1459. https://doi.org/10.1136/bmj.2.6150.1457.

Popiolek, M., Mandelblat-Cerf, Y., Young, D., Garst-Orozco, J., Lotarski, S. M., Stark, E., et al. (2019). In vivo modulation of hippocampal excitability by M4 muscarinic acetylcholine receptor activator: Implications for treatment of Alzheimer's disease and schizophrenic patients. *ACS Chemical Neuroscience*, *10*(3), 1091–1098. https://doi.org/10.1021/acschemneuro.8b00496.

Puri, V., Wang, X., Vardigan, J. D., Kuduk, S. D., & Uslaner, J. M. (2015). The selective positive allosteric M1 muscarinic receptor modulator PQCA attenuates learning and memory deficits in the Tg2576 Alzheimer's disease mouse model. *Behavioural Brain Research*, *287*, 96–99. https://doi.org/10.1016/j.bbr.2015.03.029.

Rasool, C. G., Svendsen, C. N., & Selkoe, D. J. (1986). Neurofibrillary degeneration of cholinergic and noncholinergic neurons of the basal forebrain in Alzheimer's disease. *Annals of Neurology*, *20*(4), 482–488. https://doi.org/10.1002/ana.410200407.

Rook, J. M., Abe, M., Cho, H. P., Nance, K. D., Luscombe, V. B., Adams, J. J., et al. (2017). Diverse effects on M1 signaling and adverse effect liability within a series of M1 Ago-PAMs. *ACS Chemical Neuroscience*, *8*(4), 866–883. https://doi.org/10.1021/acschemneuro.6b00429.

Rook, J. M., Bertron, J. L., Cho, H. P., Garcia-Barrantes, P. M., Moran, S. P., Maksymetz, J. T., et al. (2018). A novel M1 PAM VU0486846 exerts efficacy in cognition models without displaying agonist activity or cholinergic toxicity. *ACS Chemical Neuroscience*, *9*(9), 2274–2285. https://doi.org/10.1021/acschemneuro.8b00131.

Roszkowski, A. P. (1961). An unusual type of sympathetic ganglionic stimulant. *The Journal of Pharmacology and Experimental Therapeutics*, *132*, 156–170.

Rusted, J. M., & Warburton, D. M. (1988). The effects of scopolamine on working memory in healthy young volunteers. *Psychopharmacology*, *96*(2), 145–152. https://doi.org/10.1007/BF00177553.

Sarter, M., & Bruno, J. P. (1997). Cognitive functions of cortical acetylcholine: Toward a unifying hypothesis. *Brain Research Reviews*, *23*(1), 28–46. https://doi.org/10.1016/S0165-0173(96)00009-4.

Schliebs, R., & Arendt, T. (2011). The cholinergic system in aging and neuronal degeneration. *Behavioural Brain Research*, *221*(2), 555–563. https://doi.org/10.1016/j.bbr.2010.11.058.

Selkoe, D. J. (1991a). Amyloid protein and Alzheimer's disease. *Scientific American*, *265*(5), 68–71. 74-66, 78. Retrieved from https://www.ncbi.nlm.nih.gov/pubmed/1785042.

Selkoe, D. J. (1991b). The molecular pathology of Alzheimer's disease. *Neuron, 6*(4), 487–498. Retrieved from https://www.ncbi.nlm.nih.gov/pubmed/1673054.

Shekhar, A., Potter, W. Z., Lightfoot, J., Lienemann, J., Dube, S., Mallinckrodt, C., et al. (2008). Selective muscarinic receptor agonist xanomeline as a novel treatment approach for schizophrenia. *The American Journal of Psychiatry, 165*(8), 1033–1039. https://doi.org/10.1176/appi.ajp.2008.06091591.

Shirey, J. K., Brady, A. E., Jones, P. J., Davis, A. A., Bridges, T. M., Kennedy, J. P., et al. (2009). A selective allosteric potentiator of the M1 muscarinic acetylcholine receptor increases activity of medial prefrontal cortical neurons and restores impairments in reversal learning. *The Journal of Neuroscience, 29*(45), 14271–14286. https://doi.org/10.1523/JNEUROSCI.3930-09.2009.

Stallaert, W., Christopoulos, A., & Bouvier, M. (2011). Ligand functional selectivity and quantitative pharmacology at G protein-coupled receptors. *Expert Opinion on Drug Discovery, 6*(8), 811–825. https://doi.org/10.1517/17460441.2011.586691.

Svensson, A.-L., Alafuzoff, I., & Nordberg, A. (1992). Characterization of muscarinic receptor subtypes in Alzheimer and control brain cortices by selective muscarinic antagonists. *Brain Research, 596*(1), 142–148. https://doi.org/10.1016/0006-8993(92)91541-L.

Thal, D. R., Holzer, M., Rüb, U., Waldmann, G., Günzel, S., Zedlick, D., et al. (2000). Alzheimer-related τ-pathology in the perforant path target zone and in the hippocampal stratum oriens and radiatum correlates with onset and degree of dementia. *Experimental Neurology, 163*(1), 98–110. https://doi.org/10.1006/exnr.2000.7380.

Thal, D. M., Sun, B., Feng, D., Nawaratne, V., Leach, K., Felder, C. C., et al. (2016). Crystal structures of the M1 and M4 muscarinic acetylcholine receptors. *Nature, 531*(7594), 335–340. https://doi.org/10.1038/nature17188.

Thathiah, A., & De Strooper, B. (2011). The role of G protein-coupled receptors in the pathology of Alzheimer's disease. *Nature Reviews Neuroscience, 12*, 73. https://doi.org/10.1038/nrn2977.

Thomas, R. L., Langmead, C. J., Wood, M. D., & Challiss, R. A. J. (2009). Contrasting effects of allosteric and orthosteric agonists on M(1) muscarinic acetylcholine receptor internalization and down-regulation. *The Journal of Pharmacology and Experimental Therapeutics, 331*(3), 1086–1095. https://doi.org/10.1124/jpet.109.160242.

Thorn, C. A., Moon, J., Bourbonais, C. A., Harms, J., Edgerton, J. R., Stark, E., et al. (2019). Striatal, hippocampal, and cortical networks are differentially responsive to the M4- and M1-muscarinic acetylcholine receptor mediated effects of xanomeline. *ACS Chemical Neuroscience, 10*(3), 1753–1764. https://doi.org/10.1021/acschemneuro.8b00625.

Tsang, S. W., Lai, M. K., Kirvell, S., Francis, P. T., Esiri, M. M., Hope, T., et al. (2006). Impaired coupling of muscarinic M1 receptors to G-proteins in the neocortex is associated with severity of dementia in Alzheimer's disease. *Neurobiology of Aging, 9*, 1216–1223. https://doi.org/10.1016/j.neurobiolaging.2005.07.010.

Uslaner, J. M., Eddins, D., Puri, V., Cannon, C. E., Sutcliffe, J., Chew, C. S., et al. (2013). The muscarinic M1 receptor positive allosteric modulator PQCA improves cognitive measures in rat, cynomolgus macaque, and rhesus macaque. *Psychopharmacology, 225*(1), 21–30. https://doi.org/10.1007/s00213-012-2788-8.

Uslaner, J. M., Kuduk, S. D., Wittmann, M., Lange, H. S., Fox, S. V., Min, C., et al. (2018). Preclinical to human translational pharmacology of the novel M1 positive allosteric modulator MK-7622. *The Journal of Pharmacology and Experimental Therapeutics, 365*(3), 556–566. https://doi.org/10.1124/jpet.117.245894.

Valant, C., Gregory, K. J., Hall, N. E., Scammells, P. J., Lew, M. J., Sexton, P. M., et al. (2008). A novel mechanism of G protein-coupled receptor functional selectivity. Muscarinic partial agonist McN-A-343 as a bitopic orthosteric/allosteric ligand. *The Journal of Biological Chemistry, 283*(43), 29312–29321. https://doi.org/10.1074/jbc.M803801200.

Vardigan, J. D., Cannon, C. E., Puri, V., Dancho, M., Koser, A., Wittmann, M., et al. (2015). Improved cognition without adverse effects: Novel M1 muscarinic potentiator compares favorably to donepezil and xanomeline in rhesus monkey. *Psychopharmacology, 232*(11), 1859–1866. https://doi.org/10.1007/s00213-014-3813-x.

Venkatakrishnan, A. J., Deupi, X., Lebon, G., Tate, C. G., Schertler, G. F., & Babu, M. M. (2013). Molecular signatures of G-protein-coupled receptors. *Nature, 494*, 185. https://doi.org/10.1038/nature11896. https://www.nature.com/articles/nature11896 #supplementary-information.

Volpicelli, L. A., & Levey, A. I. (2004). Muscarinic acetylcholine receptor subtypes in cerebral cortex and hippocampus. In L. Descarries, K. Krnjevic, & M. Steriade (Eds.), *Progress in brain research: Vol. 145*. (pp. 59–66). Elsevier.

Voss, T., Li, J., Cummings, J., Farlow, M., Assaid, C., Froman, S., et al. (2018). Randomized, controlled, proof-of-concept trial of MK-7622 in Alzheimer's disease. *Alzheimer's & Dementia: Translational Research & Clinical Interventions, 4*, 173–181. https://doi.org/10.1016/j.trci.2018.03.004.

Vuckovic, Z., Gentry, P. R., Berizzi, A. E., Hirata, K., Varghese, S., Thompson, G., et al. (2019). *Crystal structure of the M_5 muscarinic acetylcholine receptor* (p. 730622). bioRxiv. https://doi.org/10.1101/730622.

Watt, M. L., Schober, D. A., Hitchcock, S., Liu, B., Chesterfield, A. K., McKinzie, D., et al. (2011). Pharmacological characterization of LY593093, an M1 muscarinic acetylcholine receptor-selective partial orthosteric agonist. *The Journal of Pharmacology and Experimental Therapeutics, 338*(2), 622–632. https://doi.org/10.1124/jpet.111.182063.

Wess, J. (1993). Molecular basis of muscarinic receptor function. *Trends in Pharmacological Sciences, 14*(8), 308–313. https://doi.org/10.1016/0165-6147(93)90049-P.

Whitehouse, P. J., Price, D. L., Clark, A. W., Coyle, J. T., & DeLong, M. R. (1981). Alzheimer disease: Evidence for selective loss of cholinergic neurons in the nucleus basalis. *Annals of Neurology, 10*(2), 122–126.

Whitehouse, P. J., Price, D. L., Struble, R. G., Clark, A. W., Coyle, J. T., & Delon, M. R. (1982). Alzheimer's disease and senile dementia: Loss of neurons in the basal forebrain. *Science, 215*(4537), 1237–1239. Retrieved from https://www.ncbi.nlm.nih.gov/pubmed/7058341.

Wilcock, G. K., Gauthier, S., Frisoni, G. B., Jia, J., Hardlund, J. H., Moebius, H. J., et al. (2018). Potential of low dose leuco-methylthioninium bis (hydromethanesulphonate) (LMTM) monotherapy for treatment of mild Alzheimer's disease: Cohort analysis as modified primary outcome in a phase III clinical trial. *Journal of Alzheimer's Disease, 61*(1), 435–457.

Wilson, I. A., Ikonen, S., Gallagher, M., Eichenbaum, H., & Tanila, H. (2005). Age-associated alterations of hippocampal place cells are subregion specific. *The Journal of Neuroscience, 25*(29), 6877. https://doi.org/10.1523/JNEUROSCI.1744-05.2005.

Further reading

Bymaster, F. P., Carter, P. A., Yamada, M., Gomeza, J., Wess, J., Hamilton, S. E., et al. (2003). Role of specific muscarinic receptor subtypes in cholinergic parasympathomimetic responses, in vivo phosphoinositide hydrolysis, and pilocarpine-induced seizure activity. *European Journal of Neuroscience, 17*(7), 1403–1410. https://doi.org/10.1046/j.1460-9568.2003.02588.x.

FSC
www.fsc.org
MIX
Papier | Fördert
gute Waldnutzung
FSC® C083411

Kolibri 360 GmbH
Ferdinand-Jühlke-Straße 7
99095 Erfurt, Deutschland
produktsicherheit@kolibri360.de

FSC
www.fsc.org
MIX
Papier | Fördert
gute Waldnutzung
FSC® C083411

Kolibri 360 GmbH
Ferdinand-Jühlke-Straße 7
99095 Erfurt, Deutschland
produktsicherheit@kolibri360.de